The
Business
of
Medicine

The Business of Medicine

Gary Gitnick, MD
Professor of Medicine
UCLA School of Medicine
Los Angeles, California

Fred Rothenberg
President, Fred Rothenberg & Associates, Inc.
Woodland Hills, California

Judy L. Weiner
Executive Administrator
Department of Surgery
UCLA School of Medicine
Los Angeles, California

Elsevier
New York • Amsterdam • London

Elsevier Science Publishing Co., Inc.
655 Avenue of the Americas, New York, New York 10010

Sole distributors outside the United States and Canada:
Elsevier Science Publishers B.V.
P.O. Box 211, 1000 AE Amsterdam, the Netherlands

Library of Congress Cataloging-in-Publication Data

The business of medicine/edited by Gary Gitnick, Fred Rothenberg, Judy L. Weiner.
    p. cm.
   Includes index.
   ISBN 0-444-01567-1 (hard cover : alk. paper)
   1. Medicine—Practice. 2. Medical offices—Management. 3. Health services administration. I. Gitnick, Gary L. II. Rothenberg, Fred. III. Weiner, Judy L.
   [DNLM: 1. Practice Management, Medical. 2. Private Practice— organization & administration. W 89 B979]
   R728.B88 1991
   610'.068—dc20
   DNLM/DLC
   for Library of Congress   91-9560
                                           CIP

Current printing (last digit):
10 9 8 7 6 5 4 3 2 1

Manufactured in the United States of America

*This book is dedicated to the members of my family.
Their support throughout my career has made it possible
to develop books. To my wife Cherna and to my children—
Neil, Kim, Jill, and Tracy—whose time was used to
prepare this text and whose patience and understanding
made this book possible; as well as to my brother Jerry,
his wife Saranne, his children, Nan and Andrea; and
my mother Ann.*

Gary Gitnick, MD

Contents

IV | **DEVELOPING AND MANAGING
A PRACTICE**

V | THE LATER YEARS

Preface

Business management for physicians has undergone significant change in recent years. Evolution of managed care and the development of prospective payment systems have greatly increased the importance of financial management. Today, both the young and the established physician must make decisions in a coordinated manner in order to preserve income and to protect future prospects. Today there are financial implications in almost all aspects of medical practice.

This book is aimed at updating contemporary management beliefs and practices as they affect a physician's business. Its goal is to provide the insights and perspectives that allow physicians to expand their own economic horizons in order to facilitate the development of their own medical practices. Whereas less than ten years ago many physicians found business activities boring and unnecessary, today's physician realizes that knowledge of the principles of business and finance are necessary for survival. Marketing and profit, concepts that were previously scorned, are now widely accepted.

The following chapters describe an approach to the development of an economically viable clinical practice. The business concepts proposed have been helpful to many physicians but they are only business concepts. The real basis for success for medical practice remains in the ability of an individual or a group to provide excellent health care service. Nevertheless, before opening an office, expanding a practice, taking on a partner, or planning retirement, the principles discussed in this book may be helpful in guiding the reader to success. The modern clinician must balance clinical knowledge, medical judgment, and business expertise if he or she is to succeed.

Readers are encouraged to use this book as a resource for future reference as well as a guide for the careful development of a medical business. The contents are designed to serve the needs of students, house staff members, young physicians entering practice, as well as established clinicians. This book provides guidelines; it does not provide all of the answers. Some situations are so individual that a single book could not possibly suffice. Overall, it is essential that the modern physician provide not only good clinical service but also develop good business strategies.

Gary Gitnick, MD

Acknowledgment

The editors wish to thank Susan Dashe for her exceptional efforts in bringing this book together. Her organizational abilities, diplomatic skills, and dedication all made it possible to expeditiously bring together chapters from a wide variety of authors, have them reviewed by associate editors and then by the editor, organize them, and deliver them in the proper order to the publisher. She directed the development of the book and encouraged all of those involved in its production. We remain grateful to her for her many efforts.

Contributors

Michael J. Alper
Executive Director, Cedars-Sinai Physicians Association, Los Angeles, California

Marsha Andersen
Director of Public Relations, Presbyterian Intercommunity Hospital, Whittier, California

Mark Babst, MPA, FACMGA
Executive Vice President, Medi-Sec, Inc., Los Angeles, California

Michael J. Benenson, MPS
President, Benenson & Associates, Inc., Woodland Hills, California

Judith E. Berger
President, MD Resources, Inc., Miami, Florida

Diane G. Brown, RN, JD
Manager Systemwide, Professional Medical and Hospital Liability Program, Office of the President, Office of Risk Management, University of California, Berkeley, California

Richard S. Chung, MD
Vice President, Medical Affairs, American Biodyne, Inc., South San Francisco, California

John R. Cochran, III
President and C.E.O., La Palma Intercommunity Hospital, La Palma, California

Robert H. Coombs, PhD
Professor of Behavioral Sciences, Department of Psychiatry and Biobehavioral Sciences, UCLA School of Medicine, Director, Office of Education, UCLA Neuropsychiatric Institute, Los Angeles, California

Paula P. Dean
Vice President, Human Resources, Scripps Clinic and Research Foundation, La Jolla, California

Victor G. Ettinger, MD
Assistant Clinical Professor, UCLA School of Medicine, Los Angeles, California

Peng Thim Fan, MD
Associate Clinical Professor of Medicine, UCLA School of Medicine, Los Angeles, California

Patricia A. Fox
Manager of Product Development, IDX Corporation, Boston, Massachusetts

Robert D. Girard, LLB
Partner, Jones, Day, Reavis & Pogue, Los Angeles, California

Gary Gitnick, MD
Professor of Medicine, UCLA School of Medicine, Los Angeles, California

John O. Goodman
President, John Goodman & Associates, Inc., Torrance, California

Peter N. Grant, JD, PhD
Weissburg & Aronson, Inc., San Francisco, California

Neal Green, MBA
President, Medi-Sec, Inc., Los Angeles, California

Rick L. Grossman, JD, LLM
Jones, Day, Reavis and Pogue, Los Angeles, California

Thomas M. Heric, MD, PhD
Assistant Clinical Professor, UCLA School of Medicine, Los Angeles, California

Paul A. Hoffstein
Assistant Dean for Clinical Practice, Executive Director of the Medical Service Plan, Office of Clinical Practice, The Johns Hopkins University School of Medicine, Baltimore, Maryland

Barbara Lichner Ingram, PhD
Graduate School of Education and Psychology, Pepperdine University,
Culver City, California

Peter E. Kane
Vice President, Administration, Medical Biology Institute, La Jolla,
California

Henry Clay Kelley, Jr., MBA, CPM
Partner and Senior Vice President, Department of Real Estate Management,
Flake & Co., Inc., Little Rock, Arkansas

Alan Koval, MBA, JD, CPA
Chief Financial Officer, St. Luke's Episcopal Hospital, Texas Medical Center,
Houston, Texas

Lawrence Leiter, MD, MBA
Henry Mayo Newhall Family Medical Group, Canyon Country, California

Orley H. Lindgren, PhD
Director, Institute for Medical Risk Studies, Professional Risk Management
Group, Sausalito, California

Barry A. Litzer
Account Executive, Dean Witter Reynolds, Inc., Woodland Hills, California

Peter C. McKenney, MBA, JD, CPA, LLM
Partner, Medical Management Group, KPMG Peat Marwick, Portland, Maine

Sherwin L. Memel, JD
Partner and Chairman, Health Law Department, Manatt, Phelps & Phillips,
Los Angeles, California

Osama Mikhail, MBA, MS, PhD
University of Texas, School of Public Health, Houston, Texas

Don Harper Mills, MD, JD
Medical Director, Professional Risk Management Group and Institute for
Medical Risk Studies, Long Beach, California

Joanne Moser, RNMN
President, Professional Office Development Company, Torrance, California

Michael W. Murphy, CPA
Partner, DeLoitte & Touche, San Diego, California

Sharon Novakoff, MHSM
Director of Business Development, Los Alamitos Medical Center, Los Alamitos, California

Robert Clifford Ossorio, MD
Medical Director, Cedars-Sinai Physicians Association, Los Angeles, California

Susan M. Ostoya
Project Manager, IDX Corporation, Alameda, California

Frank A. Riddick, Jr., MD
Medical Director, Ochsner Clinic, New Orleans, Louisiana

Noah D. Rosenberg, Esq.
President, Rosenberg and Kaplan, Beverly Hills, California

Ron Rosenberg, PAC, MPH
Managing Partner, Consulting Concepts, Inc., Salt Lake City, Utah

Haya R. Rubin, MD, PhD
Assistant Professor, Department of Medicine, The Johns Hopkins University, Baltimore, Maryland

Lester L. Sacks, MD, PhD
Senior Vice President, Medical Affairs, Beech Street, Inc., Irvine, California

Lester J. Schwartz, CPA
Principal, Zivetz, Schwartz & Saltsman, Los Angeles, California

Timothy C. Shamroy
Vice President, Fred Rothenberg & Associates, Inc., Woodland Hills, California

Westley Sholes, MPA
Deputy Director, Administrative Services, Los Angeles County Department of Health Services, Los Angeles, California

Robert A. Steinberg
Partner, Davis, Wright, Tremaine, Los Angeles, California

Drew J. Sutter, CPA
Senior Manager, DeLoitte & Touche, San Diego, California

Michael C. Thornhill, JD
Partner, Wood, Lucksinger & Epstein, Los Angeles, California

Michael John Tichon, Esq., JD
Partner, Davis Wright Tremaine, Los Angeles, California

Robin T. Tucker, JD
Weissburg & Aronson, Inc., San Francisco, California

Bernard B. Virshup, MD
Clinical Professor, UCLA School of Medicine, Los Angeles, California

Albert W. Wu, MD, MPH
Health Services Research Center, Baltimore, Maryland

Leslie C. Young, MS
Associate Consultant, Benenson & Associates, Inc., Woodland Hills, California

I | THE BUSINESS OF MEDICINE: AN OVERVIEW

1 | Introduction

GARY GITNICK, MD

Traditionally, physicians have shunned the idea of the "business of medicine" as demeaning to their role as healers. Times have changed. The practice of medicine has become so expensive and so competitive that physicians must understand the concepts and practices of business management if they are to survive as healers. Small and large practices alike need to institute systems and procedures that will not only enhance profitability, but also enable physicians to provide services to their communities in an efficient and effective manner.

We call this book *The Business of Medicine*, but it examines more than just business concepts. It focuses on interpersonal relationships, not only between physicians and their patients, but also between physicians and their employees, their communities, and government and corporate entities. The text covers the whole gamut of activities—from legal issues to office management to the design of office decor—that are relevant to the modern medical practice. While these activities may seem only tangentially related to business practices, they all affect the success or failure of a medical practice and so are bound up with the "business of medicine."

The following chapters provide a perspective on business activities as they relate to the health-care professional. The authors attempt to address real issues in modern medical practice. Management skills that have been developed in other areas of business are applied to the practice of medicine.

We have organized the book into five sections. The first, "An Overview," surveys current trends in our health-care delivery system and provides an extensive evaluation of market forces. Each chapter addresses a particular issue that has an impact both on the marketplace and on a physician's practice of medicine.

By keeping informed of the forces of change, physicians can make better management decisions. For instance, Chapter Two, "Physician Income: Historic and Recent Changes in Payment Sources, Income Levels, and Professional Autonomy," sketches a history of how physicians have been paid from the early 1900s to the present. Knowing which events have led to the current level of corporate (third-party payors) and governmental (Medicare, utilization review) constraints on physician autonomy provides a context for addressing the issues of payment in the physician's practice.

In this age of cost containment, utilization review (UR) has become a ubiquitous tool for monitoring the delivery of health-care services. Chapter Seven, entitled "Utilization Review: Old Principles and New Mechanisms," provides a thorough history and current perspective on UR as well as concrete examples of proper channels through which to register challenges and complaints.

The next section, "Going Into Practice," is primarily geared to the graduating physician and functions as a mini-primer for finding and qualifying for the right practice situation. The changing demographics of the U.S. population—smaller families, migrations to the southern and western areas, more elderly in the population—all impinge on the practice of medicine, as does the greater number of physicians. According to Thomas M. Heric, M.D., in his chapter, "Choosing Other Types of Practice: Solo v. Small Partnership v. Large Medical Group," all these factors should be taken into account when entering practice.

Changes in the health-care marketplace affect all physicians, not just those who are entering practice. Dr. Heric's chapter presents the advantages and disadvantages of each type of practice, along with pertinent questions to help the starting physician gauge the value of each situation. Because influences on the practice of medicine are in constant flux, established physicians may also find useful information in these chapters.

How does a physician go about finding practice opportunities? Should one choose a single- or multi-specialty group practice? Should one establish a solo practice, or start out as a hospital-based or clinic employee? What are the important criteria to use when considering various options? "Finding Practice Opportunities" offers guidelines that can be useful to a range of physicians, from recent graduates to those altering career paths or relocating to other geographic areas.

The following section, entitled "Establishing a Practice," deals with the nuts and bolts of setting up and running an efficient office. Leasing, subleasing, and time-share arrangements are surveyed. Joanne Moser, R.N., a professional office development consultant, provides cogent advice on working with a medical space planner to optimize patient flow and general office ambience. Critical in the design process is an appropriate assessment of your practice's present and future needs. In her chapter entitled "Office Design: How to Optimize Patient Flow, Staff Convenience, and Ambience," Ms. Moser points out the special requirements of various medical specialties and "walks through" the remodeling process, from construction plans to occupancy.

Ms. Moser's companion chapter, "Equipping and Furnishing Your Office," contains valuable checklists and information about price checking, financing, and ordering equipment. She includes discussions of colors and wall coverings and how they are affected by the light source in a room.

Next come several chapters dealing with one of the most challenging aspects of running a medical practice: managing office personnel. In "Hiring and Firing Staff," Peter Kane, vice president of personnel at the Medical Biology Institute in La Jolla, California, illustrates techniques to develop job descriptions that support your practice objectives and recruitment techniques.

The modern practice of medicine requires the employment of a variety of personnel and, consequently, the establishment of an organizational viewpoint that highlights the value of each individual's contribution. It is remarkable that in some organizations, people with mediocre abilities are highly valued, while people who are very capable and have unique skills may not be valued at all. Often it is the failure of the organization—and specifically the physician-manager—to recognize the capabilities and weaknesses of individual employees, be they physicians or office professionals. The astute physician-manager will assess his or her associates, their skills, their effectiveness, and their accomplishments based on a rational set of assessment criteria. Paula Dean's chapter, "Implementing Effective Personnel and Office Management Procedures," discusses such approaches to effective management.

Within the office organization, be it a large or small practice, communication remains the key. It has long been thought that improved teamwork and organizational effectiveness would follow directly from people communicating openly with one another on matters of importance to practice administration.

In the past, management teams have come into office practices, identified important issues, and brought people together to work out their differences. Effective problem solving could range from a meeting of two people with differing points of view on a problem, to team effectiveness meetings in which large groups of people sit down with physician-managers to plan collaborative formats for the development of effective management systems. It is remarkable how often power struggles develop among people whose interests are really compatible. By simply identifying these areas of mutual interest and need, accommodations can be reached that benefit the whole organizational structure.

The book's section about establishing a practice concludes with chapters on the maximization of reimbursements and accounts receivable and on the computerized office: evaluating the hardware and software best suited to your office information needs.

In the fourth section, "Developing and Managing a Practice," chapters address such critical issues as patient appointment scheduling, record keeping for salaries and payroll taxes, and achieving patient satisfaction. In addition, Noah Rosenberg addresses the dos and don'ts of entering the HMO marketplace. Various criteria are given for evaluating the financial viability of a health plan and of a health plan agreement. In this complicated area of medicine, there are many legal ramifications of such associations. Mr. Rosenberg addresses these issues, gives some examples of appropriate language and phrasing, and advises physicians on both the benefits and risks of HMO contracts.

Our final section, "The Later Years," deals with such concrete issues as pension plans and long-term personal financial planning as well as more complex situations, such as adding a partner or physician associate. The chapter entitled "Coping with Stress and Burn-Out," by Barbara L. Ingram, Ph.D., should be of interest to most readers. This changing world carries multiple stressors that add to an already highly stressful profession. Ironically, the personality characteristics that allow a person to remain focused through medical school and the early years of establishing a practice can be the very characteristics that allow stress to build to intolerable levels. Physicians may be required to develop new skills of personal awareness in the coming decades; Dr. Ingram's chapter offers helpful insights in this arena.

Our book concludes with a most appropriate chapter, "Preparing for Retirement," cowritten by Robert H. Coombs and Bernard B. Virshup, who conducted a survey of retiring Los Angeles County physicians and present some surprising results. In their study, many physicians cited "interference" by government and third-party payors as reasons for retiring. The most successful retirees, the authors report, were those who had developed and maintained other interests before retiring. The perspective of these thoughtful retirees is sure to offer food for thought to future retirees who are now in the full swing of their practices.

The goal of all these chapters is to provide insights and perspectives that will allow physicians and their office managers to develop and/or recast the structures of their practices to provide for long- and short-term goals. The more physicians can take command of their business, the better they will be able to deliver quality care in the next decade.

2 Physician Income: Historic and Recent Changes in Payment Sources, Income Levels, and Professional Autonomy

MICHAEL C. THORNHILL, JD

This chapter addresses three principal questions: (1) How do physicians get paid? (2) What is happening to fee-for-service medicine? and (3) How did we get to this state of affairs? In the not-too-distant past there were ready, simple, and fairly accurate answers to the first two questions, and few in the profession were greatly concerned with the third. The economics of medical practice and the sources of physician income were reasonably well defined. Fee-for-service medicine prevailed; physicians controlled their economic destiny. The "business of medicine" seemed almost a contradiction in terms.

Patients and insurers generally paid in accord with the fees physicians charged. Medicare and some private payers utilized more arcane formulas, but even they tended more to reinforce than to impair physicians' autonomy. The exceptions were not worrisome. Medicaid, industrial clinics, and health maintenance organizations (HMOs) were peripheral.

Negotiations were with one's peers, not with insurance companies. Before the onset of antitrust laws, one could refer to the local medical society's schedule in setting fees; thereafter, one could refer to unofficial sources, such as insurers' fee schedules or, as in other trades and professions, learn by word of mouth how one's peers set their fees. In any event, Medicare and Blue Cross/Blue Shield rates suggested what one's higher customary fees could be, and sliding fee schedules allowed one to adjust for patients of limited means. A physician could usually look forward to a career in solo or small group practice with comfortable earnings or even wealth, free of institutional control, provided only that he or she met the expectations of patients and peers and followed the well-established rules of the payment systems.

This golden era of high economic expectations and autonomy lasted 30 or 40 years, but it has largely passed. Today a physician may be paid (or not paid, as the case may be) in a sometimes bewildering number of ways, according to a multiplicity of rules that seem to be constantly changing.

Institutions such as insurance companies and government agencies are increasingly intrusive. Many physicians now confront two distinctly negative trends: declining real income and increasing corporate control. Traditional solo practice is no longer a predictable route to wealth, professional success, and economic security. Today the alternatives are either (1) accommodation to the new ways within the traditional private practice framework, (2) adding the role of entrepreneur or business executive to that of practicing physician, or (3) taking a salaried position.

This chapter looks at how the sources of physicians' income have changed and how the amount of such income—whether gross, net, or real (adjusted for inflation)—has grown, declined, or stagnated. It notes some of the legal and political battles that accompanied, fostered, or followed these changes in several eras, including the decades preceding World War II, the lucrative but autonomous "golden era" that followed, and finally the present, with its diverse and ever-changing ways of paying physicians. It poses, albeit simply, several answers to the question: how did the medical profession arrive at the present state of affairs?

One Explanation of the "Golden" Past

Until the 1970s, physicians could make a self-righteous but fairly accurate assertion: they had earned their autonomy and high incomes through education, training, and hard work as medical doctors and had kept insurers and other institutions at bay through assiduous legal and political efforts. Except during the Great Depression, for the first seven decades of this century physicians' real incomes grew steadily. The medical profession presided over a dramatic expansion of the health-care delivery system. When criticized, the profession could point out numerous dramatic medical advances to amply justify the persistent rise in health-care expenditures as a percentage of the gross national product. Politicians, business, and union leaders saw little reason to disturb the status quo or to deny further support through employee benefits and taxes. The nation was in the midst of a period of continuing economic growth and could apparently afford to satisfy the expectations of doctors and their patients. Despite the growing presence of other institutions such as hospitals and insurers, the medical profession was able to rebuff all challenges to its right to control the allocation of medical resources.

Prelude: The 1920s

Between 1900 and 1920, the medical profession developed as the dominant voice in public debates on health care. The American Medical Association had merely 8000 members in 1900. By 1910 its membership had reached 70,000—half of the physicians in the country—and by 1920 60% of all physicians were AMA members. Many of its wishes came true: fewer medical schools, stricter curriculum and admission standards, laws confirming the preeminence of allopathic physicians, and dramatic advances in the profession's curative powers. The ratio of physicians to the U.S. population declined from 160 per 100,000 in 1905 to fewer than 140 per 100,000 in the 1930s. (It would not significantly exceed 140 per 100,000 until the 1960s). Physicians' incomes grew dramatically. Whereas in 1900 the average annual income was (in 1928 dollars) between $1500 and $3000, by 1928 it had risen to between $5000 and $6354.

Most of this increase was paid out of patients' pockets. The large insurance companies had deemed health insurance to be unprofitable, with low premiums, too little time to invest them, and too much control vested in the insured with regard to when benefits would be due. Late in the 19th century many fraternal, mutual benefit, and industrial societies began offering disability or income replacement insurance for those unable to work because of injury or illness. Many such companies failed. This fact— not the AMA's lobbying—led to the passage of state laws restricting such forms of health insurance.

The Threat of "Contract Medicine"

A major impetus for the growth of the American Medical Association and other physicians' associations in the first decades of this century was to counterbalance some institutions arising throughout American society that threatened to reduce physicians' autonomy. A letter to the Journal of the American Medical Association in 1902 complained of humiliation and insults from wealthy corporations and government officials and of contracts offered by big corporations at unduly low fees. "As it is, if I do not accept the fees the company offers [about 60% of his customary billings], the work will go to another physician and the company knows it can get plenty of doctors to do the work for whatever they are willing to pay."

The term of opprobrium "contract medicine" was applied to a variety of arrangements that in the view of the AMA presented such evils as "lowered standards of medical services, insufficient payments to physicians and others providing the service, and domination by lay financial interests." At the beginning of the century, the most common form of contract medicine was the "lodge practice," in which a physician entered into contracts to treat society or lodge members and sometimes their families in exchange for an annual or periodic payment. The rates (eg, $1.00 per member per year) were very low, even for that era. For many young physicians, however, these arrangements were a matter of economic survival, a means to keep the office open. After World War I, the incidence of lodge practice declined. With a smaller percentage of physicians in the general population, physicians' incomes rose. Fewer were willing to accept lodge rates, and the societies were not able, either legally or as a practical matter, to underwrite fee-for-service insurance policies.

Organized medicine's efforts to avoid lay ownership or control were aided by the judicial system. State courts were often willing to ban the "corporate practice" of medicine, often with little support from state statutes, relying more on principles that echoed the rules of the AMA and state and local medical associations. The courts were much less willing to find that the AMA and other organizations had engaged in illegal boycotts. The case involving the Group Health Association of Washington, D.C., was a notable exception. The state legislatures also responded positively, enacting Blue Cross/Blue Shield and commercial insurance licensing laws that effectively barred preferred provider organizations (PPOs) until the 1980s.

The profession tolerated some forms of contract medicine or corporate practice, such as industrial clinics, so long as they did not take business away from the private practitioner. These employer-sponsored clinics, for instance, often paid physicians on a salary or per diem basis. The medical associations rarely complained if the clinic was in a remote, rural area or confined itself to industrial safety and the treatment of on-the-job injuries. If the clinic served the broader health-care needs of employees and their families, however, its physicians risked expulsion from the medical associations. Unions were also opposed, and employees in general were not enthusiastic. As a consequence, there was little expansion. Most clinics confined themselves to "return to work" services, and with the onset of the Great Depression, their numbers declined.

In the 1930s, the profession's contract medicine concerns focused on (1) service plans like Blue Cross which negotiated rates with participating providers and (2) capitated arrangements with employers, unions, or other third parties. The latter were not uncommon, particularly in the Midwest and on the West Coast (eg, the contract between Ross-Loos Medical Group and the Los Angeles Department of Water and Power). An AMA survey in 1933 reported that 20 of 224 medical groups surveyed reported offering services on a contract or periodic prepayment basis. The records of the Medical Group Management Association, and the fact that there clearly was a "wrong" answer, suggest that the number of prepaid groups was probably much higher. There were numerous reports of practitioners of contract medicine—including Drs. Ross and Loos—being denied or losing membership in medical associations, which at that time often entailed the loss of hospital privileges too.

In 1934 the AMA House of Delegates enacted "ten principles," including:

control by the medical profession over all features of medical service in any method of medical practice,

nonintervention of third parties in the physician–patient relationship,

freedom of choice by patients, and

the right to adjust fees according to a patient's means or income.

At a special meeting in 1935, the AMA announced its total opposition to commercial insurance but expressed support for voluntary health insurance under the control of medical associations.

With the expansion of Blue Cross/Blue Shield and commercial insurance, lodge practice and other forms of contract medicine declined. The exceptions were well established; for example, Kaiser Health Plan, the Health Insurance Plan of New York, and various union-sponsored clinics. However, they posed little threat to the burgeoning fee-for-service practice of medicine.

The medical profession also successfully overcame hospital rules that limited physicians' incomes. By 1910 hospitals had generally ceased to bar physicians from collecting any fees for services to inpatients. When clinical pathology and radiology were first developed, technicians often performed the services because of a shortage of trained physicians. These technicians, and many of the physicians who first performed such services, were paid by hospitals on a salary basis. A number of Blue Cross plans treated these as covered hospital services. The AMA vigorously opposed these practices, and by 1930 most hospital-based physicians were reimbursed on a professional fee basis.

The 1930s

The economic troubles of the 1930s severely affected the medical profession. Many more people were willing to defer seeing (and to defer paying) physicians. Physicians' incomes appear to have declined 40% to 50% between 1928 and 1933. A study of delinquency percentages indicates that physicians were paid after department stores, groceries, landlords, and dentists. Hospitals and physicians accepted payment through some local and state government programs and one relatively limited federal program, but not without great concern. The AMA position since 1920 had been adamantly against government-mandated or -sponsored insurance. The Great Depression, however, led many physicians to support an increased government role. The Michigan and California associations endorsed compulsory health insurance. But the AMA's supporters regained control of the Michigan association and reversed its position. Compulsory health insurance proposals foundered in California, as the California Medical Association and other interest groups could not agree on legislation. Both, however, were among the first to sponsor voluntary prepaid medical service plans (ie, Blue Shield).

The Development of Blue Cross and Blue Shield

The loss of jobs and income in the Great Depression led many Americans to forego medical and hospital care except in the most dire circumstances, in order to meet even more basic needs, such as food and shelter. To combat the resulting low census, hospitals began offering prepayment plans. The first plans, like that offered by Baylor Hospital in Dallas in 1929, only covered services in the sponsoring facility and were not particularly successful. The first community-wide plan offering choice of multiple hospitals was introduced in Newark, New Jersey, in 1933. Similar plans were established in Washington, D.C.; Cleveland, Ohio; St. Paul, Minnesota; and Sacramento, California, in the next year. Endorsed by the American Hospital Association, these became known as Blue Cross plans.

In 1939 the California Medical Association sponsored the first statewide physician prepayment plan: California Physicians Service. Because of suspicion in the medical community that the increased patient volume from such plans was offset by the reduction in fees required of participating physicians, growth of the Blue Shield plans was slower. It increased, however, as the success of the Blue Cross plans became apparent. The AMA did not officially oppose development of Blue Cross and Blue Shield plans. Rather, it took public positions against medical practice by organized groups of physicians associated with hospitals and profit-making health insurance.

The Expansion of Health Insurance

The Blue Cross and Blue Shield plans grew because they filled an unmet need. At the end of the Great Depression, only 9% of the U.S. population had some form of health insurance. World War II and the subsequent economic expansion of the United States brought about more employer-paid coverage as well as greater ability and desire of individuals to have health coverage, and the number of plans grew rapidly.

The major insurance companies began offering health insurance in the aftermath of World War II. From 1946 to 1956 the number of persons with hospital insurance grew from 42 million to 116 million, and by 1960, to 132 million. Blue Cross/Blue Shield plans represented more than 65% of the 1946 figure and about 45% of the later totals. The percentage of physicians' income derived from insurance grew rapidly, from less than 7% of private expenditures for physician services in 1948 to about one-third of such expenditures in 1960. From 1949 to 1965, real earnings of physicians increased on average 5.1% annually, from $11,519 (in 1957–59 dollars) to $25,533.

The Impact of Medicare

Enacted in 1966, Medicare had an immediate and dramatic effect on physicians' incomes. Expenditures for physician services to those over age 65 increased 43% in fiscal years 1967 and 1968, compared with a 19% increase for those under age 65. Physicians' fees in general increased 7% on average in each of those years, compared with increases of only 3.6% during 1964 and 1965. Further, Medicare did nothing to encourage corporate practice.

Physicians in solo or small group practice continued to vastly outnumber salaried physicians, and the degree (and rewards) of specialization increased.

1971 Wage and Price Controls

Physicians' fees continued to increase at an average of 7% per year through 1971. In August 1971 the Economic Stabilization Program placed price controls on physicians' services and other goods and services. The stated objective was to limit the inflation of all prices to no more than 2.5% per year. In 1973 and 1974 the program severely limited fee increases. Nevertheless, gross revenue of general practitioners increased by 11.9% and 12.4% in 1973 and 1974, respectively; surgeons' fees increased by 10.1% and 15.6% in those years, and those of internists by 12% and 19.3%. Physicians apparently responded to price controls by increasing the complexity and the number of services.

Leveling Off and More Pronounced Disparities: Physician Income After 1975

A 1987 AMA report shows that although the average net income (before taxes, after expenses) of physicians increased from $55,300 in 1975 to $119,500 in 1986, after adjustment for increases in the consumer price index the real income grew only 0.5% per year, to a 1986 average real income of $58,700. (In contrast, physicians' nominal net income had increased an average of 7.3% per year.) Further, it shows that the rich got richer and the poor got poorer: for 61.7% of pediatricians, 60.5% of physicians in general and family practice, 57.2% of those in internal medicine, and 54.7% of those in psychiatry, 1986 real income fell below the 1976 median. These specialties also reported the lowest net income. Obstetrics and gynecology came out slightly ahead: for 51.6%, 1986 real net income exceeded the 1975 median. Among surgeons, 58.4% had 1986 real income above the 1975 median; 72.1% of anesthesiologists had a higher real net income, as did 62.2% of radiologists.

The 1989 *Medical Economics* survey shows that the growth of physicians' earnings fell short of the 4.4% general inflation rate in 1987 and 1988, and that physicians' real income declined in 7 of the last 10 years. It also shows that the range of earnings has grown very wide. Although those who lost ground to inflation in 1988—anesthesiologists, general surgeons, neurosurgeons, and general practitioners—were not those who did so in the 1986 AMA 10-year survey, it probably was a short-term correction rather than a trend favoring family practitioners, internists and pediatricians.

The disparity between physicians' and surgeons' earnings has long been noted. The relative-value scales developed by various medical associations (enjoined by the Federal Trade Commission but used by many payers) exacerbated the gap. The resource-based relative value scale (RBRVS) may bring the earnings of cognitive practitioners closer to those who primarily perform surgery and other procedures. Private payors are likely to adopt similar payment systems.

The Impact of Managed Care

Results of recent *Medical Economics* surveys illustrate the growing impact of managed care. In 1986, HMOs typically represented 15% or more of the gross income for participating physicians who had been in practice one or two years, whereas for those in practice between 20 and 30 years, the percentage was only 8%. By 1989, HMOs represented between 13% and 15% of gross revenues for their participating physicians, regardless of the number of years in practice. The median gross income participating physicians derived from HMOs was $26,810 in 1988, a 60% increase over the 1985 figures. One out of 10 HMO-participating physicians received $100,000 or more, and 22% received $60,000 or more from HMOs in 1988. The median income from HMOs and PPOs combined was $35,330.

The impact varies according to specialty. Cardiovascular surgeons are the most likely to contract with HMOs. Obstetricians have the highest median income from HMO participation—$39,810—slightly ahead of orthopedic surgeons. Family practitioners and internists, who along with pediatricians act as primary care physicians or "gatekeepers," have among the lowest rates of participation in HMOs and PPOs (between 40% and 48%). For those who do participate, HMO payments are significant. In 1988, a typical participating family practitioner derived 18% of gross income from HMOs and 11% from PPOs. The comparable figures for internists are 13% and 7%, respectively. Capitation has been much more popular among the larger medical groups. For solo practitioners and groups of up to nine physicians, HMOs represented between 11% and 13% of gross income, and only 15% for groups of 10 to 24 physicians. The percentage jumps to 23% for groups of 25 to 49 physicians and to 25% for those of 50 or more.

The Status Quo: Sources of Physician Income

Physician income now derives from a variety of sources: some new, some traditional and others (eg, RBRVS), that are potentially revolutionary.

Self-paid Medical Expenses

The percentage of physician revenues that is self-paid (paid by the patient, without reimbursement by an insurer) decreased greatly with the expansion of health insurance. It still represents more than 30% of all physician income, however.

Salary and Profit-Sharing Arrangements

In the past, as in the present, the portion of physicians' income derived from salary rather than from a fee-for-service or other basis has remained fairly constant. Salaried positions are generally limited to interns and residents, younger physicians in medical groups, and employees of public health agencies and the Veterans Administration. In recent years this percentage has probably increased. Principal reasons are the growth of large medical groups—which is in turn due to their large census of capitated HMO patients—the erosion of the corporate practice doctrine as a barrier to hospitals and other institutions employing physicians, and the growing economic pressures against solo practice.

Partnership income represented at least 10% of physician income in 1965. Productivity incentives have been a common feature of medical group compensation since as early as the 1930s, when the popular "Duluth" formula developed. Now medical groups often determine the pay of physician employees as well as their partners or shareholders.

Capitation and Other Managed Care Incentives.

The development of managed care has led to a variety of incentive arrangements. One is capitation, a monthly or other periodic payment based on the number of individuals for whom the physician is responsible for providing or arranging for health care services. Capitating physicians for primary care services is a prevalent feature of independent practice association (IPA) model HMOs. It is sometimes also used to compensate referral specialists such as oncologists, orthopedic surgeons, and cardiologists. Capitation arrangements with primary care physicians often include risk and/or incentive provisions to discourage unnecessary hospital admissions, specialist referrals, and diagnostic tests. Negotiations in capitated or deeply discounted arrangements frequently carve out exceptional services, that is, those for which capitated physicians may be paid on a fee schedule basis, or a specialist paid on a more customary basis.

All-Inclusive Fees

So-called flat-fee arrangements are also encountered more often in managed care. A common example is found in obstetric care: a physician agrees to provide all prenatal and postnatal care and to attend the delivery for a normal or uncomplicated pregnancy in exchange for an all-inclusive fee. Sometimes the same rate also applies to normal caesarean sections. Hospitals and surgical teams increasingly offer all-inclusive rates, especially for cardiac procedures.

Hospital Contracts

Compensation of hospital-based physicians is a subject in itself. Although by 1930 fee-for-service arrangements had superseded salary positions, the economic terms by which anesthesiologists, radiologists, and pathologists practiced continued to differ greatly from those of office-based physicians. Thus they are often excluded from statistics on private physician income. Management agreements between hospitals and hospital-based physicians often provide for payment on a revenue-sharing basis.

As competition accelerated in the 1980s, hospitals began offering more incentives to encourage physicians to admit patients to their facilities. These arrangements included practice relocation agreements and a variety of supervisory or management positions.

Capitation

Capitation was part of the lodge practice and group practice prepayment plans early in the century. It was also a part of proposed national health insurance plans, including the Progressive Party's pre-World War I proposal and those by Senator Edward Kennedy and others in the 1970s.

Amendments to the Medicare law in 1986 called for the study and possible prohibition of physician capitation arrangements by Medicare risk contractors because such arrangements might reward physicians for denying necessary health care services. Studies by the General Accounting Office and the Physician Payment Reform Commission, as well as a recent position statement by the largest national HMO trade association, the Group Health Association of America, indicate that a blanket prohibition is unlikely. Medicare will probably continue to permit capitation when the payment for a Medicare beneficiary's specialist care and testing does not all come out of the primary care physician's pocket, and when the risks of higher-than-anticipated physician and hospital costs are spread fairly and within reasonable limits (eg, stop-loss) over a large number of practitioners.

Conclusion: The Current State of Affairs and Prospects for the Future

The question of how the medical profession reached this state of affairs, in which its autonomy—both economically and professionally—is threatened, is susceptible to a variety of simplistic but fairly accurate answers. One is that health-care costs have finally reached and exceeded the affordability limits of the institutional payers, both private and public, especially in the current era of limits on the U.S. economy. Another is that the medical profession is now the victim of its own success. According to this view, for too long physicians have been free from economic considerations. As a consequence, fee-for-service medicine has become intolerably costly to the institutions that have long acquiesced to the medical profession's autonomous decision making. State and federal agencies, insurers, employers, and other institutions (including some devised by or for physicians) have responded by tinkering with the system. They have asserted greater control at the expense of the individual practitioner. The entrepreneur may still flourish (or fail) on a more or less grand scale. The "superstar" will still prosper. Most physicians who wish to preserve as much as possible of medicine's traditional rewards will need to adapt to multiple and ever-changing payment rules; they will have to learn how to best identify and manage the business issues that now, inevitably, play a major role in the practice of medicine.

Suggested Reading

American Medical Association. *Voluntary Prepayment Medical Plans.* AMA, 1957, p. 9.

Gonzales, M. L., and Emmons, D. W. *Socioeconomic Characteristics of Medical Practice 1987.* Chicago: American Medical Association, 1987.

James, Norman. "The Flowering of Managed Care." *Medical Economics* (March 5, 1990): 89.

Owens, Arthur. "Earnings: Are You One of Those Losing Ground?" *Medical Economics* (September 4, 1988): 131.

Starr, Paul. *The Social Transformation of American Medicine.* New York: Basic Books, 1982.

Stoline, Anne, and Weiner, Jonathan. *The New Medical Marketplace.* Baltimore: Johns Hopkins University Press, 1988.

Todd, F. H. "Organization." *JAMA* 39 (October 25, 1902), p. 1061.

3 Fee-for-Service Medicine, Preferred Provider Organizations, and Health Maintenance Organizations

ROBERT CLIFFORD OSSORIO, MD,
AND MICHAEL J. ALPER

The delivery of health care is rapidly changing in the United States. New technology has allowed physicians to perform diagnostic and invasive procedures not even dreamed of a decade ago. Along with these quantum leaps in technology have come equally significant changes in the way health-care services are reimbursed to professionals. Both public and private insurance are undergoing profound changes. This chapter will review the dynamic changes occurring in health insurance coverage, some of the causes of these revolutionary changes, and specifically the differences among the three predominant reimbursement systems that currently exist.

Why Do These Different Systems Exist?

The costs associated with health care in the United States are staggering. Expenditures are projected to be $647.3 billion in 1990 (12% of the gross national product), $999.1 billion (13.4% of GNP) in 1995, and $1529.3 billion (15% of GNP) at the start of the next century. The annual per capita costs are expected to increase from $2,511 in 1990 to $5,551 by the year 2000. This represents a growth rate approximately three times the current rate of inflation. This situation is unsustainable and unaffordable for public, corporate, and family budgets. The cost impact on the two largest health insurance programs—the government-funded Medicare program and corporate-sponsored health benefits—is unquestionably approaching crisis proportions.

New technology introduced in the past decade has allowed for major advances in diagnostic, therapeutic, and invasive services. The use of this technology has become the standard of care in most communities. Physicians, who need to provide the best care available, tend to make use of new technology as soon as it becomes available. Patients, upon hearing of these new wonder drugs, procedures, or diagnostic tests, demand the most up-to-date therapy. The American public has a fascination with and strong expectation for the best, newest, most advanced health care.

The research and development costs for this technology must be recouped by increased fees from both vendors and providers of these services. Introducing a new technology requires support of the development as well as training providers in its use. These extremely expensive items are usually paid for by the patient receiving the care. The supply-and-demand cycle, which usually helps to control costs, does not seem to affect health care as quickly as it does other industries.

Malpractice and product liability litigation has also increased the cost of health-care services. The direct cost of defense and settlements in these suits is obviously very expensive. However, these costs are generally passed on to physicians in the form of increased malpractice premiums or liability insurance premiums. The sizable indirect costs, such as physicians giving up their practices or declining to perform certain procedures, has not yet been measured adequately.

Medicare costs rose relentlessly at twice the general rate of price increases throughout the 1980s, despite Congress imposing a variety of budgetary cuts and freezes and increasing the out-of-pocket expense to program beneficiaries. Medicare is projected to cost the government $110 billion in 1990, compared with approximately $300 billion for defense and $264 billion for Social Security. Government projections show that if current spending patterns hold, Medicare will become the most expensive government-supported program by the year 2010. Estimated year 2010 outlays will be $739 billion, surpassing Social Security expenses (approximately $736 billion). It is difficult to imagine where an additional $600 billion—twice the entire present defense budget—will be found.

Employers have also felt the impact of health-care cost increases. Most Americans receive health insurance as an employer-sponsored benefit. In fact, almost 85% of those under age 65 are covered through employer plans. However, only 46% of employers with 10 or fewer employees offer health insurance. Group health premiums increased at double-digit rates throughout the 1980s, rising 17% to approximately $2748 per employee per year in 1989. The total costs for health benefits are projected to surpass $3200 per employee per year in 1990.

Employers' increased health-care costs have had an unprecedented disruptive effect on management and labor relations. The percentage of strikers who walked off the job because of health-care benefits issues more than quadrupled during the late 1980s. Disputes over medical coverage motivated 18% of strikes in 1986 and 78% of strikes in 1989. The 1989 strikes are estimated to have cost the economy $1.1 billion in lost wages. These cost increases have caused the development of various health-care delivery models, all of which are intended to address the problem.

Physician Reimbursement Models and Their Effects on Health-Care Costs

Fee-for-Service Medicine

The catch phrase name for this model of reimbursement system is self-explanatory. In fee-for-service (FFS) medicine, a physician sets a fee for a particular service and expects to receive payment in that amount. At some point in time, every physician will establish fees for his or her most commonly performed procedures. How the fee is established varies among physicians, geographic areas, and community standards and is influenced, to some extent, by supply and demand.

Premiums for FFS medicine are usually based on the experience of the insurer and/or the insureds during previous periods. Benefits to an insured usually provide for coverage up to a maximum percentage of billed charges (typically 80%) after the insured has met a deductible. This "80/20" coverage has traditionally been referred to as *indemnity insurance*, because the insured is indemnified for any costs above a certain level (the deductible).

Many physicians have relied on relative value schedules for setting their fees. Standard values (units) are defined for a multitude of procedures usually grouped by service category (eg, medicine, surgery, or pathology) and a conversion factor (dollars per unit of service) is applied to these units to establish a fee. In theory, this will result in more complex procedures being reimbursed at higher amounts. However, much controversy exists regarding the way in which the units have been established. The medical community is anxiously awaiting the establishment of a resource-based relative value schedule (RBRVS), which it hopes will more accurately reflect the complexity of procedures.

Physicians have discretion in what tests, procedures, or examinations they will perform. Generally, no external utilization review mechanisms exist. Physicians may admit patients to hospitals without any preauthorization process or concurrent review. This traditional health-care delivery system yields a high level of physician satisfaction.

Essentially, FFS medicine has evolved to accommodate a "what the market will bear" mentality. Providers have continued to increase their fees at rates necessary to cover increased overhead and malpractice insurance and to sustain a life-style. Absolutely no controls exist in this environment. In fact, the more a physician can bill, the more likely he or she is to be reimbursed at a higher level.

FFS medicine has taken the blame for much of the increase in professional health-care costs. Information has been trickling in since the 1950s that there is wide variability and, most probably, unnecessary use of resources across physician practices. In the 1970s John E. Wennberg, MD, an epidemiologist at Dartmouth College, developed a valuable technique called *small area analysis* that could compare the incidence of medical procedures in similar locales. Since the 1980s he and others used this methodology to demonstrate that practice patterns can vary markedly among physicians. These variations have been attributed to professional uncertainty, differences in training, and provider-induced increases in utilization for monetary gain. Some experts have concluded that if the practice patterns of physicians at the lower end of this spectrum could be adopted nationwide, national health expenditures could decline by as much as 30%.

In the latter half of the 1980s, as the pressures to reduce costs increased and new information on the causes of runaway costs proliferated, intense scrutiny was focused on physicians. Congressman Fortney "Pete" Stark claimed that physician ownership-referral arrangements encourage overutilization and add significantly to the cost of care. He championed legislation that became part of the 1990 Budget Reconciliation Act, which no doubt will be the beginning of a series of future restrictions on physician ownership-referral arrangements. Dr. Arnold S. Relman, editor of *The New England Journal of Medicine* and a leading spokesperson within the medical community, said this type of legislation was the only way to stop a trend that was "bad for the public and unethical for the profession."

The Development of Managed Care Systems

Preferred Provider Organizations (PPOs)

The lack of payors' control over provider reimbursement led to astonishing developments in the late 1970s and into the 1980s. Given that a large portion of those covered by commercial health insurance receive this benefit from their employers, corporate America became a dominant force behind these changes. Initially employers attempted to shift some of the premium increases to employees as a means of containing costs. It became readily apparent to most corporations that this strategy alone would not yield a significant reduction in costs; decreasing utilization would have a greater impact on cost savings. This would require a partnership among employer, employee, insurer, and provider.

This partnership developed into what is now loosely called *managed care*. The first system implemented on a large scale under the managed-care umbrella was the preferred provider organization (PPO). PPOs are characterized by limiting the number of providers to those provider panels that generally accept discounted FFS payments. Providers are attracted to these programs because they most resemble traditional indemnity programs, and they hope that the reduction in reimbursement will be offset by higher patient volume. The fees are negotiated between the provider and payor, usually utilizing community standards. Generally the fee paid is all that the physician is entitled to collect; no balance billing of the patient is allowed.

In 1988, approximately two thirds of PPO physicians were paid using a maximum allowable rate for procedures. This meant that the insurer would allow only up to a predetermined amount established for specific procedures. One third of PPO physicians were paid a discounted rate, usually expressed as a percentage of billed charges. The average physician discount was 22% of usual and customary fees.

A PPO may be formed directly by any group of providers using established referral patterns among members of the group. A very popular development has been the formation of PPO networks. These are generally developed by a third-party administrator (TPA) or an insurer. Relationships are developed with physicians in wide geographic service areas, allowing the PPO network to market the organization as a single entity to any interested party.

PPO insurance programs are, from the patients' perspective, similar to indemnity in that they usually have a deductible and low or no coinsurance for patients who use a network provider. Patients seeking care outside the network will have a moderate to significant increase in their out-of-pocket expense.

PPOs usually attempt to control costs by requiring outside utilization review of many services. This may take the form of prospective, concurrent, and/or retrospective case management. Most commonly, second surgical opinions and preauthorization of elective hospitalizations are required to ensure coverage. Many physicians are skeptical of these requirements and their actual cost-saving benefits. Initially much resentment existed between PPO physicians and the PPO utilization review staff. As utilization review has become more common, most physicians have accepted it as a fact of life, and better cooperation has evolved.

PPO systems control costs only by reducing fees for specific services. Providers still have an incentive to perform more services than may be indicated; the more frequently a patient is seen, the more a provider will collect in total fees. Decreased utilization (with the hope of better controlling costs) can only be suggested by the external utilization review process. PPOs have been used as a way to accustom patients to managed health care systems, with which they hope to save additional premiums and out-of-pocket dollars.

Health Maintenance Organizations (HMOs)

Health maintenance organizations underwent a tremendous increase in enrollment during the latter half of the 1980s. The popularity of these programs can be traced to their reduced premiums and out-of-pocket expenses as well as the patient's feeling of receiving health care in a comprehensive system. More than 32 million people—approximately 12% of American workers and their dependents—belonged to HMOs at the beginning of 1990.

All HMOs express a policy of preventive medicine and offer more preventive health-care services than do other reimbursement models. It is hoped that this emphasis on wellness and prevention will allow for earlier detection of problems and encourage HMO enrollees to live healthier lifestyles.

HMOs are attractive to employers because of their emphasis on prevention and low premiums. HMOs vary in their premium structure but are either community- or experience-rated. Experience rating has become increasingly attractive to employers because it can help control their premium costs by encouraging healthy employee life-styles.

The major attribute of any HMO is its limited panel. HMOs are essentially closed systems, requiring patients to receive care from a contracted provider to ensure coverage. Emergency care rendered by a noncontracted provider is usually the only service covered outside the plan. Patients sacrifice some freedom of choice in order to receive essentially free care. Most HMOs require copayments of approximately $5.00 per office visit, and no deductible, for in-plan services.

HMOs can be classified into four provider models: staff model, group model, network model, and independent practice association model. In a staff model the physicians are employees of the HMO. These physicians generally do not maintain private practices and see only those patients enrolled with the HMO. Very often, these HMOs own or operate their own offices, clinics, urgent care centers, acute care facilities, and extended care facilities.

In the group model, HMOs will contract with an established multispecialty group. These groups may consist of physician partnerships, affiliations, or even employed physicians. The group model is attractive to the contracting HMO because the physicians already have established relationships both among themselves and, generally, with other providers in the community. A network model utilizes the same principles, but includes two or more multispecialty groups.

The independent practice association (IPA) is the newest and fastest-growing model in terms of enrollment. An IPA is an organization—usually a professional corporation—formed by physicians who each has a private practice. Usually the link among the physicians is affiliation with one or more hospitals in common. HMOs will contract either individually with the IPA's physicians or with the IPA as an entity. This arrangement is attractive to physicians because they maintain their individual private practices yet they get many benefits from affiliating with other physicians. It is also attractive to patients because the patient sees the physician in the physician's private office and has some choice as to which physician to see.

In the group, network, and IPA models, the provider organization is paid a per-capita amount for all medical services. The range of services for which the organization is responsible is negotiated between the group and the HMO. Some 70% of HMOs use a capitation system as the basis for payment of participating physicians, according to the latest study by Interstudy. Most HMOs using capitation systems place providers at risk for costs incurred by their enrollees.

The central point of care in these systems is the primary care physician (PCP): generally a family practitioner, internist, or pediatrician. The PCP acts as a gatekeeper, performing a whole spectrum of primary services and channeling appropriate services to contracted specialists. Two thirds of the HMOs included in the Interstudy survey pay PCPs on a capitated basis, placing them at financial risk for costs above the capitation amount.

Utilization review programs play an integral part in this system. All HMOs require prospective reviews for specialty and inpatient services, as well as concurrent review of inpatient stays. This review may be done by a committee from the IPA or group, by the HMO, or a combination of the two. Physicians generally are more receptive to the idea of utilization review performed by their peers than by an HMO. Peer systems can take into account community standards and are able to address concerns on a more personal level.

The typical HMO system may look much like Figure 3.1. Premiums are paid by various employer groups to the HMO. The HMO contracts with an IPA or multispecialty group to provide a full range of professional services. The IPA or group in turn contracts with its providers to act as PCPs or specialists. The IPA is paid a percentage of the medical premium collected by the HMO (capitation). Patients enroll with a particular group, and in the case of an IPA, the patient selects a specific PCP. The IPA pays a percentage of its revenue to the PCP as capitation. If a patient requires service outside the realm of the PCP's skill or service covered by the capitation payment, the PCP requests that the utilization review committee consider a referral request for specialty services. If the request is approved by this peer com-

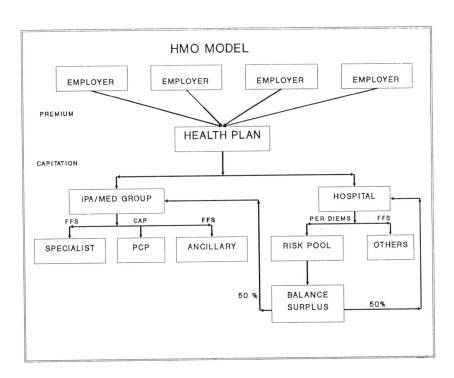

mittee, the member is sent to a contracted specialist, who may be paid either a reduced fee-for-service amount or capitation.

A similar utilization review process is usually employed to control elective hospital admissions. Generally a hospital risk-sharing arrangement exists, with any surplus in the risk pool being shared by the physicians.

Variations on this model exist. Two thirds of HMOs place PCPs at financial risk; one third capitate both PCPs and specialists. Nearly 80% of the HMOs using capitation hold individual physicians at risk for PCP services. Approximately half also place the individual PCP at some degree of risk for specialist services used by their patients. Many also capitate PCPs for hospital services. More than half of those HMOs using capitation pay individual physicians directly, whereas about one third pay physician groups or affiliated organizations. More than half of the HMOs paying capitation offer stop-loss or reinsurance coverage to protect capitated providers from catastrophic cases.

Medicare HMOs have been encouraged by Congress as a way to control costs. However, the growth in these plans has been a disappointment, with only slightly over 1 million enrollees at the end of 1989. The government will be trying to improve the situation through increased payments to HMOs and providers. Most of the activity has taken place in only a few established plans. Ten HMOs enroll about 60% of all Medicare enrollees. Of those ten plans, three large HMOs—Kaiser Foundation Health Plans of Oakland, California; Humana, Inc., of Louisville, Kentucky; and FHP, Inc., of Fountain Valley, California—have enrolled 435,000 Medicare patients or about 40% of the program's 1 million participants. If the present payment reform strategy does not work, no doubt additional efforts will be made to encourage Medicare recipients to shift to HMO programs.

The government's Physician Payment Review Commission will make necessary and appropriate recommendations, and politicians will be forced to evolve an increasingly more equitable and cost-effective Medicare reimbursement system. Well before the year 2000, Medicare may look like a mixed-model HMO, with a variety of managed care delivery systems. This will probably include direct contracting with individual physicians or small groups of physicians. In this case the contracts may be unilaterally imposed by the government.

Changes in HMO Models

To overcome the reluctance by both patients and providers to select closed or limited provider systems, hybrid models are being developed. These open-ended or point-of-service plans allow patients to choose at the time of service to receive care either within the HMO network with HMO benefits or from a non-plan provider with PPO-type benefits.

In the early part of the 1990s, much of the growth of HMOs, which is expected to extend to one quarter of the U.S. population, will probably be led by these open-ended plans. As standard HMO growth slowed in the late 1980s, open-ended programs picked up some of the slack.

These programs are extremely attractive, from the employer's perspective, combining the flexibility of a combination of HMO and PPO benefits with HMO premium structures. In the late 1980s, fee-for-service plans had rate increases of 25% to 40%, while 9% to 17% increases were implemented by HMOs. Employers are not satisfied with either of these levels of increases and are looking at open-ended programs as a better solution.

From the physician's perspective, participation in superior managed care programs has several advantages over fee-for-service systems. In a managed care program, physicians are not paid on a fee-for-service basis, but are paid more based on how effectively they deliver health care. Savings developed from facility and ancillary incentive or risk pools can be distributed to physicians. Additionally, these programs are capable of developing support systems and improving the delivery system design to dramatically improve the effectiveness of health-care delivery. Managed care programs can more expeditiously apply effectiveness guidelines and establish risk management controls to ensure more appropriate usage of services, especially new technologies. Throughout all managed care programs, appropriate concerns about quality can be addressed by implementing peer support and quality assurance mechanisms.

Conclusion

According to surveys of employee benefits in medium and large firms by the U.S. Bureau of Labor Statistics, premiums paid by employees for contributory plans have escalated faster than has the medical care inflation rate. In 1986, 46% of employees were required to contribute to their own coverage, compared with 29% in 1982. In addition, monthly premiums for contributory plans have increased 44% since 1982 for individual coverage.

Workers covered by plans with cost sharing by the employee and employer paid 6.6% of their after-tax earnings for health premiums in 1988. It is predicted that if current trends continue, the figure could rise to 27% by 1998, clearly a prohibitive amount for most employees.

Looking ahead to the 1990s, continued double-digit health-care cost inflation threatens our country with escalating labor unrest and the eventual destruction of employer-provided health insurance as the major vehicle for providing health coverage. This will result in further shifting of costs to those who are insured, further increasing premium dollars for those programs. This will probably influence more employers to develop self-funded insurance programs for their employees. Although this mechanism will tie the employer's cost to actual experience, it further fractures the insurance pool, making it difficult to spread insurance risk across larger populations.

Physicians need to understand these changes in reimbursement models. The differences among fee-for-service, preferred provider organizations, and health maintenance organizations become increasingly important as they affect the practice of medicine. To support physicians in their task of managing health care efficiently and effectively, the 1990 Federal Budget Reconciliation Bill provided funding and established an Agency for Health Policy and Research, which will guide and coordinate clinical effectiveness research and practice guideline development.

The practice of medicine must now include a long, hard look at the business of medicine. How each physician practices has a direct impact on the cost, outcome, success, and development of health-care delivery systems, which in turn affect the physician, insurer, employer, and patient.

Suggested Reading

Relman A. S. Dealing with conflict of interest. N Engl J Med 1985; 313:751.

4 | Government Regulation and the Health-Care Industry

WESTLEY SHOLES, MPA

Of the many problems health-care professionals face today, the ever-rising tide of regulations governing the industry ranks among the most frustrating. As the industry has grown and become more complex, the rules governing every aspect of health care have also changed. This chapter examines the regulatory system as it relates to the health-care industry with a special emphasis on how this system affects physicians.

The goal of this chapter is to provide a general understanding of how government regulates the health-care industry. The discussion will include past and present factors influencing the regulatory environment; trends that offer insight into what might lie ahead will also be reviewed.

This chapter is divided into three major sections: the first describes the legislative–regulatory process. The second section examines two additional roles government plays in the health-care industry that influence the regulatory process: that of financier and provider. These two roles and the interplay among all three are keys to understanding what happens in the regulatory process and why. Figure 4.1 depicts the various ways in which government is involved in health care. The third section will conclude the chapter with some general observations on what possibly lies ahead.

Some definitions and parameters are in order so that this subject can be adequately covered within the scope of one chapter. I will use the term *government* to mean federal, state, and local agencies collectively; however, unless specified to the contrary, my examples will be federal. The term *laws* will generally mean federal or state statutes passed as a result of the legislative process. *Regulations* will be used to mean instructions or procedures developed by governmental agencies to implement laws that have been passed. *Regulatory agencies* will refer to those agencies charged with oversight responsibilities for their areas of focus.

Dr. Typical Physician and the Regulatory System

Before we begin our review, let's look at a scenario of a hypothetical day in the life of Typical Physician, M.D., henceforth called Dr. TP.

It's 8:00 a.m. and Dr. TP is checking on a patient admitted from the ER last night, only to find the patient is without medical insurance and unfortunately does not qualify for Medicaid. Government regulations do allow

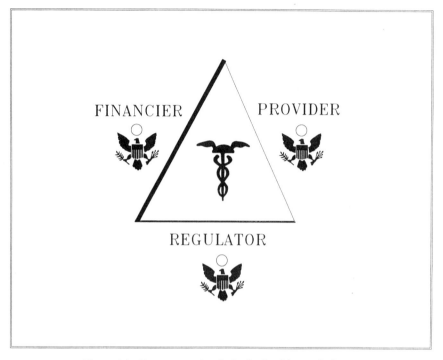

Figure 4.1. Government's role in the health care industry

for a token payment to the hospital, but not to the physician. The patient is too ill to transfer. Even if the patient could be transferred, the county hospital does not expect to be able to accept transfers for the next three days. Dr. TP is stuck with another patient for whom there will be no reimbursement.

10:00 a.m.: The hospital administrator is once again briefing physicians on the possibility of reimbursement below their usual fees because of new federal government regulations called DRGs.

12:00 noon: Dr. TP enters the office, and the manager expresses exasperation over the latest reimbursement rules from the state Medicaid agency. There is yet another level of justification required for reimbursement.

7:00 p.m.: At a meeting of the local medical society, a lively discussion is held on a regulation being proposed by the Health Care Financing Administration—the federal fiscal watchdog for Medicare and Medicaid—that would limit a physician's ability to refer patients to facilities in which the physician has a financial interest.

Later that evening, as Dr. TP reflects on the events of the day, he wonders, "Who makes these rules and regulations, and what are the motivating factors?" Although the foregoing scenario is hypothetical, it reflects the growing number and complexity of government regulations and their impact on physicians and other health care providers.

The Legislative-Regulatory Process

Most regulations govern how legislation is to be implemented. Let us first review how legislation comes into being.

Sources of Ideas for Legislation

Members of Congress and their staff are the most common source of ideas for legislation. Ideas can respond to a particular problem, reflect new ideas, or address a need to change existing legislation.

Private groups are another primary source of ideas for legislation. For the most part these groups—for instance, the AMA—represent special interests. Ideas are reflected in policy papers and through discussions with legislators and/or their staff. In some cases these groups might actually draft proposed legislation to present to a legislator to sponsor. In other cases, the executive branch might take the initiative for legislation. Generally, this occurs after the president or other key official in the administration has expressed a policy direction. This situation also requires the selection of a legislator or legislators to sponsor the bill. The route a bill takes from conception of the idea to passage into law is complex and often very time consuming; a general overview of that process follows. A graphic depiction of the process is shown in Figure 4.2.

Once the intent of the legislation has been defined, language is developed and the bill is introduced in either the House or the Senate. Congress basically functions under the committee structure, the heart of the legislative system. Once a bill is introduced, it is immediately referred to the appropriate committee or committees indicated by the nature of the bill. Many committees have a direct or indirect impact on health care; however, the eight committees listed in Table 4.1 are the most significant.

Committee membership is established at the beginning of each congressional session and is determined by the proportion each party represents in the total membership of the chamber as well as how each party assigns individual members. Seniority is a key factor in committee placements.

The chair of a committee is a pivotal figure in the legislative process because the chair determines the bills to be considered and the pace at which the process proceeds. This is particularly noteworthy since only a small fraction of introduced bills are actually passed.

Committees are generally categorized as *authorizing* or *appropriations* committees. Authorizing committees create laws that set forth what a program is intended to do and the maximum amount of public money to be spent for implementing the program. Authorizing responsibilities for most health issues are spread among four committees: Senate Finance; House Ways and Means; Senate Labor and Human Resources; and House Energy and Commerce (please see Table 4.1). Appropriations committees determine how much can be spent on previously authorized programs during a specific time frame.

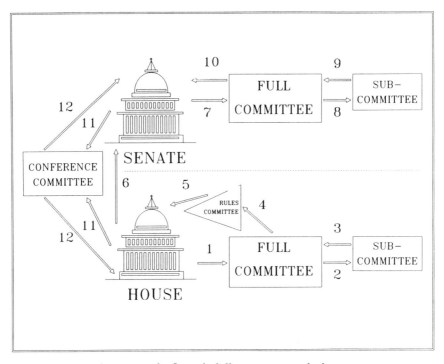

Figure 4.2. The flow of a bill originating in the house

Table 4.1 Eight Committees Having the Most Impact on Health Legislation

---

[a] Senate Finance Committee
   Subcommittee on Health for Families and the Uninsured
   Subcommittee on Medicare and Long-Term Care
[a] House Ways and Means Committee
   Subcommittee on Health
[a] Senate Labor and Human Resources Committee
   (Has no health subcommittees)
[a] House Energy and Commerce Committee
   Subcommittee on Health and Environment
Senate Appropriations Committee
   Subcommittee on Labor, HHS, Education, and Related Agencies
House Appropriations Committee
   Subcommittee on Labor, HHS, Education, and Related Agencies
Senate Budget Committee
   (Has no health subcommittee)
House Budget Committee
   (Has no health subcommittee)

Source: Isaacs, Joseph C. *Congress and Health,* National Health Council, Inc., July 1989

   [a] Authorizing committee.

Table 4.2 depicts the responsibilities of the major health committees. It differentiates between control over dollars and control over programs and illustrates the interrelated committee responsibilities.

It is important to understand how input is obtained by legislators. It is virtually impossible for legislators to know everything about every bill; therefore, Congress authorizes each committee to have professional and/or technical staff to assist in committee activities. For the most part, a group of technical and/or subject matter experts are the primary staff advisors to legislators. These individuals play a role in the legislative process that some believe is second only to the legislators themselves. It is interesting that the number of staff working for health-related committees in 1969 was approximately five; today that number has increased almost tenfold.

If the legislation successfully passes through the committee system, it is sent to the full chamber for action. The process described previously is repeated in the other chamber, and if the legislation is passed, it will be sent to the president for signature. If it is not passed or if amendments are made, the proposed legislation then goes to a conference committee consisting of members of both chambers. If the conferees are successful in resolving differences, the bill is then sent to the president for signature. If not, the bill dies.

The Regulatory Process

A number of bills passed by Congress significantly affect the health-care industry. For example, in the 100th Congress, 521 of the approximately 11,300 bills and resolutions introduced were health related. Each of the bills passed will be followed by a myriad of regulations to ensure legislative intent is carried out.

Once legislation is passed, the complex process of developing implementation rules and regulations begins. (Please see Figure 4.3 for a conceptual overview of this process.) The process is usually assigned to the agency

Table 4.2 Jurisdiction of Major Health Committees

| Committee | (Fiscal Year 1989 Estimates) | |
	% Health Dollars	% Health Programs
Senate Labor & Human Resources	10%	75%
Senate Finance	90%	15%
Senate Appropriations	59%	90%
House Energy and Commerce	56%	80%
House Ways and Means	65%	10%
House Appropriations	59%	90%

Source: Isaacs, Joseph C. *Congress and Health,* National Health Council, Inc. July 1989

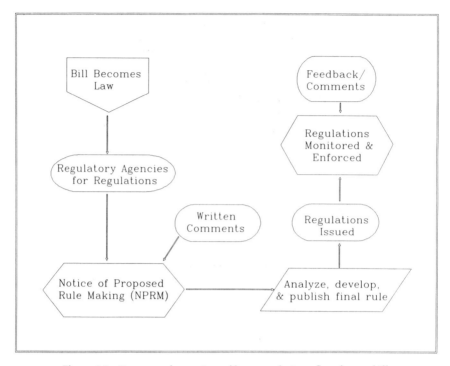

Figure 4.3. Conceptual overview of how regulations flow from a bill

with oversight responsibility for the program created by the legislation. Individuals involved with government-related programs greatly influence this process, and the resulting impact is not limited to new legislation but continues as opinions on legislative intent change and/or as new, related legislation is created.

In the health-care industry, the Health Care Financing Administration (HCFA), a unit under the Department of Health and Human Services, plays a major role in writing regulations for health-related legislation. These regulations often determine what services patients receive under federally-sponsored programs and how much providers will be paid. Because of this, the activities of the Health Care Financing Administration are of major interest to providers. This is clearly reflected in the many publications dedicated largely to interpreting the numerous regulations proposed by the HCFA. Many of the principal accounting firms that deal with health-related issues provide these publications as a courtesy to their clients.

Despite HCFA's ostensible role as a fiscal watchdog, political views regarding health care are often a significant factor in the selection and appointment of the HCFA administrator. This selection is also closely scrutinized by Congress.

The Multidisciplinary Role of Government in Health Care and How It Affects the Regulatory Process

The regulatory role of government in the health-care industry is multi-dimensional. It includes all levels of government: local, state, and federal. A significant percentage of federal and state legislation involves the health-care industry and sets the stage for how health care is delivered in this country. Regulations issued to implement legislation affect almost every aspect of a physician's work. For the most part, national health policy—to the extent the reader considers the United States as having a clear health policy—is manifested through the aggregate effect of health legislation and its ensuing regulations.

At the state level, regulations on matters such as licensing and quality control get close and continuous review. At the local level, counties or cities usually regulate or carry out state or federal requirements on matters such as communicable disease reporting. Figure 4.4 depicts examples of the three levels of government and responsibilities.

In addition to being the regulator, the second aspect of the multidimensional involvement of government in the regulatory system is its role in the health-care system as a payor for benefits and as a provider.

Figure 4.4. Multidimensional role of government in health care

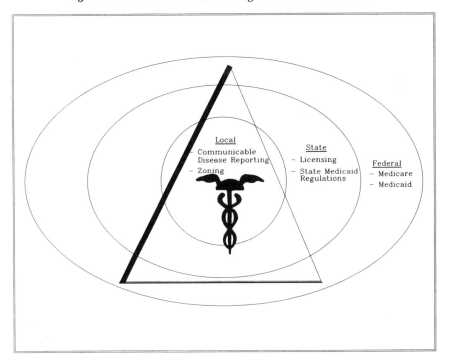

Let us now explore government's role as a financier and then as a provider.

Government as a Financier

The cost of health care in the United States is staggering:

Health care expenditures in the United States were slightly over $500 billion in 1987.

Tax dollars from all levels of government accounted for approximately 41% of health-care expenditures, or approximately $207 billion.

The federal tab was about 70% ($146 billion).

The 1987 expenditures were approximately 9.8% above the 1986 level; this represents a greater than tenfold increase over 1965.

The 1987 expenditures represent 11% of the U.S. gross national product (GNP). This is up from slightly less than 6% in 1965. However, the Health Care Financing Administration estimates a rise to about 15% of GNP by the year 2000 if current trends continue.

The United States spends the highest percentage of its GNP (11%) on health care; Canada is next, with 8.6%.

It is projected that 1990 will end with health care expenditures near $660 billion.

The sources of these data are various documents published by the Health Care Financing Administration. Please see Fig. 4.5 for graphic depictions of these data.

The federal government is currently the largest single payor for health care; consequently, its role as a financier greatly influences the regulatory process. Prior to the 1920s, there was minimal government regulation of health care. The first moves in this direction came with the reform of the physician licensing process. The World War II years saw a great increase in the number of trained health-care professionals along with great advances in health-care techniques.

In 1965, with the passage of Medicare followed quickly by Medicaid, the focus of the regulatory process shifted to a primarily fiscal role. Although initially opposed by medical establishment physicians, hospitals and health-care providers quickly recognized the tremendous potential— medical as well as economic—of these new programs. Today most hospitals and many physicians derive a significant share of their income from Medicare and Medicaid.

These new federally sponsored programs grew quickly, and costs to the government soon exceeded initial cost estimates. Because the government has been forced to allocate an ever-increasing share of the federal budget to health, it has tried to arrest what some have described as a "cash hemor-

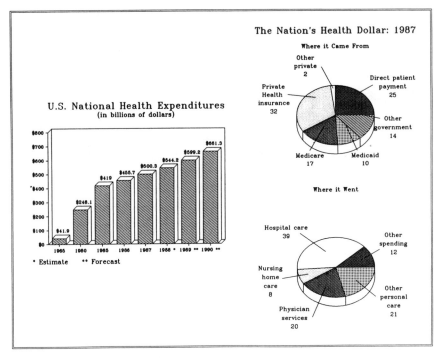

Figure 4.5. Selected statistics on U.S. health spending

rhage." The ever-increasing array of regulations is a direct function of this phenomenon.

Control mechanisms began to be developed by federal and state agencies; over the years, they have developed into what we have today: a large bureaucracy seemingly unable to find a reasonably effective mechanism to keep control over costs while still maintaining the initial goals of the programs.

A recent report by the Health Care Financing Administration included data from the Office of the Actuary on calendar year 1986 Medicare payments to hospitals. It states, "These payments increased 2.5% from calendar year 1985 to 1986. The small size of the increase, which is less than any other major service, is probably attributable to the Medicare prospective payment system. Physician payments ($18.8 billion) rose 8.6% in the same period, and outpatient services ($5.0 billion) rose 17.1%".

Prospective payment has had an arresting effect on expenditures on the hospital portion of the ledger; however, the Part B costs, which are mainly physician charges, have increased approximately eightfold since 1975. Because roughly 75% of these payments come from the federal treasury, Part

B will certainly be a ripe target for Congress and the regulators to implement more restrictive rules.

Government as a Provider

In 1985, 28% of hospitals in the United States were run by local or state governments, and the federal government ran approximately 8%. This, added to the local government's role as the provider of last resort, makes government a major player in the provider arena. Exact estimates of the costs incurred by local government for health care are complicated by the fact that many local governments provide preventive health or public health services. It is ironic that state and local governments often feel the fiscal pinch of federal regulations much more than does the private sector, given that more patients in public systems are covered by Medicare or Medicaid—assuming that the patient is covered at all.

What Lies Ahead

What will the regulatory climate be in the near future? It is likely that there will be more—rather than less—regulation of health care as we move into the 1990s. This is not to suggest more is better; it is rather a pragmatic forecast based on the current environment of general frustration with the lack of a clear federal agenda or policy direction. Following are factors that support this view.

Direction From the Top

Many observers of the health-care industry are bemoaning the lack of federal direction and leadership for a national health policy. Some believe the myriad of bureaucratic entanglements caused by increased efforts to solve our problems through regulation are worsening the situation rather than helping. At the same time, there seems to be acceptance that for now we will maintain and refine the tools currently in place or under consideration.

In his recent commentary, "Financing Health Care: A View From The White House" (*Health Affairs* 8 [Winter 1987]), William L. Roper states:

> As America enters the 1990s, many believe that major problems exist within our health care system. Despite recent incremental changes, the growing belief is that further modest change will not be sufficient and that fundamental health care system overhaul is needed. I believe that the next steps are to determine what the fundamental reform should be and how best to bring it about.

Roper points to cost of care, access to care, and quality of care as key issues that must be better addressed. He further discusses the trade-offs necessary to accomplish the goals leading to reform and suggests there is an insufficient mandate from the public to move the president to take action significantly different from our current course.

Blendon and Donelan, writing in *Health Affairs*, seem to echo Ropers' observation in a discussion on the importance of health in the 1988 election. They concluded that although the candidates' stands on health issues were important, they were insufficient to influence the outcome of the election.

More of the Same

These two observations suggest a continuation—in the intermediate future—of an incremental search for relief through a variety of approaches. Further, increased regulations will continue to be the instrument of choice to gain relief, by design or through default.

Some influential forces in the industry seem to be gearing up for a continuation of the current environment. The American Hospital Association's 1990 policy statement contains four major goals. One of these, "Public Policy Development," has seven subgoals, of which six specifically mention Medicare and Medicaid issues.

Another noteworthy observation is *Hospitals* magazine's forecasts on health care in the 1990s. In a discussion on hospital Medicare margins, Alden Solovy stated, "The amount of money that hospitals earn treating Medicare patients in the 1990s will depend on the results of the continuing struggle between health policy and budget policy. If health policy is the clear winner, hospital Medicare margins could rise to 5% by 1995. But if budget policy wins, they could fall to -10%."

Conclusion

Government regulation of the health-care industry has grown over the years from a relatively minor role, primarily involving public safety, to a complex system of rules dealing with all aspects of the health-care delivery system. The driving force today continues to be the welfare of the public; however, fiscal and medical policy considerations now influence the current regulatory process.

The process by which government regulates the health-care industry is now very complex and includes local, state, and federal agencies. Two additional roles the government plays—the role of health-care provider and the role of financier—are major factors contributing to the development of regulations.

Henry David Thoreau believed that the government that governs least governs best. In 1942 George Bernard Shaw wrote in *Doctor's Dilemma*,

> That any sane nation, having observed that you could provide for the supply of bread by giving bakers a pecuniary interest in baking for you, should go on to give

a pecuniary interest in cutting off your leg, is enough to make one despair of political humanity.

History shows where we in the health-care industry have come from. Observers may not agree on where we are today, and clearly, there is not a consensus on where we should be.

Acknowledgments

Acknowledgment is gratefully extended to Carol Fox, Jack Love, Stuart Williams, Estela Sandoval, and Della Stern for their technical assistance in preparing this chapter.

Suggested Reading

"Abstract." *Wall Street Journal* (April 4, 1989), Section B.

"A Hidden Health-Care Tax." *Boston Globe* (March 10, 1989).

"An Interview with Pete Stark." *Nursing Economic$* 5 (July–August 1987):151–156.

Benda, Chuck, "HHS Inspector General's 'Safe Harbors' May Be Stormier Than You Think." *Minnesota Medicine* 72 (April 1989):229–231.

Berk, Marc L., Monheit, Alan C., and Hagan, Michael M., "How the U.S. Spent Its Health Care Dollar: 1929–1980." *Health Affairs* 7 (Fall 1988):46–60.

Blendon, Robert J., and Donelan, Karen, "The 1988 Election: How Important Was Health?" *Health Affairs* 8 (Fall 1989):6–15.

Brink, Stephen D., "Health Care in 1990s: A Buyer's Market." *Hospital & Health Services Administration* (September-October 1986):16–28.

Coile, Russell C., Jr., "The Mega Trends—And the Backlash." *Healthcare Forum Journal* 33 (March-April 1990):37–41.

Deloitte, Haskins, & Sells, *Health Care Review* 7 (August 1988).

Deloitte, Haskins, & Sells, *Health Care Review* 7 (December 1988): .

Deloitte, Haskins, & Sells, *Health Care Review* 8 (March 1989): .

Deloitte, Haskins, & Sells, *Health Care Review* 8 (April 1989): .

Deloitte, Haskins, & Sells, *Health Care Review* 8 (December 1989): .

Deloitte, Haskins, & Sells, *Washington Briefs: A Perspective on Health Care* (March 22, 1989): .

Easterbrook, Gregg, "The Revolution." *Newsweek* (January 26, 1987):40–74.

"Expenditures for Health Care in the United States." *GHAA News* 31 (March-April 1990):27–28.

Freudenheim, Milt, "Calling for a Bigger U.S. Health Role." *New York Times* (May 30, 1989), Section D.

"Good Health-Care News." *Los Angeles Times* (May 30, 1989), Section II.

Gross, Jane, "What Medical Care the Poor Can Have." *New York Times*, (March 27, 1989), Section A.

Hanson, Kate, "The New Reimbursement Regulations." *Nephrology Nurse* (September-October 1983):17,20.

Health Care Financing Administration, *Health Care Financing Program Statistics: Medicare and Medicaid Data Book*. Washington, D.C.: U.S. Department of Health and Human Services, 1988, HCFA Publication No. 03270.

"Health-Care Market Operates on Bad Economic Principles." *Atlanta Journal* (December 5, 1989), Section A.

Hedlund, Carel T., "Why is HHS-HCFA Losing in the Courts?" *Health Span* 6 (January 1989):9–13.

Hiatt, Howard H., and Berwick, Donald M., "Health-Care Crisis: Instead of a Cure, A Sicker Patient." *Boston Globe* (April 2, 1989).

Isaacs, Joseph C., (Ed.), *Congress and Health: An Introduction to the Legislative Process and Its Key Participants*, 8th Ed. One Hundred-First Congress, Government Relations Handbook Series. Washington, DC: National Health Council, Inc., July 1989.

McCarthy, Carol M., "The AHA's Priorities for 1990." *Hospitals* 64 (January 5, 1990):40–43.

Merski, Paul G., "U.S. Health Costs Could Triple by the Year 2000." *Christian Science Monitor* (October 25, 1989).

Miller, Jeremy N., "Public Hospitals: The Legal Obstacles of Entering into Joint Ventures." *Healthcare Financial Management* (March 1986):44–48.

Neal, Thomas R., Mercer, John S., and Valentine, Robert L., "Medicare Reimbursement Issues." *Topics in Health Care Financing, Legal Issues in Health Care Joint Ventures* 13 (Fall 1986):41–56.

Oberg, Charles N., and Polich, Cynthia Longseth, "Medicaid: Entering the Third Decade." *Health Affairs* 7 (Fall 1988):83–96.

"Political Trends and Health Care Reform." *Nursing & Health Care* 10 (April 1989):178–179.

Reinhardt, Uwe E., "Perspectives on Physician Payment Reform." *Group Practice Journal* (March-April 1988):7, 10–13.

Roper, William L., "Commentary: Financing Health Care: A View From the White House." *Health Affairs* 8 (Winter 1989): 97–102.

Solovy, Alden, "Health Care in the 1990s: Forecasts by Top Analysts." *Hospitals* (July 20, 1989).

5 | Hospital Corporations and Their Changing Impact

JOHN R. COCHRAN III

In 1989 there were 5500 nongovernmental hospitals in operation in the United States. Of these, 1389 were operated by not-for-profit multihospital systems. Another 1104 were operated by investor-owned multihospital systems. This represents 45.3% of all hospitals, a dramatic change in hospital ownership and operation from 1980, when only 30% of U.S. community hospitals were part of systems.

The rise of hospital corporations parallels several key events in the development of the American hospital system. This chapter will link the growth and development of hospital corporations to several key events and explore the impact of multihospital corporations on physicians and their relationships with hospitals. Implications for the future also will be discussed.

1900s to 1940s

Hospitals were independent, free-standing facilities, largely operated by not-for-profit groups such as religious organizations or fraternal orders for the benefit of their communities. Because technology, including laboratory testing, diagnostic imaging, surgical interventions, and antibiotic drug therapies, were either underdeveloped or in their infancy, hospitals provided little more than basic nursing care and surgery. Because of relatively limited technology, physicians practiced primarily in office settings and used the hospital in limited ways. Diagnostic tools and treatment options were limited, and relatively few patients survived hospitalization.

Costs for hospitalization were relatively low, and much of the care was paid for through charitable funding. Health insurance was not in place, so the need for sophisticated business skills and organizational structure to manage hospitals did not exist.

1940s to 1960s

The discovery of antibiotic drugs, the development of modern anesthesia and surgery, and the introduction of diagnostic laboratory and imaging procedures created the need for more complex hospitals. The cost of the new equipment and the scarcity of personnel trained to use the equipment led to the concentration of these programs in hospitals. The hospital thus became the vehicle that attracted capital and personnel to provide the newly created services.

The scarcity of medical facilities after World War II heavily influenced the creation of the Hospital Survey and Construction Act of 1946 (Hill-Burton), which marked the beginning of extensive federal subsidy to both develop health resources and facilitate access. Other expansionary policies followed. Huge budget growth at the National Institutes of Health led to an enormous increase in medical research and technological advances as well as policies supporting growth in the supply of physicians and other health professionals.

Tax policy in the 1940s encouraged the development and growth of private health insurance plans and provided a steady flow of new funding to expand and enhance the hospital as the central focus of diagnostic and treatment resources.

The rapid infusion of new funds and growing complexity of services created a demand for organizational structures that could receive increasing funds, manage a growing and diverse work force, and deal with the complexities of the new health-care arena.

Academic programs in hospital administration began to train nonphysician managers to operate the hospital. By the mid-1960s, most hospitals were still free-standing, controlled by local community boards of directors. Physicians assumed growing responsibility for evaluating the qualifications of other physicians to use the increasingly complex and specialized equipment and procedures. This trend gave rise to the organized medical staff, the vehicle used to grant or deny doctors the right to use the hospital. Hospitals, mainly nonprofit, were still immune from professional liability for doctors' actions, and physicians viewed the hospitals as their workshops.

1960s to 1970s

Growing societal concerns about access to the products of medical research and technology created a demand for further federal intervention in order to ensure access for the aged and the poor. This led to the creation in 1965 of Medicare and Medicaid. Funding from these programs, coupled with federal funding for new hospitals, training of new physicians, and the encouragement of technology diffusion, led to a sevenfold increase in real federal spending for health care between 1950 and 1970. Health-care spending rose from 4.4% of GNP in 1950 to 7.4% in 1970. The late 1960s were described as the "transition from unquestioned payment to concern with the seemingly endless increase in expenditures for health services."

Enormous financial resources from federal and private insurance drew attention from highly successful businesspeople from other industries, who recognized that hospitals were being transformed from charity-funded organizations to large businesses. Leaders within the industry also recognized the change and called for reforms. Carl M. Platou wrote in *The Harvard Business Review*, "It has become apparent that community service is not in itself a sufficient incentive to insure the quality of operation required to meet the health field's problems of rising costs and uncoordinated delivery efforts. Reorganization of the health field into coordinated systems is inevitable. Within the next decade hospital management must commit itself to new corporate patterns".

Paul M. Ellwood, a leading thinker in the field, wrote in *The Harvard Business Review* in 1973, "The hospital industry is characterized by uninformed consumers, lack of management skills and small and inefficient delivery units".

New corporate structures emerged to capitalize on and provide new capital funding and economies of larger-scale operations. Many of these new structures were created by religious, charitable organizations as they attempted to deal with the growing costs and resultant financial risks. By 1980, there were 44 Catholic hospital systems, 29 Protestant hospital systems, and 45 secular hospital systems. The largest system in 1980 was operated by a large conglomerate known primarily for its construction and steel divisions—Kaiser Permanente.

At the same time, the growing need for capital to expand and provide new technology led to the development of investor-owned hospital groups. Buying free-standing hospitals and building new ones, investor-owned groups operated hospitals for the business opportunities they presented—a transformation of purpose from the earlier, charitable roots.

Physicians, feeling the impact of the change to groups of hospitals, investor-owned hospitals, and multihospital systems, were able to participate in the economic growth as part owners and investors. Systems in this early stage, however, did not seem to affect the physician's view of the hospital as a workshop.

Government, large purchasers of health care, and insurers welcomed the emphasis these new systems placed on business skill, which they hoped would restrain the rapid cost growth. Dr. Thomas Frist, chief executive of a large system, Hospital Corporation of America, wrote in a 1983 *Harvard Business Review* article, "The entry of large hospital management companies has been a healthy stimulus to a complacent, obese, and fragmented industry. Costs and productivity are the two most important issues facing the hospital industry."

1970s to 1980s

In the 1970s and 1980s government and insurers began initiatives to contain the growth in costs through such regulatory approaches as utilization review, rate controls, and control over technology diffusion through capital expenditure review. Most of these efforts applied to hospitals and did not significantly affect physicians' ability to continue their free-standing practices. During this period, hospital systems expanded through acquisitions, dealt with the variety of controls over rates and services, and generally became bigger and more sophisticated. By the early 1980s, all constituencies realized the regulatory approach was effective neither in improving access to care nor in emphasizing economy and efficiency.

In 1983, acknowledging that systemwide cost containment through regulation was failing, the federal government turned to a more focused, tactical approach aimed at limiting its own expenditures. The federal government also encouraged cost containment within hospital systems by creating financial incentives for newly developed health maintenance organizations (HMOs) to participate in Medicare. Enactment of prospective payments based on diagnosis (the prospective payment system, or PPS) forced hospitals to take financial risks never before taken. This increased responsibility to assume and manage financial risk across large groups of patients was a job previously carried out by insurers. Federal policy also encouraged private purchasers and insurers to create HMO and other managed care plans, which required totally new relationships between hospital systems and doctors.

No longer could the hospital view itself as the doctors' workshop. The hospital and doctor were forced to begin the difficult process of aligning their financial fortunes. New risk-sharing arrangements arose in which insurers transferred their financial risk to hospitals and doctors. The magnitude of financial risk and the complexity of the information and management skills needed to function in this environment further strengthened the roles of hospital systems.

Concurrently, the congruence of the increasing costs of operating physician practices and the competitive environment and oversupply of physicians created more need to develop management and clinical systems for physicians. Hospital systems were forced to implement marketing plans in order to keep their institutions functioning and profitable. Of necessity, larger, more efficient entities needed to be developed to deal with lower payments and higher risk. For the first time, physicians and hospitals had financial incentives to work together to reduce patients' lengths of stay and overall costs, as a result of federally stimulated HMO growth. This caused fundamental changes in the hospital-doctor relationship: the physicians' financial future was increasingly tied to that of the hospital, and vice versa.

The hospital also has become increasingly legally responsible for the practice of independent physicians because of the removal of immunity to suit and the placing of liability on boards of directors for doctor practices. New mechanisms have developed to measure and evaluate the clinical performance of physicians. Growing pressure is being placed on both doctor and hospital to function as one when it comes to performance and outcome measurement. Data on both hospital and doctor performance are being collected, analyzed, and published to inform the consumer and the purchaser of the value a particular group of hospitals and doctors provide for the funds they receive.

Excess capacity, costly new data systems, financial risks related to fixed price payments for services, and the growing demand to provide a coordinated system are increasing the influence of hospital corporations over all portions of the delivery system. The solo practitioner will face greater, more difficult challenges in surviving without a hospital system affiliation and a group-type setting.

Today hospital corporations assist physicians to develop new practice models with which to reduce practice overhead. These models frequently require physicians to form closer ties with insurers and employers in order to provide access to their patients and market the combined doctor-hospital entity.

The sharing of financial risk between hospitals and doctors is making it necesssary for larger groups of physicians to spread risk in an affordable manner. Shared risk has encouraged corporate medical practices such as medical groups, independent practice associations, and large partnerships to flourish.

The Year 2000

Multihospital systems will dominate hospital care provided in the United States because of (1) transfer of the risk of losses from patient care from insurers to hospitals and their doctors and (2) the necessity to manage this risk across large numbers of patients and facilities. Physicians with managed care contracts will influence the hospital corporation of the year 2000 by their control of patient referral and flow and by continuing their role in evaluating who is permitted to utilize costly and scarce technology in the hospital and how effectively services are being provided.

Payments will be funded by a nationally based payment mechanism that will ensure minimal access but leave operations in the hands of the private sector. Multiple private health plans will still exist to provide market choices supplementing the minimal benefits provided under the national scheme.

A physician trying to determine which hospital to join in this environment will need to evaluate new and challenging factors: reputation, stability of finances and management, location, market position, vision and strategy for the future, and the role of the parent corporation in gaining access to patients for its affiliated physicians. The concentration of high-risk and high-technology procedures in large centers will limit practice opportunities for those specialists who perform procedures such as transplants.

Hospitals and their doctors will develop their corporate structures to resemble HMO groups such as Kaiser, with large groups of hospitals and their doctors joined together to assume risk and manage care. There will be few hospitals in the United States that will be better funded, better managed, and more stable as a result of the implementation of universal access. The evolution of hospitals from poorly funded charities with very little technology or management skills into sophisticated systems with major risk contracts will complete this process.

Physicians will enjoy a greatly enhanced position in the new health-care corporation of the year 2000. Medical director positions and leadership roles for the combined doctor-hospital entities will evolve when clinical and business skills are merged into the health-care delivery system corporations.

Suggested Readings

1. Historical Growth of Hospital Corporations

Ellwood, Paul M., "Healthcare—Should Industry Buy or Sell It?" *Harvard Business Review* (July 1973).

Goldsmith, Jeff C., "Outlook for Hospitals—Systems are the Solution." *Harvard Business Review* (September 1981).

Platou, Carl M., "Multihospital Holding Companies." *Harvard Business Review* (May 1972).

2. Future View of Hospital Corporations

Longest, Beaufort B., "American Health Policy in the Year 2000." *Hospitals and Health Services Administration* (Winter 1988).

6 Medical-Legal Issues in Today's Practice

PETER N. GRANT, JD, PHD,
AND ROBIN T. TUCKER, JD

Physicians entering the practice of medicine today are facing a substantially different practice environment than did their predecessors. The business of medicine has become highly regulated, and the law and lawyers affect almost every area of a physician's practice. The physicians of the baby-boom generation are facing increased competition as well as growing cost containment pressures, discounted or capitation payment, and Medicare fee freezes. After a physician establishes a practice and obtains the appropriate licenses and certifications, he or she must then focus on building strong relationships with his or her patients, with other providers of health-care services, and with health benefit payors in order to flourish in the newly competitive health-care environment.

A number of legal constraints are placed on a physician's relationships with patients. Laws regarding informed consent and the right to refuse or withdraw from treatment affect a physician's treatment options. Third-party payors and employers are taking an increasingly active role in patient care determinations, causing physicians to confront the ethical dilemma of divided loyalties between the patient and the payor.

Physicians' relationships with other providers have become increasingly complex. The emergence of alternative delivery systems requires physicians to be savvy business negotiators in addition to being well-informed practitioners. Physicians are as likely to be employees in the new health-care environment as they are to be employers. Physicians have turned to joint ventures and integrated practice models to retain their competitive edge. However, physicians must be wary of the antitrust issues surrounding their newly formed business combinations in light of the federal antitrust authorities' aggressive posture in the health-care field.

Finally, federal and state governments have taken a more active role in physician peer review. The development of federal peer review organizations (PROs) under the Medicare laws has brought with it myriad regulation, reporting, and disclosure requirements. Federal and state laws have been enacted to foster the peer review process in the provider setting; yet at the same time the law of many states has granted greater hearing rights to physicians. Now, more than ever, physicians' clinical decisions are questioned, challenged, and scrutinized at every level.

Professional Licensure and Certification

The primary prerequisite to enter into medical practice is obtaining appropriate licensure. A physician should focus not only on his or her own licensing requirements, but also on the licensing requirements for any employees or independent contractors working with the physician.

Typically each state has a basic medical practice act, which defines medical practice and the permissible scope of action for other health practitioners. Broad authority to use various techniques, ranging from surgery to the prescription of drugs, is bestowed on the medical doctor and the doctor of osteopathic medicine. Unlawful practice of medicine is generally made a criminal offense, and courts may be empowered to issue injunctions. Medical practice acts generally establish a board or other entity to oversee the examination and registration process and to take disciplinary actions, such as revocation or suspension of licenses. In addition to licensure, a physician may wish to consider applying for one or more specialty boards.

The Physician's Relationships with Patients

A physician's relationship with his or her patients is fraught with legal and ethical obligations. Historically the physician-patient relationship was based on paternalism. The physician was deemed to have full authority to make medical care decisions in the best interest of the patient. In the last 25 years, the philosophical underpinning of the physician-patient relationship has shifted toward a focus on patient autonomy and patient rights.

Contractual principles at the foundation of the physician-patient relationship require that the physician meet a certain standard of care in treating the patient and in terminating the physician-patient relationship. The physician is obligated to comply with informed consent requirements in making determinations about the course of treatment and must respect the wishes of the patient in determining the ultimate choice of care. Physicians are now faced with situations where patients choose death over life-sustaining treatment and must be prepared to administer to the patient's spiritual—as well as physical—needs, in complying with these requests.

Initiation of the Physician-Patient Relationship and the Obligation to Continue Patient Care

The physician-patient relationship is essentially a contractual one. By coming to see a physician, submitting to a physical examination, and returning for follow-up visits, the patient accepts the physician's offer of medical care in exchange for a promise to pay a reasonable fee for the services. In return, the physician is generally obligated to provide the patient with all required follow-up care.

Although the patient can formally discharge a physician by simply not returning, or by choosing another physician, the requirements for the physician to terminate the relationship are not as straightforward. The level of care required of a physician in terminating the relationship depends on the medical status of the patient. Generally a physician is expected to give timely notice of the intention to terminate the relationship so that the patient has the opportunity to obtain substitute medical care. The notice should include the physician's statement that he or she intends to terminate the relationship on a specific date in the future, and that the patient should seek other medical care. This can be done in writing or orally. If the physician chooses to send the patient a letter, it is best to send it by registered mail, return receipt requested.

Whether the notice will be viewed as timely depends upon the surrounding circumstances and the perceived difficulty the patient may have in finding alternative medical care. Should a physician fail to give the patient timely notice of the termination, the physician is open to a charge of abandonment. Some of the circumstances that have supported a legal finding of abandonment include premature discharge from a physician's care; failure to give instructions on what to do or whom to call should unexpected symptoms occur; failure to supply any, adequate, or competent coverage on the physician's days off or at vacation time; and failure to give either the covering physician or the patient the requisite information about the other.

Informed Consent

Laws regarding informed consent affect the way patient care is rendered. The doctrine of informed consent imposes on a physician the duty to explain the procedure to the patient and to warn of any material risks or dangers inherent in or collateral to the therapy, before the patient is subjected to medical treatment. Additionally, complying with the consent requirements in the case of minors can be complicated, and the rules vary from state to state. Complete disclosure is not required in some circumstances, and under emergency circumstances no consent is required. A physician must also remember that inherent in the doctrine of informed consent is the right to withhold consent.

Standards of Informed Consent

The patient must be given the opportunity to make an intelligent and informed choice about whether or not to undergo treatment. The duty to disclose requires the physician to reveal to the patient the nature of the ailment, the nature of the proposed treatment and the desired outcome, the probability of success of the contemplated therapy and its alternatives, and the risk of unfortunate consequences associated with such treatment or the alternatives. Failure to obtain the patient's consent (or the consent of a legal representative) or failure to inform the patient of the consequences of refusing treatment may subject a physician to a claim of negligence.

Consent of minors. The laws regarding the consent of minors vary depending on the state and on the type of treatment sought by the minor. The age of majority is generally prescribed by statute in each state. In some states, a parent or guardian must give consent for the minor; in others, both the parent *and* the minor must consent to the medical treatment.

Minors who have moved out of the parent's or guardian's home, have graduated from high school, have married, or have been pregnant may be considered emancipated and may be able to give effective consent to medical care for themselves, even though they have not reached the age of majority. However, it is not entirely clear that an emancipated minor may refuse medically necessary treatment. In some states, a minor may consent to care to determine the presence of or to treat pregnancy, venereal disease, and other reportable diseases. In addition, the existence of a requirement of parental consent for a minor to obtain an abortion varies widely from state to state.

Therapeutic privilege. Courts have recognized that a physician may, under certain circumstances, withhold information from a patient that would otherwise require disclosure, provided that the physician has determined that disclosure would be harmful to the patient's health and well being. This *therapeutic privilege* may apply if the patient is extremely apprehensive and emotional about his or her condition and the physician believes full disclosure would be likely to cause such great anxiety that treatment would be hindered or psychological injury would be suffered. Where the privilege is invoked, the physician should provide the nearest relative or relatives with the information that is withheld from the patient. The family, however, may *not* dictate that any information be kept from the patient. It should be noted that withholding such medically relevant information from patients is increasingly frowned upon by courts.

Refusal of treatment. Generally, medically competent patients have the right to refuse treatment or to withhold or withdraw consent for treatment. A physician must be prepared to determine whether a patient is capable of making that decision. A patient who has been administered large amounts of medication, or who is in extreme pain or shock, may be unable to appreciate the significance of a decision to refuse care. The physician must assess the patient's capacity to comprehend information, to respond to questions based on it, to think clearly, without confusion or disorientation, and to act in a rational manner. Patients must also be assessed in light of their social environment, their family pressures, and their relationship with the physician.

Emergency exception. In response to the complications involved in obtaining consent in emergency medical situations, an exception to the informed consent requirement has been recognized. When a patient does not have the mental ability to reach an informed choice and treatment appears to be immediately necessary to prevent deterioration or aggravation of the patient's condition, consent is not required. In some jurisdictions, the legal next of kin is authorized by law to give permission on behalf of the patient in emergency situations.

The emergency exception may not be applicable if the patient has previously refused treatment. Generally, a competent patient who refuses treatment but later lapses into incompetence (eg, the patient's bleeding reaches a point at which the patient goes into hypovolemic shock) should not be treated under the emergency exception because the subsequent incompetence does *not* invalidate the patient's original refusal of treatment. Careful attention should be given to the laws surrounding refusal or withdrawal of treatment, which are discussed below.

Most physicians view informed consent as most important in the tertiary care setting, where discrete procedures are performed, the risks to the patient are significant, and the values placed on alternative forms of treatment are weighty. It can also be assumed that the specialist physician performs a limited number of procedures and can be expected to know the precise risks, benefits, and alternatives for each. However, the primary care physician performs a multitude of procedures, and in many cases the risk to the patient is minimal. Nevertheless, no legal premise supports a distinction between the consent requirements in these two settings.

A California case, *Truman v. Thomas* (1980) 27 Cal.3d 285, 292, held that the defendant doctor had breached his duty to his patient when he failed to inform her of the risk involved in her failure to authorize and undergo a pap smear test. The court stated: "If a patient indicates that he or she is going to *decline* a risk-free test or treatment, then the doctor has the additional duty of advising of all material risks of which a reasonable person would want to be informed before deciding not to undergo the procedure." Better incorporation of informed consent in the primary care setting has strong advocates.

Refusal and Withdrawal of Life-Sustaining Treatment

Because of medical technological advances, courts in a number of states have had to grapple with the issue of when to uphold an individual's *right to die*. Physicians are routinely confronted by decisions to withdraw life-sustaining procedures, including nutrition, from a patient. Some states treat the withdrawal of life-support systems differently from the withdrawal of food and water. Although these decisions must be made by the patient or surrogate in conjunction with the physician, hospital ethics committees and occasionally the courts may also be involved. Little—if any—training in medical school prepares a physician for this type of life-and-death decision.

In most situations, a competent patient's decision to forgo any and all life-sustaining treatment must be honored. Additionally, a surrogate may authorize—and perhaps compel—discontinuation of treatment for an adult person without decision-making capacity who is terminally ill or irreversibly unconscious. The next of kin is presumptively the surrogate, unless there is a guardian or the patient has previously designated a decision maker, typically through a document called a "durable power of attorney for health care." The parent—or if there is no parent, the guardian—may refuse treatment for a minor patient who is terminally ill or irreversibly unconscious, if the minor has indicated agreement prior to impairment. However, there are restrictions concerning such decisions for infants under certain federal laws and state child abuse laws.

The general standard of care dictates that the diagnosis and prognosis of terminal illness or irreversible unconsciousness be documented by the attending physician and, in most situations, confirmed in writing by at least one other physician. Decisions to withhold or withdraw treatment should, in nearly all situations, be pursuant to a written order by the physician.

Numerous states have attempted to address the issue of the right to die by enacting laws regulating living wills, which give individuals the opportunity to consent to the withdrawal of treatment before their mental competency can become an issue. If a patient has a validly drafted living will, the decision to uphold the patient's wishes may be easier to carry out. When the physician disagrees with the patient or surrogate, based on grounds other than the prognosis or diagnosis, the care of the patient should be transferred to another physician acceptable to the patient. The obligation to transfer care of the patient is mandated by the living will laws of many states.

Duty to Treat the AIDS Patient

Generally, physicians do not have a duty to accept patients they do not wish to treat. However, state antidiscrimination laws have carved out numerous exceptions regarding refusals to treat certain persons. The increase in the number of patients with acquired immunodeficiency syndrome (AIDS), and the corresponding demand for physicians to treat them, could force the courts to find a public policy duty to treat such patients. The Washington State Human Rights Commission has interpreted its antidiscrimination statute protecting handicapped individuals to apply to AIDS-based discrimination in dental offices, doctors' offices, hospitals, and nursing homes. California and New York have municipal antidiscrimination ordinances that expressly prohibit such discrimination by health-care providers.

The American Medical Association's Council on Ethical and Judicial Affairs has stated that physicians may not ethically refuse to treat a patient who has AIDS or has tested positive for human immunodeficiency virus (HIV). Individual state medical organizations have not felt bound by the

AMA's pronouncement, and some have specifically endorsed a physician's right to refuse to treat AIDS patients. For instance, the Arizona State Board of Medical Examiners and the Texas Medical Association have decided that physicians may ethically refuse treatment to patients with AIDS.

Hospitals that receive Medicare, Medicaid, or Hill-Burton funds, and possibly tax-exempt facilities, are prohibited from discriminating against AIDS patients. The question remains as to whether the facility has a duty to require members of its medical staff to treat HIV-infected patients. Although the answer varies from state to state, the clearest case is presented with hospital-based physicians. An argument can be made that if a facility has a duty to treat an HIV-infected patient, that duty extends to a contract physician, who has been given the exclusive right to render certain services at the facility; noncontractual physicians, who nonetheless practice within a defined specialty, present a more difficult question. At least one California opinion has held that where a physician controls scarce health resources in a community, that physician is operating as a quasi-public enterprise, and may have a greater duty to provide care than would otherwise be the case. (See *Leach v. Drummon Medical Group. Inc.* (1983) 144 Cal.App.3d 362.) The public policy issues may revolve around the physician's specialty and the availability of alternative sources of care.

The Physician's Relationships with Other Providers

Today the physician's relationships with his or her primary professional colleagues and institutional affiliates are quickly evolving. Traditionally physicians in the United States have engaged primarily in solo or small-group practice and have related to other physicians through loose referral networks. The emergence of alternative delivery systems, such as health maintenance organizations (HMOs) and preferred provider organizations (PPOs), has forced physicians to reconsider their practice settings and delivery systems.

The physician's relationship with the hospital is changing as well. Formerly an institution in which the physician practiced, now the hospital frequently is the physician's business partner. A debate has even emerged regarding the fundamental nature of the hospital medical staff: Is it part of the hospital or a separate legal entity?

Partially and Fully Integrated Practices

Increased competition, the growing costs of providing care, and the need for more effective contracting with HMOs and PPOs have encouraged some physicians to consider integrating their practices in a variety of ways. Such new medical practice entities range from the loosely organized physician PPO to more tightly organized individual practice associations (IPAs) and *clinics without walls* and, finally, to fully integrated medical group practices.

Although the IPA is currently the most frequently adopted partially integrated practice model in the more competitive geographic markets, the clinic-without-walls model is being experimented with in several locations. Under such a scheme, member physicians continue to practice in their separate locations, but they consolidate their entire practices into a single legal entity that employs all of its members and fulfills the same functions as the traditional group practice. The entity takes on the responsibilities of leases and support services, as well as providing for malpractice insurance and employee benefits. All of the professional revenues of the participating physicians are revenues of the group. The economic integration allows the group to take advantage of significant economies of scale, and to adopt uniform fee schedules for all patients without running afoul of the antitrust laws.

In restructuring their medical practices, physicians must be aware of the restrictions imposed by a number of areas of the law, including corporate-practice-of-medicine laws, tax laws, antitrust laws, and state facility licensing statutes. Although corporate-practice-of-medicine laws are often ignored, such statutes are still on the books in many states. These laws prevent a physician from being employed by a business corporation. State and federal tax laws also play a role in determining the form of entity selected by physicians for their practices and any health care ventures in which they might participate. Tax and labor codes control the types and amounts of benefits provided by the physician's business, and state licensing laws may control the types of ventures in which the physician may own an interest.

Hospital-Physician Joint Ventures

Another response to competition among health-care providers has been the physician joint venture or the hospital-physician joint venture. By pooling economic resources, physicians compete with new or potential market entrants in the areas of urgent care, ambulatory surgery, imagery, and so on. Recent changes in both the statutory and regulatory framework of anti-referral laws have made it more difficult to engage in these types of joint ventures. In addition, many states have enacted antireferral statutes.

Although it has become increasingly difficult for physicians to invest in health-care facilities to which they might refer patients, there are still forms of investment that may have positive advantages for the physician. Investments in medical office buildings may still provide attractive returns on investment while facilitating the integration of physician practice groups. Hospital-physician joint ventures can still be structured in a manner that does not violate the antireferral laws. Some of the other legal issues that must be reviewed by a physician entering a joint venture are antitrust issues, reimbursement considerations, tax implications, and the applicability of Internal Revenue Code Section 414(m), which requires certain joint-venture entities or investors to be considered as one employer for purposes of their employee benefits plans.

The Hospital-Medical Staff Relationship

Generally, the most important provider relationship that a physician has is with a hospital. The tension between a hospital's need to determine which physicians may practice within its facilities and the physician's right to practice there has created a web of common law and statutory protections relating to the hospital-medical staff relationship.

As a general matter, a physician has a right to fair treatment should his or her application for medical staff membership and clinical privileges be denied or right to practice at a hospital be curtailed or completely withdrawn. Basic fair procedure in this context is established by various state laws. However, at a minimum the physician must be generally accorded a right to a hearing on the matter.

Peer Review

Traditionally the hospital medical staff was a primary source of peer review in each local community. The scope of physician peer review has expanded far beyond the traditional medical staff setting.

Congress has created its own peer review system under the Medicare regulations. Independent peer review organizations (PROs) were established nationwide. PROs can deny payment to a physician for Medicare services on the basis of medical necessity, professional standard of care, or appropriate setting. Denials of payment based on the provision of substandard care carry with them a requirement of notice to the Medicare beneficiary that the care rendered was substandard.

The implementation of the PRO review process not only created a system for review of a physician's care decisions after they have been rendered, but also requires the physician to seek approval prior to rendering care in certain situations. Additionally, PPOs and HMOs often have their own peer review process. The rules and regulations governing these peer review bodies are contained in both federal and state law. Physicians are encouraged to consult counsel if peer review proceedings are initiated against them.

Through the reporting requirements under the Health Care Quality Improvement Act of 1986 (HCQIA), physician peer review actions can now be reported to state licensing authorities, increasing the significance of such actions. One purpose of HCQIA is to attack the problem of incompetent physicians moving from state to state. HCQIA also expanded the hearing rights of physicians. Pursuant to HCQIA, a National Practitioner Data Bank is being established to receive, correlate, and disseminate information on disciplinary actions taken against physicians. Hospitals will be required to request the information in the data bank when credentialing physicians. In addition, information regarding a judgment or settlement of a malpractice claim against a physician must be reported by payors or insurance companies. Pursuant to amendments to the Medicare and Medicaid Patient and Program Protection Act of 1987, the data bank may take a proactive role in disseminating information to state Medicaid fraud control units, peer review organizations, state attorneys general, and other law enforcement agencies.

In the hospital setting, provisions in HCQIA have increased the responsibility of hospitals to conduct peer review. The increased liability on the part of hospitals that fail to police the quality of care provided by their physicians has naturally created tension between physicians and hospitals in the peer review process. To protect physicians who participate in peer review in hospitals, numerous state laws have established immunity from liability for peer review decisions. In an effort to protect the rights of physicians, HCQIA provides due process safeguards for physicians involved in a peer review process. Under the terms of the federal law, California and Maryland have replaced the HCQIA protections with their own peer review systems, ostensibly to provide even broader due process protections for physicians.

Summary

The current level of review and regulation of an individual physician's practice has created a legal mine field for the unwary practitioner. Physicians are exposed to licensing, tax, labor, antitrust, and general corporate laws in the transaction of their businesses. In addition, Medicare regulations, state and federal peer review requirements, and developing ethical rules continue to affect the way a physician provides care.

Medicine as a learned profession has given way to the demands of medicine as a business. The pressure to control costs imposed by the government, third-party payors, and employers is forcing physicians to find alternative methods of delivering their services. The regulatory environment, however, is controlling the manner in which physicians can choose to provide care. A physician entering practice should be aware of the multitude of laws that apply to the practice of medicine. A physician should consult legal counsel before entering a transaction or selecting a form of entity to avoid many of the pitfalls inherent in today's health-care environment.

Suggested Reading

Quimby, Charles W., *Law for the Medical Practitioner*. City: AUPHA Press, 1979.

Rozovsky, Fay A., *Consent to Treatment: A Practical Guide*. Boston: Little, Brown, and Company, 1984.

7 | Utilization Review: Old Principles and New Mechanisms

LESTER L. SACKS, MD, PHD

Utilization review (UR) is a system for allocating resources, focusing on health care under the control of the physician. The primary issue addressed in any UR system is cost containment. Originally review mechanisms were structured to deal with government-funded programs such as Medicare, Medicaid, and maternal- and child-care programs. The concept of UR has since been expanded to include all provider services, from ambulatory care to inpatient hospital care.

History and Overview

As early as 1965, the federal government mandated a UR system for Medicare. However, no specific criteria were developed for the process. As a result, there was little cost control in this system, which left criteria for review up to each group. In 1972, Congress developed a system called the Professional Standards Review Organization (PSRO), which helped to create national normative values and standards for the review process. These programs were established to control federal contributions to medical care and were principally directed to inpatient hospital care. According to the PSRO guidelines established by the U.S. Department of Health and Human Services, the government would reimburse providers for medical services rendered (1) only when and to the extent medically necessary, as determined in the exercise of reasonable limits of professional discretion; and (2) in the case of services provided by a hospital or other health-care facility on an inpatient basis, only when and for such period as such services cannot effectively be provided on an outpatient basis consistent with professionally recognized health-care standards or more economically in an impatient health-care facility of a different type, as determined in the exercise of reasonable limits of professional discretion.

As a result of PSRO, UR grew to puberty and currently encompasses not only programs for inpatient hospital stay, but also outpatient or ambulatory review mechanisms. The outpatient reviews occur as "bill review," and inpatient utilization is generally preceded by prior authorization requirements.

Utilization review has been an outgrowth of cost containment directed to the need to reduce unnecessary medical care. Its aim is to put a cap on medical costs, to determine whether medical care is actually required, and to ensure that the level of care is appropriate. In the past decade, an entire industry evolved to meet the UR needs of the marketplace. A variety of vendors provide these services to health-care insurance companies, health maintenance organizations (HMOs), and preferred provider organizations (PPOs).

Initially, UR was purchased by major employers as an adjunct to the claims payment process. When it proved successful, the claims payor was required to incorporate UR as part of its payment process.

Formats of UR

By definition, UR evaluates the necessity, appropriateness, and efficiency of the use of medical services, procedures, and facilities. This description is applicable to all provider services.

Utilization review occurs in three basic formats:

1. Prospective: review of the necessity of care prior to the provision of services
2. Concurrent: review while care is being provided
3. Retrospective: review after the care has been rendered

All the major UR companies offer services addressing these three formats. However, each vendor serves the industry differently based on its strength in the designated areas of preadmission certification, second opinion surgery programs, case management, discharge planning with home services, and retrospective review reporting. These services evolved because the major payors were either unable or unwilling to perform these services themselves.

A menu of UR services is being offered to the health-care industry. These include:

1. Case management: controlling medical costs by managing and guiding the care process, rather than simply letting it take its course
2. Discharge planning: developing an appropriate plan of post-hospital care to help guide the medical outcome in a cost-effective way
3. Preadmission certification: authorization review to determine necessity of hospital admission.

Essentially, payors purchase these UR services in order to contain costs. However, it is also essential that the money saved by UR exceeds the administrative cost of the program.

How the UR System Functions

The question "How does utilization review work?" is frequently asked. According to author Stephen Casady, the "sentinel effect" provides the initial deterrent to overprovision of services. In other words, our performance frequently can be altered if we perceive we are being monitored or observed. However, this answer is too simplistic. If an observed behavior continues, a physician might develop creative adjustments in the quantity of services in the name of "quality of care."

For a UR system to function effectively, the review should be performed according to well-documented, appropriately researched, objective criteria. The criteria need to be quantifiable and subject to scrutiny. For example, to state that the delivered care was inappropriate is, in itself, inappropriate. We need to know the standards to be used for making such a determination, whether there are specific protocols used for the duration and frequency of the treatment patterns, and how these patterns were formulated. Data flow is essential to update any criteria governing the issue of quality care.

Quality care is best judged by measuring the outcome. It is possible that the same outcome can be achieved by an alternative care that has been demonstrated to be cost effective in previous cases. Thus by demonstrating alternatives, cost containment can be achieved without relying solely on deterrence by a sentinel effect.

The utilization of personal health services involves three elements:

1. The purpose of the utilization of the service (why services were required)
2. The type of service required
3. The organization setting (how the service is accessed): HMO, PPO, or nonmanaged care.

For each of these three categories (purpose, type, and setting), quantifiable measures have been established and updated. These measures address the issues of level of service, frequency of service, and duration of service attributed to each of the standard accepted diagnoses. According to Paul Torrens, M.D., patterns of utilization can be statistically judged and identified, based on the ICD-9 (International Classification of Disease) diagnostic codes, and this results in quality assessments.

The entire process of UR must continually adjust to advances in medical technology. For instance, although magnetic resonance imaging (MRI) is a costly technology, it has been quite effective in patient management. Because patient management is not a static activity, the UR process must address such technological changes in the medical marketplace.

In addition, when utilization patterns are analyzed, it is imperative to distinguish between the concepts of health needs and wants. A *need* for specific medical service is generally perceived as such both by the individual and by established protocols governing medical judgments. *Wants* refer to the quantity of health services individuals feel they should have, based on their own perception of need.

How UR is Implemented

In the beginning of this chapter, I identified the basic concepts of UR. I will now shift the focus to examine current implementation of the UR program. What began as a device for monitoring health-care costs in hospital environments has mushroomed into a multifaceted, complex system affecting the entire health-care delivery system. That is to say, all services are monitored, from hospital to ambulatory services, to entitlement programs or workers' compensation programs.

There are several approaches to the implementation of UR programs. Managed care concepts generally approach UR from the perspective of retrospective review. However, the more technically advanced companies have added prospective and concurrent review to their menus of service. If one applies the basic assumption that UR is the true focal point or foundation for cost containment, then it follows that *any* services provided by a managed health-care company would or could be a function of UR.

An HMO or PPO can be a tool for cost containment, provided that it is governed by utilization review protocols. One example of such a protocol guards the entrance into the health-care system by establishing appropriate gatekeeping controls through the provider of services. This is a prospective activity, because the primary care provider must request additional health-care services on behalf of the consumer of services. The ability, by contract, to negotiate or establish provider fees also allows further control or incentives for both the provider and the patient, thereby directly affecting the needs and wants of the individuals requesting health care. In essence, simple barriers are created which affect the decision as to whether or not the care is appropriate.

At some future point, the provider of service bills the payor. In turn, the payor does a bill review and bill audit, which can identify patterns of care. Subsequently, if the billing activities are outside the normative range, it is probable that there will be further review of the services. Thus retrospective review has been accomplished. This closes the loop and completes the cost-containment process.

The UR process can also function in the workers' compensation arena, because workers' compensation laws provide access to all reasonable medical treatment or remedies necessary to cure or relieve the effects of work-related injury or disease. To effectively utilize workers' compensation, stringent criteria regarding the primary care site and its policies of utilization must be applied before the facility is given a contract for services. It is imperative in such a situation to identify the utilization of service pattern of the contracting provider.

The following paragraphs will give examples of how UR is implemented in prehospital review, continued stay review, and retrospective review programs.

Prehospital Review Program

Medical costs of workers' compensation constitute 50% to 60% of the benefit dollar, and hospital costs account for approximately half of all medical costs.

A recent study by the Workers' Compensation Research Institute indicates a shift of the billings of medical care providers and suppliers from other benefit programs to workers' compensation. HMO providers sometimes inappropriately label health benefit cases as work related and subsequently bill workers' compensation for the services provided. This may result from ineffective utilization and billing reviews within the workers' compensation system.

The prehospital review and concurrent stay programs are designed to stem the growth in hospital costs. A prehospital authorization for all admissions predefines medical necessity, setting, and initial length of stay. The sentinel effect of this program alone is responsible for a significant reduction in admissions.

The concept of prospective review, originated by the HMO, addresses utilization prospectively. The individual's needs are identified and the wants are generally deferred. The cumulative data generated by the HMOs are significant and have contributed greatly to the prospective and retrospective review processes. These statistically evolved protocols have helped define community standards of care.

For example, if a payor's current utilization pattern for hospital care is 800 days per 1000 persons in the population, the payor would find that any UR would reduce the 800 days to approximately 600 days per 1000 persons. By introducing a well-managed PPO into the picture, that number could be reduced to about 400 patient days per 1000 persons. Introduce an HMO and the activity would be further reduced to approximately 325 days per 1000 persons. These estimates are based on values reviewed from utilization patterns for the year 1986. However, these figures can be misleading, because dollars saved on inpatient hospital stays may be spent elsewhere in outpatient services.

Continued Stay Review

In a continued stay review program, the patient's attending physician is contacted 24 hours prior to the preauthorized discharge date to confirm the discharge. If an extended stay is required, the new data are reviewed and a revised discharge date is authorized. This process keeps length of hospital stay to a minimum while responding to changing situations necessary to maintain quality medical care.

Retrospective Review

Retrospective review is provided for any hospital admission that circumvents the preadmission program. The billing and the medical record, accompanied by appropriate discussion with the attending physician, may be required in order to determine the appropriateness of the care provided. The quality of treatment should not be compromised, and medical decisions regarding authorization, length of stay, and treatment settings should be reached through the interaction between a review physician and the patient's attending physician.

Population Demographics

The implementation of UR services cannot be addressed without accounting for the changing demographics of the population and for inflation factors affecting health-care delivery. The need for health services increases rapidly after the age of 40, and the United States is now observing the aging of the baby-boom generation. Stephen F. Coaty of Health Economics Corporation pointed out in an article published in 1987 that "America is in the early steps of one of the sharpest changes in demographic structure in history." He also indicated that the cohort older than 65 is growing more rapidly (on a percentage basis) than is any other age segment of the population.

Legal Issues

Implementation of UR systems presents potential legal liabilities. Attorney Stephen Sturgeon has written extensively about these issues. According to Sturgeon, as employers become more aggressive in mandating control of medical costs, especially in the self-insurance marketplace, their liability exposure increases. The UR process itself is a planned reduction of medical services. If the services are reduced or withheld inappropriately, then the risk of liability is increased.

Sturgeon points out that if the standards of care are well established by proper utilization data, then the threat of negligence can be challenged with this defense. If the physician knowingly executes poor medical judgment by not challenging the UR when he or she knows it is inappropriate, the physician—not the employer or the UR company—is liable.

A UR company can be held liable and legally accountable when inappropriate medical decisions result from defects in either the design or implementation of the cost containment mechanism and if the decisions are mandated capriciously by the review company.

Challenging the UR System

All providers of medical services have had the experience of having services rendered for the care of a patient denied and/or challenged. Physicians often feel angry or frustrated because they feel the person from whom they are requesting the service authorization does not actually know the patient and is not sophisticated enough to recognize what the physician is doing to care for the patient.

The most important way for the provider to avoid these situations is to make certain that the need for the services requested is well documented. The diagnosis must be complete and consistent with the evaluations performed. It may be helpful for physicians to keep in mind that those administering the review services and programs do not have personal experience with the patient. If the information about the patient's condition is scanty or inappropriate, the physician may receive a notice denying an additional hospital stay or a service in an ambulatory setting. If the physician is able to precisely document charts and requests for service, denials will be infrequent.

If a physician sends a request for service without addressing the information requested by the reviewer, the case cannot be appropriately reviewed. Neither the review companies nor the agencies are attempting to practice medicine. They do not control the treatment patterns, and they base the appropriateness of treatment only on the usual customary standards. The physician must "paint a picture" of the case so that the reviewers have all the information they need to make a determination.

If you are certain your request was appropriate or that the service rendered was necessary for the diagnosis stated, you, as the provider, have rights. You can challenge the system. The following are suggested steps for making a challenge.

1. Write a letter to the office that denied your request or refused to pay for the service rendered. Explain why you performed the test or examination to corroborate the identified diagnosis or diagnoses. Use the ICD-9 codes for the diagnosis and Current Procedural Terminology (CPT) or Relative Value Study (RVS) codes for procedures.
2. Request a return letter explaining why benefits were disallowed.
3. If the communication that you receive in return does not satisfy you, request a physician review. All UR companies provide access to physician review processes. There is no cost to you.
4. Again, if you are not satisfied with the explanation given during the physician review process, call the review company directly and ask to speak with a physician reviewer. You can also ask to speak to a peer specialist. Generally, when you reach this level of challenge, the situation or challenge is remedied.

The process of challenging denial of inpatient services is basically the same as the steps above. However, you must follow the rules designated by the hospital's UR committee.

Summary

The UR process evolved from the Medicare-Medicaid mandate to control hospital costs in the mid-1960s. Cost containment through UR now has a firm footing in the health-care delivery system. The present approach to UR encompasses ambulatory patient care as well as inpatient hospital care.

The basic processes of UR are prospective reviews, concurrent reviews, and retrospective reviews. The health-care industry has become creative in its definitions of these basic activities, resulting in the expansion of the basic principles. PPOs and HMOs have flourished under the expansion of these concepts.

Legal issues are raised routinely because the UR system can be perceived as withholding medical services. If appropriate data are used in making decisions, the likelihood of any negative or adverse outcome is negligible.

Physician participation in the UR process is imperative. The physician's role as guardian of the patient's welfare must continue. In addition, however, physicians able to interact with the UR system in a planned, constructive manner will have a positive and profound impact on the entire expanded UR process.

Suggested Reading

Health and Human Resource - PSRO- PL 92-603 Title V.

Casady, Stephen, "Utilization Review Claims Processing: Cost Containment and Managed Care Plans." *Auto Supply* (October 1987).

Toreens, Paul, *Introduction to Health Care Services.* New York: John Wiley and Sons, 1982.

Beech Street, Inc., "Managed Health Care Corporations." *Review of Utilization Process Manual* (July 1989; archives).

8 | Sources of Health-Care Financing: Impact on the Patient, the Hospital, and the Physician

OSAMA I. MIKHAIL, MBA, MS, PHD AND
ALAN F. KOVAL, MBA, JD, CPA

This chapter addresses the key financial characteristics and dynamics of the U.S. health-care system. In particular, the sources of financing (payment) and their impact on three of the major components of the health-care delivery system (the patient, the physician, and the hospital) will be described.

The U.S. health-care system is undoubtedly the most complex and costly health-care system in the world. It is a system of extremes with an abundance of technology, sophisticated treatment modalities, and massive commitment of national resources, and yet 15% of the population is uninsured. Moreover, with 70% of health-care expenditures directed at 10% of the population, the distribution of expenditures raises questions about appropriateness of spending and equitable allocation of resources. The U.S. system is consequently a much-criticized one, with ongoing, intense debate as to its future direction and need for restructuring. At the center of this debate is the nature of the financing, payment, and reimbursement for health-care services.

Unlike the consumption of most goods and services, the payment for "consumption" of health-care services involves a third-party payor (insurance company, self-insured employer, or government) in 75% of personal health-care services delivered. The existence of third-party payors as a major source of health-care financing and their influence on health-care delivery adds significant complexity to the transaction between the recipient of care (the patient) and the providers of care (in this case, physicians and hospitals). Thus to understand the nature of health-care delivery and associated decisions, it is essential to understand who the third-party payors are, their role in the health-care process, and the impact they have on patients, physicians, and hospitals in the delivery of health care. Clearly this brief chapter can give only a glimpse into the sources of financing and their impact on the patient, physician, and hospital.

The Structure of the Health-Care System

The U.S. health-care system is a complex array of providers, consumers, distribution channels, and payors. For the acute care component of the system in particular, the provider segment includes approximately 500,000 physicians involved in patient care, with 80% to 85% in a specialty practice. The rise in the number of physicians per 100,000 population, from 148 in 1965 to 237 in 1987, has been accompanied by recent debate as to the appropriate balance between primary and specialty physicians, the distribution of physicians across specialties, and whether in the aggregate this trend has created a surplus of physicians. Clearly the answers are not simple and a detailed analysis at the specialty level would be necessary to begin to address these complex issues. Nonetheless, the number of physicians has been increasing at a faster rate than has the general population and is projected to continue to grow in the face of increasing costs of health care.

The other major provider in the acute care system is the hospital. In terms of operating bed capacity, the hospital industry is composed of four major segments: (1) not for profit, (2) for profit, (3) federal government, and (4) state, local, and county government (see Table 8.1). The hospital segment of the health-care system, however, has been in a decline since 1984

Table 8.1 U.S. Acute Care Hospital Beds, by Ownership—1989[a]

Not-for-profit hospitals	
Religious systems	146,000
Secular systems	70,000
Free-standing hospitals	435,000
Total	651,000
For-profit hospitals	
Multi-hospital systems	102,000
Free-standing hospitals	19,000
Total	121,000
Total private beds	772,000
Federal government hospitals	
Veterans administration	48,000
Armed forces	18,000
Other federal	3,000
Total federal	69,000
State, local and county government	169,000
Total government beds	238,000
Total beds	1,010,000[b]

Source: Bernstein Research, *The Future of Health Care Delivery in America* (New York: Sanford C. Bernstein & Co., April 1990).

[a] Excludes psychiatric beds.
[b] National occupancy—67%.

with diminishing utilization (influenced by reimbursement pressures) leading to shrinking occupancy, reduced number of beds in operation, and hospital closures.

Health-Care Expenditures

Although the health-care delivery system encompasses more than acute care, it is the largest component of the health-care system. Other components of the health-care system, such as allied health services, public health, and long-term care, will not be addressed in examining the principal sources of financing. As an overview, however, Table 8.2 depicts the scope of national health expenditures and the relative size of the various sources of payment.

For the $442.6 billion of personal health care expenditures in 1987, the sources of payment break down as shown in Table 8.3.

The size and growth of the U.S. health care system has become an area of growing concern as increases in national health expenditures outpace inflation and consume ever-increasing percentages of GNP (see Table 8.4).

The estimates for 1989 and beyond do not anticipate any relief under the current framework for health-care delivery and reimbursement. Of additional concern is the comparison of expenditures as a percentage of gross domestic product (GDP) relative to that of other countries with developed health-care systems (see Table 8.5).

Table 8.2 National Health Expenditures by Type of Expenditure ($ Billions)

Type of expenditure	1987	1988
Personal health care		
Hospital care	$194.7	$212.8
Physicians' services	102.7	115.3
Nursing home care	40.6	44.1
Drugs and medical supplies	34.0	36.9
Dentists' services	32.8	35.6
Other health services	12.1	13.4
Other professional services	16.2	18.2
Eyeglasses and appliances	9.5	10.5
Subtotal	$442.6	$486.8
Program administration and net cost of insurance	25.9	29.4
Government public health activities	14.7	15.5
Total Health Services and Supplies	$483.2	$531.7
Construction	8.3	9.1
Research	8.8	9.5
Total National Health Expenditures	$500.3	$550.3

Sources: Health Care Financing Administration, *Health Care Financing Review* (Washington, DC: U.S. Dept. of Health and Human Services, Winter 1988); and Health Insurance Association of America, *Source Book of Health Insurance Data* (Washington, DC: Author, 1989).

Table 8.3 1987 Personal Health Care Expenditures by Type of Payor and Type of Expenditure ($ Billions)

Source of payment	Total personal care	Hospital care	Physicians' services	Nursing home care	Other health services
Personal health-care expenditures	$442.6	$194.7	$102.7	$40.6	$104.6
Direct payments	123.0	18.5	26.3	20.0	58.2
Third-party payments	319.6	176.2	76.4	20.6	46.4
Private health insurance	139.1	71.9	44.6	0.4	22.2
Other private funds	5.3	2.2	0.1	0.3	3.0
Government	175.3	102.2	31.8	19.9	21.5
Medicare	81.2	53.3	22.3	0.6	5.1
Medicaid	46.0	17.8	4.4	11.8	6.0
Other	48.1	31.1	5.1	1.5	10.4

Sources: (see note to Table 8.2).

Sources of Health-Care Financing

The current system of financing health care is a complex combination of public and private payments. The majority of the population relies on private health insurance, with corporate employers serving as the largest purchasers of this insurance to cover employees, retirees, and their dependents. In 1965, with the creation of the Medicare and Medicaid programs, government joined corporations as a major purchaser of health care. In spite of these major sources of financing, the population as a whole reflects substantial gaps with respect to adequate coverage and financing of needed health-care services. Of the total population, "there are some 37 million Americans who are uninsured, 70 million more who are underinsured, and 23 million who are served by Medicaid, who are not guaranteed access to or equity in medical treatment" (In *Medical Alert*, a staff summary of congressional testimony on "The Future of Health Care in America," Oct. 1989, Joint Economic Committee, Subcommittee on Education and Health).

By the early 1980s, in response to accelerating utilization of health-care services and a medical services inflation rate higher than the overall inflation in the economy, payors sought to introduce mechanisms that would contain and reduce the growth in consumption and cost of health-care services. In particular, the federal government, faced with escalating Medicare payments and a growing budget deficit, introduced a new reimbursement mechanism in 1984 and a utilization review process. Insurance com-

Table 8.4 National Health Expenditures: % of GNP

1980	1981	1982	1983	1984	1985	1986	1987	1988
9.1	9.4	10.2	10.5	10.3	10.4	10.7	11.1	11.3

Sources: (see note to Table 8.2).

Table 8.5 Health Expenditures as % of GDP, 1986 (Selected Countries)

United States	11.1%
Canada	8.5%
Germany	8.1%
Japan	6.7%
Netherlands	8.3%
Sweden	9.1%
Switzerland	8.0%
United Kingdom	6.2%

Source: Health Affairs, International Health Care Spending and Utilization Trends, Fall 1988; and Health Insurance Association of America, *Source Book of Health Insurance Data* (Washington, DC: Author, 1989).

panies raised premiums at double-digit rates (in some years 20%–30% increases) to keep up with ever-increasing utilization and cost of claims. Corporations, in turn, faced with rapidly increasing cost of health-care benefits, sought to increase deductibles and copayments by employees and began to change their benefit packages from defined benefit to defined contribution plans. Consequently, individuals saw their contribution to health-care payments increase dramatically.

The other major development during this period of escalating health-care costs was the growth of alternative delivery systems (ADS), later referred to as *managed care* in the form of health maintenance organizations (HMOs), preferred provider organizations (PPOs), and so on. These emerging wholesale buyers of health-care services functioned as distribution channels and relied on large-scale purchases of care and inefficiency of the current system to drive down, to some extent, utilization and cost of services. The principal form of pricing (for HMOs) was a capitation rate: a comprehensive, periodic rate per individual covered that generally required no out-of-pocket expense to the individual for a broad array of health care services. The constraints on the individual were reflected in the choice of providers that were qualified or approved by the HMO through contractual agreements. By the end of 1988, 32 million persons were covered by HMOs. The PPOs operated somewhat differently in that their arrangements with providers were based on discounted fees (eliminating the risks inherent in capitation-based plans) and their members generally had greater choice of providers and financial incentives to utilize preferred providers.

As these forces and trends work their way through the health-care delivery system, the major sources of financing (payors) fall into two categories: private insurance and Medicare, along with a collection of other, relatively minor, sources.

Private Health Insurance

A variety of medical insurance plans protect against the financial cost of illness or injury. Health insurance is offered by commercial insurance companies, the Blue Cross and Blue Shield plans, and prepaid health plans, including health maintenance organizations. A number of corporations are self-insured: they directly fund the cost of medical services provided to their beneficiaries.

Traditional indemnity insurance reimburses the patient for medical costs incurred without restricting the choice of provider(s) of care. Prepaid health plans, however, either operate their own facilities or make arrangements for services with selected providers, usually at reduced fees. In addition to individual coverage, group policies (contracts) are purchased by employers to provide health-care coverage to employees, retirees, and their families.

Under any form of private insurance, part of the payment for health-care services may be the responsibility of the individual. If that amount is fixed, it is referred to as a *deductible*. If the insurance company reimburses only a percentage of the cost, then the arrangement is referred to as *coinsurance*, and the individual is responsible for the noncovered portion. Coverage is typically divided into four categories: hospitalization, surgery, regular medical expenses, and major medical expenses (protection against catastrophic charges).

The Medicare Program

Medicare is a federal insurance program that finances health-care services for individuals older than 65 years and for severely disabled persons. It is funded largely from general tax revenues, premiums paid by enrollees, and a portion of Social Security payroll taxes.

Medicare has two components. Part A provides coverage for inpatient hospital care, some stays in skilled nursing facilities, and home health care. Part B pays for physicians' services and hospital outpatient care. Because Medicare was designed to cover primarily acute care needs, it does not cover certain medical services, such as long-term nursing home care, outpatient drugs, and dental services.

Initially, Medicare paid for covered hospital services by reimbursing expenses actually incurred. However, as mentioned earlier, the cost of the program increased so substantially over the years that in 1984, Medicare introduced the prospective payment system (PPS) for inpatient hospital care. Under PPS, hospitals are paid a fixed amount per discharge regardless of actual costs incurred. The payments are based upon diagnostic related groups, or DRGs. All diagnoses are currently assigned to one of 490 DRGs. Each DRG has an assigned weight or index number that reflects the relative amount of resources required on average to provide hospital care to patients with that diagnosis. Hospital stays (and costs) that exceed certain norms are termed *outliers*, and an additional payment is made for these cases. As might be expected in moving from cost-based reimbursement to fixed-price reimbursement, the financial performance of hospitals was significantly and dramatically affected. Because of the manner in which PPS was phased in, many hospitals experienced short-run improvements in financial performance; however, over time prospective payment has placed significant downward pressure on hospital net income.

For physicians' services, Medicare currently sets rates using the "customary, prevailing, and reasonable" (CPR) system. Payment for each service provided is the lowest of the physician's actual charge, the physician's customary charge for that service, or the prevailing fee in the community. Physicians can elect to sign "participating" agreements whereby they agree to accept the Medicare payment rates for services rendered to Medicare patients. These physicians are said to *take assignment*. If a physician chooses not to accept the Medicare rate as full payment for services provided, the physician bills the patient for the balance of the charges that Medicare did not pay. Medicare payment rates are currently about 5% higher for participating physicians.

From 1980 to 1988, Part B costs increased 17% per year, with physician services constituting approximately 72% of Part B expenditures. In 1989, Congress enacted legislation to replace Medicare's CPR payment method with a resource-based relative value scale (RVS) starting in 1992. This new fee schedule for physicians is intended to consider a physician's time and effort in treating a patient, geographic location, and practice expenses. As a result, cognitive-oriented physicians, such as those in family practice, receive higher fees, whereas procedure-oriented physicians, such as surgeons, receive less for their services. Fees for rural physicians increased relative to those for physicians in urban areas. This legislation also contained a mechanism for controlling the annual increases in total Medicare payments to physicians.

Other Sources

Medicaid is a health-care program jointly funded by the federal government and the states to pay for medical services to the poor. The individual states administer the program and determine eligibility and services to be provided. Medicaid generally covers inpatient hospital and nursing home care, clinical treatment, doctors' fees, and various home or community health programs. Since 1988, courts in several states have declared the Medicaid system invalid because hospitals receive insufficient (below cost) payment for treating Medicaid patients, a violation of federal law.

State and local governments may also establish hospital districts and public and community health programs financed by local taxes. These local tax revenues are used to employ health-care workers, including physicians (often in affiliation with medical schools), who deliver care at government-owned- and -operated facilities to the indigent and those unable to purchase needed health care services.

State workers' compensation statutes protect workers and their dependents against injury, disease, or death occurring in the course of employment. Benefits are generally financed by insurance purchased by the employer and usually includes hospital and other medical payments.

The federal government operates a system of veterans' hospitals and also finances a number of programs that provide health-care benefits to military retirees and dependents of military personnel at private (nongovernment) facilities.

Finally, health-care providers themselves have traditionally rendered voluntary, free care to those unable to pay. From a financial perspective this has been explained or described as part of a phenomenon called *cost-shifting*: charging more to those who can afford to pay in order to subsidize those patients who either cannot pay at all or are inadequately covered.

The Impact on Physicians, Hospitals, and Patients

Physicians

The emergence of payors as more aggressive participants in health-care decisions and the purchase of health-care services has led to downward pressure on the demand for health-care services (including physician services). This pressure has been magnified by the growing number of physicians relative to the population. The combination of these two trends has intensified competition among physicians and lowered income expectations.

In addition to these economic pressures (and more disturbing to physicians) is the "intrusion" of payors into the traditional physician-patient relationship by constraining physicians in their practice of medicine. With approximately 80% of the average physician's revenues coming from federal and private insurance, physicians find themselves increasingly monitored, questioned, and needing to comply with bureacratic procedures in prescribing and proceeding with medical treatment for their patients.

This growing bureaucratization and perceived intrusion into the physician's practice of medicine is leading more physicians to abandon solo practice in favor of group practices and HMOs. According to the AMA (as reported in the February 18, 1990 *New York Times*), "for the first time, more physicians were employees than were self-employed."

Certainly the pressure from payors is not the only cause of physician disenchantment and frustration—malpractice litigation and competition are among other factors—however, it is a major contributing factor. The same issue of the *New York Times* also reported the findings of a Gallup poll conducted in 1989 on behalf of the AMA. In particular, the article noted that "40% of the doctors interviewed said that based on what they now knew about medicine as a career, they would definitely or probably not enter medical school if they had a career choice to make again." The increasing prevalence of this attitude has been accompanied by a 25% reduction in medical school applications over the past five years.

In summary, as a result of payors (sources of financing) involving themselves in health-care decisions in order to contain costs, physicians are having to cope with (1) payor and physician surplus-induced economic pressures, (2) limitations on their autonomy in dealing with patients, (3) changing organizational structures for medical practice (staff model HMOs, IPAs, etc.), (4) new forms of business relations (contracts with managed care firms, Medicare assignments, discounted fees, etc.), and (5) new administrative procedures (preadmission certification, utilization review, etc.).

Hospitals

The hospital industry has undergone tremendous change since the advent of the Medicare prospective payment system in the mid-1980s. Initially hospital occupancy rates decreased substantially as fewer persons were admitted and patients were discharged sooner to complete their recovery outside of the hospital. With technological developments and economic pressures on hospitals, many surgical procedures that had been performed on an inpatient basis were converted to outpatient procedures. Outpatient surgery grew at double-digit rates as more procedures were performed without the patient ever being admitted to the hospital.

During the last five years, Medicare and Medicaid payment rates, which have largely been set in response to the significant federal budget deficits and state budgetary considerations, have not kept pace with inflation. This situation, combined with a population of "sicker" patients and the introduction of new, expensive technologies, has resulted in reduced hospital profitability and cost shifting to other payor groups. Managed care firms, including HMOs, have sought discounts and financial risk-sharing arrangements in return for providing patients to hospitals. This in turn has further exacerbated the financial pressures and the potential for cost shifting (or, from the payors' perspective, discriminatory pricing).

Hospitals have reacted to these pressures in various ways. The increased competition for patients has resulted in more aggressive efforts to recruit physicians onto the medical staff, the creation of joint-venture and other business arrangements between hospitals and physicians, and the adoption of "bonding" strategies whereby a hospital seeks to secure the loyalty of its medical staff through programs specifically designed to assist the physicians in their practices.

Operationally, hospitals have implemented programs to lower costs including staffing reductions, enhanced purchasing practices for equipment and supplies, and the elimination of unprofitable programs, often involving expensive services such as trauma care that are desperately needed by the community. New services have been added and expensive equipment acquired in an effort to be competitive. Utilization review mechanisms have been established to review doctor's decisions on admitting patients and length of stay. More sophisticated business procedures, including cost accounting and case-mix management systems, have been installed.

The focus of current efforts by hospital management is to achieve a closer collaboration with their medical staff in treating patients. Quality—entailing the questions, "What is it?" and "How can it be measured?"—is becoming the competitive battleground. Procedures are being developed to ensure that various types of illnesses are treated within prescribed guidelines to achieve the desired outcomes in a cost-effective manner. Ambulatory surgery centers and other entrepreneurial business arrangements have developed outside of, and in competition with, the hospital.

Patients

The impact on patients of the more aggressive posture adopted by payors has been felt primarily in terms of increasing out-of-pocket payments (deductibles and copayments) and restrictions on the patients' freedom of choice of provider, particularly in managed care plans. Through the 1970s, patient out-of-pocket expenses for health care grew at approximately 8% per year; however, in the early and mid-1980s out-of-pocket expenses grew at approximately 10% per year, with the trends indicating continuing substantial increases in such expenses. Thus convenience (access) has diminished and the financial burden has increased for the patient. These two factors have led to a more demanding and informed patient population that is insisting on a larger role in treatment decisions. In effect, patients are beginning to act more like consumers. As might be expected, this has the potential to create tension in the traditional physician-patient relationship.

Corporations, representing large groups of patients through their health-benefit plans, have experienced dramatic increases in health premiums in recent years that have added significantly to their costs. These increased costs have been singled out as contributing significantly to the decline of American competitiveness on the world scene. In response, corporations have moved toward greater direct sharing of costs with employees through a variety of mechanisms. There is also a growing trend for these employers to become self-insured, direct purchasers of health-care services through contracts with providers that eliminate the middlemen. The response of corporations to their increasing cost of health-care benefits has been of particular concern to retirees who perceive that their retirement health benefits are in jeopardy.

For the indigent, who rely on Medicaid, public hospitals and health services, and charity care, little short-term relief is in sight. Hospitals, in particular, facing declining profitability, will be less inclined to offer voluntary free care. Without increased taxes, neither Medicaid nor public health services will be able to expand coverage and improve access.

The Health-Care Delivery System: Seeking Equilibrium

The impact of the sources of financing on the components of the health-care delivery system did not develop in a vacuum, but grew out of the underlying structural characteristics and dynamics of the health-care system in the late 1970s and early 1980s. In that time, health-care costs and utilization grew at ever-increasing rates, consuming a growing percentage of the gross national product. Throughout that period there was a growing perception that the health-care system, as defined by the interaction among physicians, hospitals, private insurers, and the government (Medicare), was highly inefficient and wasteful and growing out of control. In the late 1970s, wholesale buyers of health-care services, which had been on the scene for some time in the form of HMOs, began to grow rapidly, leveraging their purchasing power, placing pressure on providers, and restricting members' choice in order to squeeze inefficiencies out of the system. In the early 1980s the federal government (through Medicare) sought to gain some control over federal health expenditures by redesigning the reimbursement system for Medicare (DRGs).

The result of these combined pressures led to a decline in hospital utilization in the Medicare and managed care populations. Providers (particularly hospitals) faced with excess capacity became more competitive, resulting in significant deterioration in financial performance initially, with some improvement toward the late 1980s as providers became more efficient. In compensating for pressure from managed care and government payors, providers (hospitals and physicians) raised prices to the privately insured. The insurance companies, in turn, tightened their procedures and raised premiums and deductibles. This led to dramatic increases in corporate costs of health benefits and out-of-pocket expenses for individuals. Physicians were also economically affected but not as severely as were hospitals. The greater impact on physicians was in reduced autonomy and deterioration in the traditional physician-patient relationship.

The health-care system still has excess acute-care capacity, with costs continuing to grow at what is generally regarded as an unacceptable rate. Societal issues of access, coverage, and quality are emerging as health-care issues of primary concern, as are health-care delivery issues of long-term care and disease prevention.

Consequences of the Financing System on the Future of Health-Care Delivery

What changes will occur in health care as a result of these pressures, particularly with respect to the key problems of high cost and access to care? Costs will continue to escalate, consuming a greater percentage of GNP (projected to be 15% by the year 2000), and a large segment of the population will be denied access to care. Some initiatives, however, are under way to address these issues.

The complete overhaul of the health-care system is a distinct possibility. Major reform is being debated and studied, but dissatisfaction with the present system is probably not yet great enough to support this effort. However, concepts such as universal health insurance and a national health plan are gaining greater acceptability. Such reform could take the form of a national health system with a centralized single payor, providing a basic set of health-care benefits to all. Another possibility is a continuation of the existing combination of private insurance and government programs, expanded to provide broader coverage. Discussion of alternatives will be a high priority over the next several years.

Managed care enrollment in HMOs and PPOs will continue to grow in the 1990s with a commensurate decrease in indemnity insurance coverage. The open-ended HMO is currently the fastest-growing product in this market. When subscribers need medical care, they can elect either to stay in the network of physicians and hospitals that has contracted with the HMO or to pay a higher deductible and coinsurance to use providers of their choice. As the subscribers' out-of-pocket costs increase, they are more likely to seek services within the system. Direct contracting by employers with providers for health-care services to their employees, usually at reduced rates, is also developing rapidly as employers seek to hold costs down by eliminating the overhead associated with an HMO. Direct contracting, in many respects, is emerging as the next generation of managed care. In the process, physician autonomy and patients' freedom of choice will be further eroded, and individuals will have to pay a greater share of their health-care expenses.

Advances in medical technology often stimulate demand for costly procedures such as organ transplants or enable life to be sustained in terminally ill patients. Today, more than one third of Medicare spending for a typical American occurs during his or her final year of life. The aging population will cause these expenditures to increase substantially. Yet millions of Americans do not receive basic health services such as prenatal care and inoculations against contagious diseases because they are unable to pay for them. These circumstances have created an implicit rationing of medical care without addressing the significant ethical and social issues that are created by the present health-care financing system. The state of Oregon has taken the lead in this area by attempting to rank health-care services by cost-effectiveness and likelihood for success. These rankings are used to determine which services are covered by the state's Medicaid program. It is doubtful that the nation can meet all of the health-care needs of every person, so some rational process to allocate available resources must be found.

A major initiative over the next few years will involve quality of care: how to define and measure it. Consumers of medical services, whether they are patients or payors, have no way to compare the value of services received from various physicians and hospitals. Efforts to develop physician practice protocols based on type of illness and case management processes to determine if the desired medical outcomes are achieved in a cost-effective manner have begun and will continue. Hospitals and physicians will, of necessity, have to learn to work closer together, and the financial incentives to do so will have to be created. Employers and other-third party payors will select providers based on quality and effectiveness.

Further changes will occur in the payment mechanisms. It was previously noted that Medicare has adopted a relative value scale for reimbursing physicians. The present system of cost-based reimbursement for hospital outpatient services will be replaced by ambulatory DRGs and a second generation of inpatient DRGs instituted to more closely align the payment for services to the underlying cost and severity of the illness.

We Have Met the Payors. . .

We cannot end this chapter leaving the possible impression that the payors (the sources of financing) are totally independent entities functioning according to their own agendas and exerting arbitrary pressures on the health-care system.

Ultimately, the sources of financing stem from the consuming public. Thus to paraphrase Pogo's immortal words, "We have met the payors and they are us." For after all, the sources of payment (private insurance, Medicare, Medicaid, etc.) are themselves dependent on financing capacity; private health insurance is dependent on premiums paid by subscribers, and government-funded programs are dependent on tax revenues. Direct payment for services by patients, including self-pay, deductibles, and co-payment, is dependent on individual income.

In the end, the fundamental questions emerging from the 1980s are what the nation can afford in terms of health care, and how health-care resources should be distributed across the population.

9 | Leaving Academia and Setting Professional Goals for Private Practice Success

PENG THIM FAN, MD

Change is not made without inconvenience even from worse to better.
(Samuel Johnson)

One is often besieged by trepidation at the prospect of change. You may have just embarked upon a modestly successful academic career and have enjoyed the fruits of early recognition in your teaching and research. You feel the excitement of the scientific chase; and even though medicine has become more like a trade, you enjoy the comforting warmth of collegiate life which it still provides, in however attenuated a fashion: a taste of Cardinal Newman's lofty "idea of a University." What would tempt you into the sordid world of commerce? What qualities that have sustained you in your academic advancement are relevant to the marketplace of private practice?

An academic career has many rewards: for instance, the feeling of being constantly surrounded by youth, fresh outlook, and new ideas. In addition one is challenged on clinical rounds by house staff and students who worship at the altar of the latest journal articles, and in the laboratory by peers who are continually outpacing one in skill, speed, insight, and cunning. Laboratory research can be what Natalie Angier has called the *natural obsession*: the relentless pursuit of a germinating idea, a sense of wonder that science actually makes sense of the complexity of life, and that the pieces of the puzzle that made up "the immune response" truly fit together into a "fearful symmetry."

Life in academia can be urbane and pleasant. There is time to travel and visit colleagues in other states and countries or to take a few months to gather thoughts and plan projects. One is not bothered by a night-call schedule that interrupts evenings and sleep, and is free from the business of medicine, at least as it pertains to office rents, employees' salaries, billing, collections, prepaid health plans, and chasing delinquent accounts. Clinical medicine is practiced at the state of the art, both in the caliber of fellow consultants and in the array of high-technology equipment at one's disposal. If a clinical abnormality in a patient is interesting there is a research laboratory to work out the details or the luxury to design one's own studies to elucidate the problem.

Table 9.1 Pros and Cons of Academia

Pros	Cons
An educational environment of scientific creativity and new ideas	Conflicting priorities and multiple obligations and responsibilities
Availability of resources and the latest medical terminology	Pressure to "publish or perish" and attain tenure or undergo a forced departure within a fixed time frame
Diversity of health professionals available for consultation and exchange of information	Dealing with the requirements and inflexibilities of a large bureaucracy
Availability of house staff and fellows to provide front-line care of patients and handle routine paperwork	Decreasing availability of grant support for research
Protected time to conduct research projects in the laboratory	Tedium of constant grant submissions
	Ever-increasing paperwork
Time flexibility to attend professional meetings and educational conferences	Slow decision-making process and dependence on "decision by committee"
Referral base and reputation of a university medical center	Lack of control over one's time and commitments
State-of-the-art medicine	Limited income potential
Guaranteed salary and benefits package	

Of course, this is an idealized picture of academic life. Table 9.1 points out some of the pros and cons of academia. There is endless drudgery of grant visions and revisions, submissions and rejections, each attempt less intelligible than the one before and with a smaller scope and smaller chance of funding. There is the constant psychological pressure to perform easily publishable research, curriculum vitae inflation that clutters up the medical literature. One is tempted to perform safe experiments with predictable and pedestrian, but publishable, outcomes. At times, academicians give up aspirations for a higher synthesis because they recognize that nothing is as deadly to a young career as a "reach that exceeds your grasp." One may realize that as a physician, one is not trained well enough to pursue the really interesting questions in immunology and that the days of the inspired amateurs, like Watson and Crick, are probably over.

Those in charge of a clinical section or division are plagued by the mountain of paperwork that is the product of every bureaucracy. They sit on many committees, holding meaningless discussions. Finally, the two personal aspects of academic life that can propel you into private practice are the realization that you are rapidly losing your basic clinical skills, in spite of a reputation of being a good clinical teacher, and that you can work yourself into a blind end in research. Short of going through several arduous years of acquiring new laboratory skills and insight—most likely at a distant institution—one can be condemned to a career of mediocre research. The added responsibility of children can give further impetus to move along.

Perhaps you have reached a similar impasse in your academic career. As you toy with the idea of entering private practice, there is one central question you need to ask yourself: how much do you enjoy being a doctor? Do you like taking histories, examining patients, counseling your patient about his or her illness, planning treatment, concerning yourself with such mundane aspects as diet and exercise, sorting out psychological and social influences, dealing with families and relatives, and providing comfort when your patient dies? A university clinician who has an outpatient clinic practice and makes occasional inpatient hospital rounds is not going through the same experience as the private physician in primary or consultative care. It may be a chore or an exhilarating experience for you to gather your data first hand rather than through the filter of medical students and house staff. It may be very disconcerting for you to find out that you are the only one on whom your patient and his or her family can rely. Caring for patients may be an interesting diversion in academic medicine, but it is the essence of private practice.

A higher salary is a major incentive to pursue a successful private practice; other authors in this book will more competently show you how to reach that goal. The principal reward and unadulterated delight of private practice is experiencing the basics of being a doctor. You meet people from all walks of life and can interest yourself in their small and large problems. Your pulse quickens to the odd comment and out-of-place symptom in an otherwise too-familiar history, and the discovery of an unusual clinical sign brings back all the sense of wonder and mystery that first propelled you into the study of medicine. You discover that classic textbook descriptions of even common diseases are often wrong and that you fall back constantly on your carefully nurtured skills of observation, interrogation, and physical examination. Sometimes the results achieved can be as dazzling as those of a Sherlock Holmes. Dr. Gerald Weissman has captured the essence of clinical sleuthing in his wise and compassionate book, *They All Laughed at Christopher Columbus: Tales of Medicine and the Art of Discovery.* The age of the skilled clinician is not yet over. As he said, "Come along, Watson, the game is afoot."

Some of your accomplishments in academic medicine may be of value in private practice. The following advice is offered:

1. If you are a subspecialist, try to practice your subspecialty exclusively rather than dilute it with some general practice. You may take a lot longer to establish yourself, but you will be happier in the end. If you are lucky enough to secure a part-time job in your university during this transition period, then stick with being a subspecialist. Unless you have the intellect and energy of an Aristotle or a da Vinci, you will not be able to practice state-of-the-art internal medicine. A subspecialty narrows the focus and allows you to provide the most knowledgeable care, and it reduces the literature base that you have to master and keep current. More importantly, it is the attention to detail and nuance that can give you the margin of success in the management of a complex and chronic illness. The good subspecialist learns early on that all medical knowledge is tentative and that criteria and rules have little relationship to the individual case. True

mastery comes from repeated encounters with a very restricted palette of diseases. Osler may have had romantic notions of the omniscient generalist, but it is an illusion in late 20th-century medicine. Paradoxically, an exclusive subspecialty practice has a better chance to grow in a crowded medical arena than does one that mixes general internal medicine with a subspecialty interest; as an exclusive subspecialist you are more likely to obtain referrals from your general colleagues, because they are less concerned about the possibility that their patients would stay with you for all their medical care and not return to them.

2. Establish your practice near your medical school. Reputation travels poorly, and the contacts you have made with local physicians during your tenure will prove invaluable as you develop your referral base. Your university connections allow you to conduct collaborative clinical research and continued teaching in the university, and involvement in the activities of your department keep you current. If you are forced to relocate, it follows that you should establish a close relationship with the medical school in your new community as soon as circumstances allow.

3. Bring your special skills with you. If you are renowned for treating a certain disease, then that should be publicized. If you have developed new techniques that are clinically useful, then perhaps they can be adapted to private practice. Many large community hospitals that aspire to the status of regional health-care centers are very supportive of such efforts.

4. Consider group practice. Many large groups relish the added cachet of an academic reputation in their new associate. Sometimes several academicians in the same specialty can create an immediately formidable presence in the community by coming out of academia to practice together. Your group will define state-of-the-art care in the local community and provide an alternative to a more distant and impersonal university referral. In a period of intense anxiety about the future of the medical marketplace, many experts have predicted that the large multispecialty group will have the best chance of survival against the HMO juggernaut in the 1990s.

5. Go where you are needed! There is nothing more discouraging than to see a large number of superbly trained specialists clustered within a few miles of each other in the choicest part of town. The fierce competition greatly reduces the likelihood of your practicing only your subspecialty. In the long run, such a practice location damages your clinical judgment. You will be forced—for reason of livelihood—to hold on to patients with minor ailments who should have long ago been referred back to their primary doctor. This is accomplished either by exaggerating the seriousness of their complaints or by overtreating them with costly and complicated regimens that require frequent follow-up visits. Respected former academicians have demeaned themselves and soiled their reputations by prescribing exotic and, often, toxic experimental regimens to (erroneously) bolster their claim to being innovative specialists. They hope that the referring physician will relinquish the patient to their care rather than be involved in monitoring such toxic and unusual treatment programs. A practice in a poorer commu-

nity and where there are fewer competitors may be less prestigious and financially rewarding, but you reap the inestimable joy of truly putting your skills to the treatment of real and serious diseases.

6. Maintain the highest standards of professional probity. Avoid financial arrangements that may compromise your clinical judgment. Initially one may perform some unnecessary procedures and laboratory studies for financial gain, with full cognizance of that motivation. In time, rationalization takes over and one is convinced either that these tests are necessary, after all, to be "complete" or that they are the regretted product of "defensive medicine." Most of us have fought similar battles within ourselves and we see through such pretenses. An exploitative reputation spreads quickly and can be very damaging.

When some academicians enter private practice they quickly forsake their allegiance to the double-blind, controlled clinical trial. Experimental regimens are used with abandon, invasive procedures are frequently done, and there is no attempt to set up a framework for evaluating meaningful clinical results. We forget the great dearth of well-done clinical studies in the midst of the current publishing glut as well as the golden opportunity for honest research that dearth represents.

The Japanese have proved to us that honest value and workmanship are the surest way to success. In the practice of medicine the doctor who listens more attentively, examines more thoroughly, and prescribes medications and tests with proper, honest restraint will do very well as long as patients are able to freely choose their doctors. Dishonest behavior will only hasten the day when all free choice is proscribed.

7. Be a staff member of all the hospitals in your community. You will gradually learn the referral patterns and the relative strengths and weaknesses of these institutions. At the beginning, the key word is *availability*. Quite often the established specialists either are too busy or have become complacent. Your ready presence in the doctors' dining room or in the emergency room may make the difference. Be prepared to serve on the various medical committees of the hospitals. Everyone recognizes such work as odious but necessary. Your diplomatic management skills acquired through long years in the subterranean passages of academia can be put to good use, and you may earn the gratitude of the hospital administration and the acceptance of the medical staff.

8. Accept every lecture opportunity. The requirements for continuing medical education (CME) have given the academician skilled at teaching a golden opportunity to widen his or her reputation. Almost every community hospital now has a CME program that needs a fresh supply of speakers. Approach your audience with respect. Try to summarize a field in depth and present the latest data with as much clarity as you can muster. Do not gloss over controversial issues or oversimplify a subject. All the listeners have to do in that instance is to read a recent review to recognize that you are insulting their intelligence. It is also important to accept opportunities to teach the nursing staff and other health professionals. Nurses, pharma-

cists, physical therapists, and laboratory technicians are also valuable sources of patient referral.

9. Give your time generously to patient service organizations. They crave the insight of someone truly knowledgeable about the diseases they have, and they badly need guidance about how the precious donations they have raised can be best put to use. In return they educate you about the resources that are available in the community for your patients and they will be happy to send you new patients once you have proved your worthiness.

In the best of all possible worlds you would probably opt for a blend of both academic life and private practice. However, good research, either clinical or laboratory, must be an all-consuming passion. Our knowledge of biology and medicine is increasing at an exponential rate, and much of it is rapidly applicable to the care of patients. Nevertheless, there is a general air of pessimism in America about the future of medicine, much of it engendered by the prospect of increasing governmental control, loss of professional freedom, and the demise of the fee-for-service method. The loss of public respect for the physician, the litigious climate, and the proliferation of HMOs and PPOs further add to the gloom. Yet private practice provides the opportunity to alleviate some suffering and improve the lot of some people. These are rich rewards in an age of lowered expectations. Modern medicine is indeed a many-splendored thing. One can study it with the awe with which Wordsworth regarded the French Revolution:

"Bliss was it that dawn to be alive, But to be young was very heaven!"

Suggested Reading

Angier, Natalie. *Natural Obsessions: The Search for the Oncogene.* Boston: Houghton Mifflin, 1988.

Weissman, Gerald. *They All Laughed at Christopher Columbus: Tales of Medicine and the Art of Discovery.* New York: Times Books, 1987.

II | GOING INTO PRACTICE

10 | The Academic Medical Practice and Faculty Practice Plans

PAUL A. HOFFSTEIN

The clinical practice of medicine by medical school faculty members has always been closely linked, indeed integral, to the fulfillment of the academic missions of the medical school. The American medical education system is grounded in bedside teaching, requiring clinical faculty members to demonstrate diagnostic skills and therapeutic procedures in the care of patients. Medical students cannot learn clinical medicine unless they actively participate in the medical care system. Similarly, a clinical faculty member cannot teach competently without continuing to practice.

In this chapter the term *faculty practice plan* (FPP) will be used to refer to the formal organization and policies for self-regulation and management of clinical practice activities within a medical school environment. An FPP does not necessarily imply group practice, the redistribution of clinical income, supplemental physician compensation, or any specific legal or organizational arrangement. Rather, FPP is a generic term describing the framework within which clinical practice is conducted. Practice plans are organizational mechanisms for the identification, documentation, use, and/or distribution of all specifically identified portions of the professional fee income generated by the participating plan physicians. An FPP provides billing, collecting, and follow-up services for the group. The FPP also offers the structure for planning the group practice activities and reporting the results to management. Finally, many FPPs operate ambulatory facilities for the faculty, contract with hospitals and managed care groups, and provide a wide array of consultative services for individual faculty and for the plan's management.

History: First Full-Time Clinical Faculty

In 1911, Dr. Abraham Flexner left the Carnegie Foundation to join the staff of the Rockefeller General Education Board. With the leverage of the Rockefeller philanthropy, Flexner promoted the funding of full-time clinical professorships. The first grant went to The Johns Hopkins University School of Medicine in 1913. At the time, the concept of full-time clinical faculty was considered too radical and was opposed by the AMA and its Council on Medical Education, as well as by most other leading medical educators.

Prior to 1951, there were so few full-time clinical faculty members in American medical schools that their numbers were not even reported. As recently as 1954, 15 of the 80 medical schools then in existence did not have full-time faculty members. Faculty practice plans provided the structure and resources to accommodate the rapid growth of full-time clinical faculty.

FPPs have existed for about 50 years and were initially very loose organizations. Hart described one of the earliest, the Duke University Private Diagnostic Clinic (P.D.C.), which began in 1931. The major impetus for the development during the 1960s and 1970s of formal FPPs was the perceived need to develop a new source of support for the institution and the growing availability of third-party reimbursement. This was followed by a heightened interest in developing new compensation arrangements for physician faculty. As practice plans grew, the constraints of university and—especially in the case of state-supported schools—government con-

Table 10.1 Factors Influencing Faculty Practice Plans

Medical care industry changes:
    Medicare and Medicaid established (1965) as sources of fee-for-service income
    Fewer dollars, more regulation, extraordinary cost-containment efforts
    A changing scope of health-care delivery represented by the development of
      horizontally and vertically integrated health-care organizations
    Emergence of health-care services as investment opportunities with the growth of
      investor-owned hospitals, surgicenters, dialysis units, psychiatric hospitals,
      emergency facilities, nursing homes, etc.
    Medical schools' need for accountability and control of clinical faculty income
    Medical schools' need for diversified sources of revenue
    A national movement toward the group practice of medicine.
Trends that began in the 1980s and will continue in the 1990s to present predictable
    and powerful forces for further change:
    The aging of Americans
    The possible oversupply of physicians
    The technological explosion and the growing need for capital
    Competition from conventional and, especially, nonconventional patient-care
      providers
    Competition from community hospitals, which are making significant investments
      in technology and offering incentives to well-qualified specialists and
      subspecialists to utilize their institutions
Changes affecting academic medical centers and their teaching hospitals which
    encouraged the development of FPPs:
    Price competition, reimbursement controls, and physician payment reform
    Competition for a larger market share from community hospitals and community
      physicians; ironically, the academic medical center's mission is to create (ie,
      train) its own competition
    Large numbers of uninsured Americans are steered to the academic medical center
      as the only source of care for this segment of the population
    The growth of managed care or alternate delivery systems with a decline in fee-for-
      service medicine and the corresponding constraints on referral and self-referral
      patterns

Table 10.2 Objectives of Faculty Practice Plans

A number of objectives have been cited for the establishment of FPPs. While there are many variations among institutions, the major purposes are:

1. To provide a mechanism for organizing and controlling the practice of medicine to provide better coordinated patient care consistent with the mission of the academic medical center
2. To provide a significant source of revenue to support the academic programs of the school of medicine
3. To ensure sufficient flow of patients for educational and clinical research programs, and to meet the financial needs of the teaching hospitals
4. To provide a vehicle to recruit and retain high-quality faculty

trol suggested the need for more formality and/or separate governance, to maintain accountability to the school while avoiding day-to-day control. The development of separate governance matured with the development of independent legal entities and tax-exempt 501(c)3 corporations, which resulted in formal, almost corporate-model, practice plans. By the mid-1980s, competition for limited patients and a diminishing profit margin propelled these practice plans to emphasize planning and other group practice strategies.

Faculty Practice as a Source of Medical School Income

Beginning in 1960, accelerating in the 1970s, and involving almost all schools today, academic medical centers have adopted FPPs to offset diminished research and education funding from historical sources, especially as government resources have dwindled. The FPP allowed institutions to develop efficient systems to increase reimbursement for patient care services and to better compete with for-profit physician groups and community hospitals.

A 1967 survey of 84 four-year medical schools reported only 22 operational plans out of 72 schools responding. Of the 22, only four had existed prior to 1945. In 1968, Hardy identified a set of nine criteria for faculty practice plans. After two decades, the nine criteria remain relevant:

1. Include all strict and geographic full-time faculty
2. An FPP should be a subdivision of the school of medicine, not a part of the teaching hospital, and not independent
3. A separate professional fee billing office
4. A full-time administrator
5. A written agreement for the use of the professional earnings
6. Limits on time spent on practice
7. Financial incentives for physicians
8. Coordinated clinical practice facilities
9. All patients must be available for teaching and research

By 1985, however, 118 plans existed at the 127 medical schools. How many are "formal" FPPs is unknown. In 1988, the Association of American

Medical Colleges (AAMC) formed a new division, the Group on Faculty Practice. One hundred twenty schools nominated both an administrator and a physician to represent their practice plan.

During the last decade, income generated by FPPs has become crucial to the fiscal integrity of most medical schools. The relative decrease of state and federal support for medical education and research and the expansion of clinical faculty over the last two decades have contributed to this trend. With rapid changes taking place in the health-care delivery system, the structures and arrangements for FPPs have been in constant flux. The forecasted environmental pressures (e.g., managed care and RBRVS) will probably ensure almost constant change through the next decade.

Traditionally, until mid-century, medical teaching occurred on ward services at teaching hospitals where there were few private physicians and where the students and house staff members, under the guidance of an attending faculty physician, assumed major responsibilities for the care of the patient. Attending physicians were community physicians acting as volunteers or part-time paid faculty. The nucleus of full-time clinical faculty was small, if it existed at all. As a result, little or no income was generated from the care of ward patients. Teaching in a few settings may still be carried on in this fashion. Since the late 1960s, federal support for entitlement programs such as Medicare and Medicaid has changed the financial picture. Patients previously classified as "service" patients are entitled to be treated the same as private patients; the only difference is that a government-sponsored program has become the third-party payor. In 1960, the 85 medical schools employed 7,201 full-time clinical faculty. By 1984 the number of full-time clinicians had grown to 43,023 and by 1989 to 55,468.

Medical schools rely on four major sources for their funds: (1) state appropriations or, for private schools, endowment; (2) tuition and fees; (3) research grants and contracts, primarily from the National Institutes of Health; and (4) income from professional services to patients. Professional service income may take the form of hospital salaries, Veterans Administration funds, and now, to the largest extent, fees for rendering medical and surgical services. At most schools in recent years, the first three sources have been decreasing, at least on a relative scale, because they have not increased as rapidly as the growth of the medical school's expenses, while the fourth has continued to rise both in absolute and in relative terms. Income from faculty practice grew from $48 million in 1968 at 95 U.S. schools (with many not reporting practice income) to $4.692 billion in 1989 at 111 of the 127 schools. Some of this sizable growth, especially before 1980, is attributable simply to organizational changes. As medical schools developed FPPs, reimbursement for patient care services, formerly paid directly to the physician, began to be recognized as income to the school. Faculty practice accounted for 4% of medical school income in 1968, 11% in 1977, and 27% in 1989. In 1989 the AAMC broadened its definition of professional fee income, which tended to inflate the latest data.

Alternative Organizational Structures for Faculty Practice Plans

FPPs may be separate legal entities or they may be part of the institution—either the medical school or the teaching hospital. Institutional involvement varies and three broad examples may include the following structures:

1. The institution collects all professional fee income and redistributes it in relatively authoritarian fashion
2. The institution retains a portion of the income, and most of the remainder is distributed to the producers of the funds
3. The institution is relatively passive and uninvolved and gets indirect or no benefit from the plan

Most practice plans tend to remain within their host institutions, usually as divisions of the school of medicine, and operate in the second option listed above, offering a school "tax" and providing partial departmental autonomy.

The historical trend has recently resulted in a number of separate legal entities, either individual, departmental, or institution-wide. Considerations of forms of separate legal entities for FPPs have developed an array of possible separate legal entities, including nonprofit (professional) corporations or charitable trusts, for-profit corporations, partnerships, and voluntary associations or business trusts.

Most independent practice plans have taken the form of multispecialty group practices organized as tax-exempt 501(c)(3) professional corporations or associations.

Form and Governance of FPPs

The wag who said, "If you have seen one practice plan you have seen one practice plan," was correct. FPPs did not develop at the nation's medical schools at the same time, at the same rate, or for any one purpose. The political environment, the ethic and aspirations of the institution, the alternative sources of funds, and the opportunities for billable patient care services all affect the form and governance of a school's medical service plan. Major environmental factors, especially at state schools, include the requirements of the university or the board of regents. Finally, the school's historical relationship with its faculty influenced the timing of the FPPs' implementation and the form and structure each plan has taken.

Wide variations exist among financial operations and earning power of various clinical departments. Surgery and radiology departments, for instance, have historically had a much greater opportunity to accumulate reserves for both personal and departmental use, whereas departments of pediatrics and psychiatry, at the other end of the scale, have found it far more difficult to earn sufficient funds to cover clinical practice salaries and still retain funds to add to the departmental budget. A practice plan may either mitigate or exacerbate the "have" or "have not" clinical departments. A good plan should support the school's mission, which means allowing the reallocation of funds to basic and clinical departments as needs dictate.

FPPs enjoy myriad governance opportunities. The composition of a governing body may be represented by a strong executive model headed by a dean or one department head. However, the majority of practice plans have large governing bodies. About half include the dean as a voting member, and all seek representation from each department, usually through the chairman. The governance system for FPPs is often dominated by a group of interested and powerful chairmen. In some instances, the dean may initially control the governance system by establishing the organization and appointing its membership, but allow the group to move toward self-governance as a strategy to promote consensus.

The governance of a plan is a highly complex matter, influenced by the size and nature of the parent university, the academic medical center, the medical school, and its departments or divisions. High-revenue-producing departments often attempt to dominate policy making. Many times the chairs of medicine and surgery departments are granted special privileges, such as ex-officio seats on the executive committees. If the definition of a *resource* is anything worth fighting about, then the FPP is a vital resource.

Of the 118 schools with recognized FPPs, 84 are organized on a nonprofit basis and are exempt from federal, state, and local taxes. The remaining 34 FPPs are for-profit corporations or a combination of professional corporations, professional associations, and nonprofit organizations. As employees, individual faculty members pay federal and state income taxes on income received through the practice plan. As with nonacademic professional corporations and hospitals, even for-profit FPPs do not pay significant taxes on their profits because every effort is made to distribute the revenues collected to the clinical faculty members and to the medical school before the end of each fiscal year.

Most medical schools have centralized their billing systems for faculty practice, leaving less than one third with decentralized billing systems. Over the past decade, FFPs have been migrating from individual-based billing (ie, a bill presented by a physician, often in his or her name) to decentralized department plans with department billing, and from decentralized to centralized billing procedures. The decentralized plans were often developed in schools where strong departmental control over the FPP existed. Both history and the structure of the billing system affect the structure of the practice plan.

Much of the push toward centralized billing offices in recent years relates to the economies of scale needed to drive down unit costs, the need for group practice management information systems, and the need for a central office to negotiate with various third-party payors, alternative delivery systems, and government agencies. The remaining resistance to centralized billing may arise from a department head's reluctance to relinquish control of the billing and collection functions and the possibly misperceived notion that cash distribution is not possible within a centralized system. The major argument against a centralized FPP is the loss of control by departments and divisions and the fear that the central office will "not care enough."

The virtues of decentralized (usually departmental) FPPs include placing billing and collecting personnel closer to the patients and the physicians. This awareness of purpose—call it loyalty or esprit de corp— may result in better communications and an understanding of specialized jargon and modes of practice. A departmental plan also provides an opportunity to reward successful business offices. Not all specialties place the same priority on clinical practice, and a decentralized FPP allows each department to vary its emphasis on practice and the accountability of the business office staff.

The centralized nature of an FPP is defined by much more than common governance and centralized billing services. In the rush to develop efficient organizations, it is important that administrators not lose sight of the first goal of group practice to provide better coordinated patient care. To that end, more centralized group practice will provide (a) coordination of patient care activities for complex cases, (b) coordination of clinical teaching activities utilizing the same complex cases, and (c) simplified maintenance of relationships with affiliated institutions.

The growth and development of FPPs has often frustrated medical school deans who have attempted to coordinate and balance the different goals of research, training, and clinical practice. For instance, the uneven growth in size and number of clinical faculty often has had little relationship to the educational needs of the medical school. The department, not the medical school, has frequently become the primary force in planning for future growth and further expansion of clinical activities. Although there are many exceptions, strategic planning for clinical practice has often been ignored. Alternatively, strategic planning has been actively or passively delegated to only *one* of the following institutions, to the exclusion of the others within the academic medical center: the medical school, the teaching hospital, or the FPP.

Coordination of the faculty's clinical activities is often achieved through standardization of administrative procedures. The need for centralization of the billing function is a fine example. However, as noted above, decentralization persists in many instances because it preserves departmental autonomy, especially protected by high-revenue-producing specialties and subspecialties. At some institutions, this decentralized authority diminishes the dean's effectiveness in setting school-wide objectives, establishing outcome standards, and managing activities of the faculty, staff, and trainees. Another manifestation of decentralization is the relatively small percentage of patient care revenues allocated to the school of medicine (ie, the dean's office). In many individual physician arrangements and decentralized department plans, the physician or the department has control over the clinical revenues with limited managerial support. In these instances, the dean's office controls only a small percentage of an FPP's budget, and a few wealthy departments may operate largely independently of the dean's control.

In the end, the organizational form of the FPP must facilitate the practice plan's ability to generate revenue, make policy decisions, and manage.

FPP at an Academic Medical Center

Ideally, the FPP should support rather than challenge, threaten, or compete with academic teaching and research. It is critical that the leadership of the faculty, school of medicine, and university understand the financial, professional, academic, personal, and other considerations that affect, and might possibly compete with, the goals of the FPP. The development of organized FPPs has been one of the major forces promoting change in academic medical centers. Just as the faculty practice plan has been a change agent, the process of developing a faculty practice plan has also been a source of internal friction. Examples of major problem areas include the following:

1. *Conflict between the hospital and the school of medicine*: Although the future of the two institutions is inextricably entwined, the emergence of an FPP may appear as a threat to the hospital. For instance, the locus of practice activity usually is a determinant of the cash flow, control, and power. Only a few teaching hospital CEOs view a cohesive clinical faculty as an asset to be promoted. This perception has not been strengthened by the practice plan's strong ties to the medical school dean's office and the distancing from the hospital CEO. In the future, the result might be conflict or a closer and more intimate relationship between the hospital and the practice plan which, in turn, may result in a series of joint ventures or other arrangements where both parties can ensure their viability.

2. *Conflict between the school's administration and the clinical faculty*: The acceptance of who "owns" the clinical income may vary. The faculty's primary goal may be to develop new and additional sources of individual salary support and to improve and expand fringe benefits. The faculty leadership may also expect the funds to be available to support the mission of their department or division. The school administration's primary goal may be to develop and use new sources of funds to support the general academic enterprise. Clinical faculty members frequently fault institutional administrators (both school and hospital) on such practice-related issues as (a) inadequate space, (b) lack of a private practice atmosphere, (c) excessive overhead allocations, and (d) the amount of the school's and department's required contribution. Administrators of teaching hospitals and schools of medicine often perceive that the clinical faculty demonstrate little desire or initiative to engage in practice activities

and do not assume sufficient fiscal responsibility. On the other hand, some schools worry about faculty being too entrepreneurial.

A reason frequently offered by schools of medicine for limiting physicians' salaries is that it will ensure that time will not be taken away from clinical teaching and research. This reasoning assumes that faculty, unless constrained, will devote all their time to remunerative clinical efforts at the expense of their other responsibilities. Others may claim, however, that busy physicians with thriving clinical practices are also the most prolific researchers and the best teachers. Whatever the case, the practice plan must not prevent the dean and chair from promoting a desirable balance between patient care, teaching, and research.

Medical schools have traditionally rewarded their faculty for excellence in research and other traditional academic activities. The priorities and interests of medical school faculties have been substantially affected by the existing reward system. If academic medical centers are to compete for patients that will produce the clinical research material, teaching opportunities, and income streams that are required, a high standard of clinical care must be achieved and a high level of interest on the part of the faculty must be developed. The school of medicine must develop mechanisms to reward and heighten the status of those physicians primarily engaged in clinical care and teaching.

3. *Conflict between clinical faculty and basic science faculty*: The idea of a salary limitation is often mentioned as a method of avoiding disparities among groups of faculty. It is easy to understand that disparities in total earnings may cause discontent on the part of academic faculty. Income disparities are market driven and an economic fact of life. On the other hand, the FPP must be a means by which clinical faculty may become more self-supporting, enabling the institution to use funds heretofore required for one purpose (eg, clinical practice), to be diverted to other projects (eg, the support of basic science efforts). In addition, a viable FPP may provide the means for the school of medicine to support economically stressed departments, both clinical and basic science. It would be counterproductive if clinical earnings were constrained only to avoid a perceived disparity of income.

4. *Conflict between procedure-oriented departments and non-procedure-oriented departments*: Generalists earn less for their diagnostic and management skills. There are natural patient referral patterns from generalists to specialists which may exacerbate the conflict in this relationship. We noted earlier, income disparities are driven by market forces beyond the scope of the school or FPP.

5. *Conflict between full-time faculty and volunteer faculty*: "Town-gown" issues, competition, fee disparities, marketing, professional buildings, satellite offices, and so on have all been cited in past disputes. Former academic faculty physicians as well as well-trained specialist and subspecialist physicians are enhancing their practices and becoming more like the

full-time physicians at the academic medical center. At the same time, FPP satellites are being developed in the suburbs to provide better services and/or follow the patients. It is likely that town-gown rifts will increase in the 1990s.

6. *Conflict between state legislatures or boards of regents and the school*: Similarly, in private institutions conflicts develop between the university board of trustees and the school. External board members are often baffled by the inability of top management to reallocate resources from the "haves"—usually the school of medicine—to a "have-not" entity. In both private and public institutions, conflicts may develop between the other campuses and schools and the school of medicine.

To mitigate the above-mentioned conflicts and the possible misperceptions that give rise to them, it is critical that the mission statement and goals of the FPP be fully understood and accepted by the faculty, including the basic science faculty as well as the major teaching hospital(s), and the board of regents or board of trustees of the university. Conversely, the institution's mission and goals, as well as its history and culture, must be well understood by the framers of the FPP. Many universities, especially state-funded ones, have as a major (if not principal) goal the training of primary care physicians to serve the community and the state; other universities have as their main mission the training of academic physicians and the support of basic and clinical research. Many schools attempt to balance these two goals, with varying degrees of success. An FPP will test the culture of the institution by placing demands and pressures on its faculty that are deemed unacceptable by some faculty or by an affiliated organization such as the teaching hospital. One common example is the development or purchase of group practices at satellite locations and the recruitment of faculty who will not spend much time at the medical school. Other examples that have stressed schools of medicine and FPPs include (a) the development of an HMO by one of the parties, (b) the lack of a two-track system to allow clinical faculty to be recognized and promoted, and (c) the development of an ambulatory care building to promote patient care services, convenient timely referrals, and longer hours of operation, which may not be supported by the mainstream faculty. A successful practice plan will attempt to satisfy the major participating groups, or at least take into account their needs and concerns.

Faculty Membership and Compensation

At academic medical centers, full-time faculty have been defined as *strict full time* or *geographic full time*, although the definitions are not always comparable and the terms are falling out of common usage. Most FPPs are developed primarily to govern income generated by the strict full-time faculty. The strict full-time faculty member has an annual salary, contracted or otherwise delineated, with the head of the clinical department and the appropriate university administration official. These negotiations are controlled by school, academic medical center, university, regional, and legislative guidelines and traditions. Salaries of strict full-time faculty usually contain a component of university-appropriated money, often called the *base* or *hard-money* salary. The remainder, to make up the projected total salary, may (a) come from patient care funds generated through faculty practice plans, (b) come from grants and contracts, or (c) be self-generated through consultations and other professional activities.

Geographic full time often referred to a part-time, paid faculty member who practiced independently but exclusively at the teaching hospital and billed and collected in his or her own name. Geographic full-time faculty had been characterized by "two paychecks." With the emergence of independent 501(c)(3) practice plan corporations, the legion of two-paycheck faculty members increased, and their new members act as if they were strictly full-time faculty. For most FPPs, the setting of the total compensation is within the purview of the chair and dean, and this alone defines the relationship as strict full-time, irrespective of the number of paychecks received.

In negotiating a salary for a strict full-time faculty member, all of the sources of faculty-generated income are taken into consideration. In some FPP systems, the annual salary agreement includes an incentive portion, often based on the base salary or total salary, and often with a maximum. The faculty member is allowed to earn an amount between the agreed-upon projected total salary (TS) and the maximum total compensation (TC). Two salary models common to many medical schools are shown in Table 10.3.

Model 1 is the simplest scheme, with the university base salary (Part A) often a function of both the faculty member's contribution to the school of medicine and his or her ability to generate other funds. For example, a surgeon may have a smaller university base salary than does a similarly ranked pediatrician, or a new faculty member may have a higher university base salary than does a senior faculty member with an endowed chair. The clinical practice income (Part B) may be either guaranteed, at risk, or, as is usually the case, quasi-guaranteed. *At risk* means that the physician is held responsible for the collection of sufficient funds to cover his or her portion

Table 10.3 Salary Models for Strict Full-Time Faculty

	Model 1	Model 2
University base salary	A	A
Clinical practice salary (either guaranteed, at-risk, or quasi-guaranteed)	+B	+B
Other (grants, contracts, endowments, etc.)	+X	+X
Total salary	TS	TS
Incentive salary (always at risk)		+C
Maximum total compensation		MTC

of the department's overhead *and* his or her own clinical practice (Part B) salary. More often, the quasi-guarantee scheme is based upon the entire department or division faculty group generating sufficient funds to cover the collective Part B salaries and other clinical practice expenses.

Model 2 expands the sources of compensation to include incentive salary. Unlike clinical practice (Part B) salary, incentive salary (Part C) is always at risk. Many institutions distance themselves from the perceived entrepreneurial aspects of incentive salary by avoiding strict formulas based on income and expense and, instead, distribute a portion of the surplus pool (often a plan's requirement is up to one half) to the department or division's faculty (ie, only the clinically active faculty). This distribution is based upon a number of mediating factors in addition to clinical practice collections and a physician's individual net surplus. These factors include education, research, and services to the division, department, and school of medicine including, for example, service on major administrative and academic committees.

Details differ from plan to plan so that the reader must add the word "usually" to all statements describing FPPs. Either Model 1 or Model 2 may be modified to have Part B income paid by an independent FPP professional corporation. In many strict full-time models, the head of the department and a university official, usually the dean of the school of medicine, must approve all salary components including the incentive salary (Part C) and, thus, the faculty member's maximum total compensation (MTC). Although a separate FPP corporation provides a high degree of legal and operational autonomy, the university traditionally maintains ultimate control over faculty compensation. If a tax-exempt corporation is the vehicle, one of the three major criteria for maintaining tax-exempt status relates to physician compensation—that is, the lack of personnel inurement and the reasonableness of the salary. The involvement of the department chair and the dean or other university official ensures that both portions of this criterion are met.

Incentive salary is often capped or otherwise controlled to avoid a potential conflict of interest with the mission and goals of the school of medicine and to preserve some degree of equity of faculty compensation across department lines. It is the responsibility of the chair and dean to maintain a balance between the tripartite goals of education, research, and patient care. One mechanism to achieve this is to aggressively tax clinical practice income to support education and research. In addition to a contribution to the university (controlled by the dean of the school of medicine) and a contribution to the clinical department (controlled by the chair), the available surplus of funds after clinical practice expenses is often shared between the department and the clinical faculty. A common distribution is 50% to the department and 50% to an incentive practice pool. For more control, institutions may cap incentive salary payments at a multiple of total salary such as 50% or 100% or 200% of total salary (TS). However, a greater financial return seems to be enjoyed in those institutions where the physicians are not rigidly subjected to ceiling limitations. At many schools, the idea of a ceiling has been altered to provide a ceiling "with a hole in the roof" so that total compensation may continue to increase past the ceiling, but possibly with differing department, division, and school taxes. One result of incentive options is that departments or specialties with above-average capability to earn clinical practice income provide relatively high salaries when compared with their clinical faculty colleagues. Specialties with more primary care responsibilities and office practice activities have little or no incentive salary opportunities and are compensated by higher-than-average university base salaries. The end result is usually salaries that are more homogeneous based upon academic rank compared with salaries of physicians in nonacademic group practices, whose salaries are more dependent on specialty or subspecialty. Faculty in office-practice specialties may receive a total compensation that equals a nonacademic group practice physician's salary, whereas higher-earning specialists may find their academic compensation to be much lower than that of their nonacademic colleagues.

The Ideal Faculty Practice Plan

Can one define an ideal practice plan? Probably not—every plan must satisfy the needs of so many constituencies. Still, some common thoughts and characteristics may be offered. First, to be responsive, the FPP should be faculty-managed in concert with the school of medicine. Second, the school of medicine should, at a minimum, control total compensation. Third, all full-time faculty must be members. Fourth, the plan should have formal, written bylaws. Fifth, the rules and formulas for income distribution must be equitable, consistent, and understandable.

The ideal plan must be devised to ensure and reward high-quality patient care. The plan should encourage the establishment of departmental reserve accounts with a planned savings algorithm and a realistic goal: for instance, three or more months' net income. The reserve account will protect against crises when departments find themselves not earning sufficient funds to meet salary and other needs. In addition, it provides seed money for new projects. In cases where a major investment is contemplated, such as for million-dollar pieces of equipment for clinical practice facilities, an investment account is also necessary. Finally, developing a clear audit trail that accounts for the practice plan dollars returned to the teaching and research enterprise is essential to demonstrate the value of an FPP. Without a clear picture of the practice enterprise as a goal, there may be a tendency to purposely use FPP funds to cover nonpractice shortfalls.

In such an ideal plan, the first distribution would be an off-the-top contribution to the school of medicine. This is the common practice, with contributions ranging between 5% and 15% of gross collections. Distribution of a larger percentage (usually 10%–25% or more) of the *net* revenue after expenses is another method; however, it is far more difficult to administer and is subject to debate by both sides. While both methods have merit, the off-the-top gross collection calculation is more predictable for the school of medicine and more understandable. The distribution after expenses may bias the tax toward the high earners and protect the low earners, but it could encourage an adversarial or police-like relationship with the dean's office. If redistribution of funds from high-earning to low-earning departments is perceived as a goal of the FPP, such allocation can be accomplished after the fact by the dean, or by varying the tax, with a lower tax for, say, office practices, and a higher tax for practices with many procedures.

Most FPP administrators and deans believe the plan should have a governing board, a full-time administrative head, and a common professional fee billing and patient information system, with close ties to the teaching hospital data base. The board should set policies, procedures, and practice guidelines to promote high-quality care.

On balance, the most flexible, consistent, and responsive program should be selected. The local environment, including the personalities of the current dean and the departmental leadership, will help direct the evolution of the practice plan, as will the demands of the university administration. A practice plan must fit the culture of the institution and allow the organization to provide self-governance within the overall mission of its medical school. Whether the FPP is organized as a formal, centralized corporation or professional association or as separate, decentralized legal entities, it must be purposely structured to allow the plan to evolve to respond to the environment and the needs of the members.

Well-designed and operated FPPs are a requisite for a healthy school of medicine. The practice plan will (a) ensure high-quality clinical teaching with the necessary breadth and depth, (b) organize the administrative and financial operations of clinics and ambulatory care centers, (c) allow the medical school to be competitive in recruiting and retaining clinical faculty members of the highest quality, (d) provide incentives to ensure high-quality patient care, and (e) produce revenue for the medical school to support clinical teaching and the other missions of the school.

Philosophically and pragmatically, an FPP is a beneficial and essential administrative element in the management program of a contemporary medical school. Practice plan governance documents tend to be living documents. While these documents frequently create a great number of legal, administrative, and financial problems that are not easily resolved, a practice plan also provides the basis for the solution of serious and fundamental issues.

In designing an FPP, there are myriad competing considerations that must be identified and then reconciled or compromised in light of the particular circumstances. Ideally, designing an FPP deserves deliberate, patient, and analytical study. Where a plan already exists, changing it requires a flexible organization with a willingness to evolve. Finally, an ideal plan calls for an understanding of the long-range aspirations and potential of the medical school and its faculty.

The Future of Faculty Practice Plans is the Future of Medicine

FPPs are often hampered by a cumbersome organization, with leadership divided among departments, the school of medicine, and the teaching hospital. Many practice plans evolved with diverse leadership and oversight by many planning and governance committees. The ability to react to an ever-changing environment will be crucial if FPPs are to continue to grow and prosper. For the past two decades, it has been the academic medical center that has been the leader in the development of new technologies and new procedures, often characterized by and criticized for high cost. Managed care programs do not favor academic medical centers because of their alleged high prices and prefer to refer only the highest-risk tertiary care cases to a center with an FPP. Third-party payors are all watching with great interest the federal government's attempts at physician payment reform, the goals of which are to control volume and reward primary care and nonsurgical and noninterventional services. While each school has tailored the structure of its practice plan to fit its own particular environment, the trend is now toward the development of customized academic group practices with the emphasis on group practice. The school of medicine and academic medical center must also change to accept the new cadre of practice-oriented faculty.

The FPP will remain a key player only if it adapts to the threatening environment and only if it finds an appropriate niche for its special array of services. Only a streamlined and businesslike FPP, with the ability to make prompt group decisions, will succeed in the 1990s.

Suggested Reading

Association of American Medical Colleges, *U.S. Medical School Finances.* Washington, D.C.: AAMC, 1988–89, pp. 6 and 7.

Association of American Medical Colleges, *AAMC Data Book.* Washington, D.C.: AAMC, May 1990.

Bunch, Wilton H., and Siegler, A. H., "What Faculty Members Value in Practice Plans." *Journal of Medical Education* 63:799–804, 1987.

Flexner, A., *The Flexner Report on Medical Education in the United States and Canada.* Washington, DC: Science and Health Publications, Inc., 1910 (republication).

Hardy, C. T., "Group Practice by Medical School Faculty." *Journal of Medical Education* 43:907–911, 1968.

Hart, D., "The Responsibility of the Medical Profession to Medical Education." *Annals of Surgery* 145(5):599–623, 1957.

Hart, D., *The First 40 Years at Duke in Surgery and the P.D.C.* Durham, NC: Duke University Press, 1981.

Hilles, W. C., and Fagan, S. K., *Medical Practice Plans at U.S. Medical Schools.* Washington, DC: AAMC, March 1977.

Kettel, L. M., "Faculty Service Plan: A View for the Dean." *Medical Group Management,* Vol. 27, pp. 12–17, May–June, 1980.

MacLeod, Gordon K., and Schwartz, Roy M., "Faculty Practice Plans." *JAMA* 256(1):58–62, July 4, 1986.

Petersdorf, R. G., "The Evolution of Departments of Medicine." *New England Journal of Medicine* 303(9):489–496, 1980.

Petersdorf, R. G., "Current and Future Directions for Hospital and Physician Reimbursement--Effect on the Academic Medical Center." *JAMA* 253(13):2543–2548, 1985.

Siegel, B., "Medical Service Plans in Academic Medical Centers." *Journal of Medical Education* 53:791–798, 1978.

11 | Choosing Other Types of Practice: Solo v. Small Partnership v. Large Medical Group

THOMAS M. HERIC, MD, PHD

> We doctors have always been a simple trusting folk.
> Did we not believe in Galen implicitly for fifteen
> hundred years, in Hippocrates for more than two
> thousand?
> (Sir William Osler)

As the internship and residency period draws to a close, the young physician is faced with what can be the most important decision of a lifetime: where and how to venture out into practice. Virtually every medical student has a fantasized vision of the doctor: a pillar of the community whose advice and counsel is sought by all; a comforter of the sick, sharing confidences with grateful patients; respected, loved, and rewarded; a large brick house on the hill; these are the traditional but fading icons of our profession.

Interviews with currently enrolled medical students suggest that attitudes have changed. Just a generation ago the traditional rewards—financial success, high community profile, and business independence—were cherished realities. The popular medical journals are now littered with bitter letters and accusatory articles by older physicians whose expectations were not realized. Most young graduates today envision themselves in some sort of employed position: that is, working for an institution, a hospital, or a group, receiving their income in the form of salary. Most have accepted the fact that the financial compensation they receive will be less than that of their predecessors. Many emerging physicians express greater concern for other benefits, particularly shorter hours and longer vacation time.

An old Chinese proverb says, "May you live in times of change." The coming decade will see dramatic changes in how medicine is practiced. Dr. Arnold Relman described the "revolt of the payers" and the "era of cost containment." Indeed, economic and demographic factors affecting society may leave us with fewer choices in the type of professional life we wish to lead.

The 1960s saw a national commitment to expand clinical services. The survey by Jolly showed that medical school enrollment increased

56% to 16,000 per year, with academic faculty in the medical schools approaching 50,000, constituting almost 10% of all practicing physicians. This rapid expansion in the medical training system prompted the Graduate Medical Education National Advisory Committee to predict a surplus of physicians. Accordingly, federal payment to medical schools was subsequently reduced, and training grants in many specialities virtually ceased. Ringel pointed out that deficits in the Medicare program have translated into federal funding cuts to health science centers approaching 50%. Clearly there will be less room in academia for the budding physician.

Practicing physicians today must labor with diagnostic-related groups (DRGs) in their hospital practices. In their offices, competitive bidding arrangements through independent practice associations (IPAs), capitation programs, preferred provider organizations (PPOs), and a veritable alphabet soup of cost-containment mechanisms tax the most sophisticated of practitioners. The physician will struggle under a resource-based relative value scale (RBRVS) that may reward a doctor more for making diagnoses than for performing procedures. Skeptics say the net result will be to compensate everyone less. All of this heralds increased government involvement in the medical marketplace. Studies by Gabel, Cohen, and Fink suggest that the majority of Americans (82%) support federal intervention.

Regrettably, you must stuff the nostalgic Norman Rockwell pictures back into the drawer and take a hard look at some of the facts that will directly affect how you will practice medicine.

Owens profiled the patient population of the coming decade. Consider, for example, the changes in family size. Households are shrinking; the large, extended family ubiquitous at the turn of the century is now replaced by increasing numbers of childless couples, divorced persons, single parents, and people living alone. Among this latter group are the elderly. It is estimated that 50% of today's children will spend some part of their youth with only one parent. Single working parents, isolated elderly persons, working couples—all of them will find it hard to come to your office during normal business hours. Will you be in your office to see them in the evening or on the weekend?

America is aging rapidly. By 1995 persons aged 65 and over will constitute more than 13% of the population; more than half of these will be over age 75, and most will be women. In medical school, the emphasis may be on collagen vascular disease, cardiomyopathy, and cat scratch fever, but the practitioner should be prepared for dementia, dizziness, and disability. Will you be skilled in geriatric medicine?

America's population is moving. The past decade has seen a steady migration from the Northeast and Midwest to the South and West, and there is every indication that this trend will continue to the end of the century. A rapid population increase in an area may reflect expanding industry, translating into more people that are better able to pay you for their health care. Will you have the flexibility to go where the need is greatest?

And thus I dreamt that round me stood
The victims of disease,
The patients I had failed to cure,
Though some had paid my fees.
(William Snowden Battles)

For years there was an adage in medicine in which the wise old practitioner advised the young graduate, "The first thing to do is to decide where you want to be, then go there. There may be a lot of doctors there already, but if you stick with it, and if you're a good doctor, you'll build up a successful practice." This advice could now be a recipe for disaster. It is vitally important for the graduating physician to understand not only that the number of options open to physicians is markedly reduced, but also that the next decade will see an even more dramatic reduction in options open to patients. The cherished notion that seems as American as motherhood and apple pie—that all of us have freedom of choice in selecting our doctor—may in fact virtually disappear.

The months prior to leaving the teaching institution should be a period of thoughtful self-assessment. What is it that you want in medicine? How do you see yourself in ten years? in twenty years? What sort of a doctor are you? Inglehart has called teaching hospitals "the institutional high priests of the technological imperative that drives American Medicine." The training you are completing has emphasized a reliance on technology unparalleled in medical history, a technology whose exponential acceleration in cost has paralyzed our society's ability to financially cope. It will be the challenge of your practice years to apply this technology in a cost-effective manner. The differing modes of practice—solo versus association, partnership, and group—delineate the extent of your autonomy. You must steer your medical ship between the siren calls of Scylla and Charybdis; between the freedom of independence and the warm blanket of security.

The Solo Practice

The best a physician can give is never
too good for the patient.
(Oliver Wendell Holmes)

As traditionally defined, the solo-practicing physician is alone and has a direct medical and financial relationship with his or her patient. In today's environment, the doctor who is totally solo is a rarity. Physicians in extremely remote and rural areas may be alone, but most physicians work out on-call arrangements with others. Solo practice is the greatest challenge for the emerging doctor, who in addition to beginning a medical practice will of necessity have to set up a small business.

The beginning doctor may not fully realize the advantages of solo practice. McCue cautioned that being a "good physician is hard work, but success is rewarded by the love and respect of grateful patients." The solo physician usually is able to accomplish within his or her community a doctor-patient intimacy that is not possible in any other setting. Location influences this relationship. In rural settings, patients tend to be blue collar, agricultural workers, farmers, and small-business owners: people who usually establish long-lasting and trusting relationships with their physician. In busy urban practices, this intimacy of the doctor-patient relationship is more difficult to achieve. Operating costs of the urban practice are generally higher, necessitating shorter patient visits.

The outstanding and most sustaining virtue of solo practice is independence: independence in one's personal life, in business life, and perhaps most importantly, in professional life.

Personal Independence

Practicing alone allows you freedom of choice: choice of location, of your office decor, of the hours you work, and of the times you want to take a vacation. You can directly affect the amount of money you will make by working longer or shorter hours, and you need seek no one's permission for more leisure time.

Business Independence

You can select the number and type of employees that work for you and determine their salaries, benefits, and working hours. You control expenses in your office and can make decisions regarding your fee structure, the amount of charity work that you will do, and whether you will give discounts or free service to friends and colleagues.

Professional Independence

You establish the type of doctor that you want to be, how your telephone calls will be answered, how your medical records will be kept, where your patients will be hospitalized, what medicines you will prescribe, how laboratory procedures will be handled, and so on. All of these functions will be the direct product of your decisions and will weave the fabric of your professional life. As an independent practitioner, you may elect to incorporate into your practice laboratory, x-ray, and specialized diagnostic and therapeutic services. In some private practices these ancillary services can generate more income than do patient visits. The beginning physician should realize, however, that with entrepreneurship, one approaches the ethical boundaries of the profession. Care must always be taken not to undermine the primacy of the patients' needs in favor of business decisions.

Solo practice has its down side: risk. Business skills are required, more so today than ever before, given the rapidly changing financial environment. In solo practice, usually you are your own business manager, and you will have to make financial decisions directly affecting your patients and employees.

Many solo physicians feel isolated. Collegiality may be lacking in a small community, and there may be no one, other than your spouse, to whom you can confide your problems and your successes. The solo practitioner in the urban setting may find ample communication with other physicians in a large medical building or may be involved in various programs and committees at a nearby hospital.

Few laypersons truly understand the stress that a doctor experiences. For the solo practitioner, bottling up this stress can be a major problem.

The solo practitioner faces an enormous burden if he or she attempts to be on call all of the time. In the urban setting, solo practitioners typically work out coverage systems with one or two other physicians. It is not uncommon for as many as six or eight physicians to form such an arrangement. This can be impractical for the rural doctor, and before committing to such an obligation, one should reflect carefully.

Last is the disadvantage of cost. The solo practitioner must equip an entire office, and, depending on the nature of the practice and speciality, expensive equipment may be required. In the past, banks were eager to make such start-up loans, but the current economic climate has caused lending institutions to be wary. Before leaping into solo practice, estimate what your costs will be and determine how many patients you will have to see to cover these costs.

Some helpful hints for the would-be solo practitioner are discussed in the following paragraphs.

1. Carefully examine the location where you want to practice. Is it medically overserved or underserved? Can you fit in? Will you be welcomed by the medical community? Will you be welcomed by the business community? Are your services needed? In many rural areas, hospitals and city governments are actively looking for physicians and may provide a number of financial and business incentives for you to practice there. In the classified sections of most medical journals you will find advertisements of companies that perform physician placement; interview with them, and examine the type of practices and the locations they offer. Remember that the immobility of the physician in practice is rarely appreciated by the doctor in training. Where you go initially is where you may remain. It may be prohibitively expensive for you to move later on, so choose wisely.

2. Before committing yourself, talk to other doctors. You may at first be intimidated going to a doctor's office and explaining that you are a new medical graduate thinking of setting up practice nearby. However, most physicians will make you feel welcome and take time to talk to you. Listen to their advice but be cautious, remembering that it may be self-serving.

3. Establish yourself with an accountant. If you are in solo practice, you will need a business system setup from day one. An experienced accountant can tell you how other doctors run their practices and, moreover, can give you insight into how the medical community in the area is doing. An

accountant can also introduce you to a banker, another key step in establishing your business. You will probably need operating capital, and for this you will probably need to borrow. It is important to establish relationships as soon as possible. Again, examine yourself: are you the type of individual that can go out and make new business relationships? This quality is essential for the solo practitioner.

4. When you furnish your office, spend the minimum. Do not burden yourself with debts you do not need. Expensive wallpaper, the latest examination table, and so on can wait until you are better established. Many patients are put off by a lavish waiting room, knowing full well who will have to pay for it. If you need a piece of expensive equipment, perhaps you can lease it. Keep track of all operating costs as you accumulate them. You do not want to be surprised at the end of the month when the bills come in.

5. Hire an experienced secretary or office nurse. This can be the single most important thing you do when you begin your practice. An experienced person working in your office will know other doctors in the area, the successes and pitfalls that others have experienced, and how to get you quickly on a businesslike footing so that you can concentrate on the professional matters that you do best.

6. Socialize. If there are other physicians around you, you must seek them out, meet them, and tell them about yourself. They may be very busy or secretly resent your appearance in their community, but it is up to you to win their support and respect. If the other physicians see that you are bright, competent, and eager, you may well find the excess patients in their practices being referred to you. It is especially important in rural settings to meet the business community. Join one of the local service clubs, or at least offer to speak. Participate at local school functions. Offer your services at a football game or other event. There are many ways to elevate your profile in your community, and it is absolutely essential that you do so as soon as possible.

7. Be available. The new physician has time available, time to see that extra patient that the busier colleague down the road cannot. Be available to a nearby emergency room. Meet the emergency room doctors. Be helpful, open, and supportive, and you will find them calling you with new patients.

To the starting physician, all of this may seem overwhelming, but one should take solace in the fact that hundreds of thousands of physicians have faced the same situation and have built successful and rewarding practices. Solo practitioners may be declining in numbers in this country, but this fundamental form of medical practice remains for many the most enjoyable and rewarding.

The Association and Partnership

Here's good advice for practice: Go into partnership with nature; she does more than half the work and asks none of the fee.

(Martin H. Fischer)

Physicians may practice together in a formal or less formal relationship. In the description that follows, these two entities are combined, but in fact they constitute a wide spectrum of relationships among physicians. A true partnership can and should be defined in a legal contract. This contract can address such matters as how revenues are to be divided among the partners, professional liability, retirement, pension plans, employee responsibilities, and a mechanism for dissolution of the partnership upon death, disability, or retirement. A partnership document should be prepared by an attorney experienced in medical practices. "Good fences make good neighbors," says the proverb, and likewise, a good contract can protect the parties involved. Spelling out remedies for all of the problems that might arise is extremely important. In the past, many physicians who went into practice together neglected to create formal partnership documents. Years later, unexpected developments—such as the financial drain on a now-successful practice by the disability of one partner or the needs of a surviving spouse—can threaten insolvency. Planning for these contingencies in advance, agreeing on a mechanism for partnership dissolution, and proper insurance coverage for the inevitability of death are important to consider at the commencement of the partnership.

Because of these formal constraints, many physicians elect to go into associations. These are much simpler relationships in which each individual practitioner acknowledges his or her own practice as sole and separate property but agrees through a formula to share overhead and expenses. Even in this instance, it is advisable to have a written document spelling out what each associate believes the agreement to be. Associations can work well for an entire practice lifetime. If any equipment or furnishings are purchased jointly, it is advisable to have a mutually agreed-upon, written buy-out agreement in the event of the termination of the association.

The patients and their medical records are an important consideration. In the typical association, each doctor has a separate practice with patients and medical records. It may be cost effective, however, to combine these medical records in one file system. Typically, billing records are also combined in associations. To avoid acrimony and litigation at the dissolution of the association, it is important to establish a mechanism by which each patient is identified with one of the associated physicians. Even with the best of intentions, identification of the patient's doctor can sometimes become difficult, as when an associate covers for you during your vacation and cares for one of your patients through an acute episode of illness. Your patient may elect to transfer to the care of your associate, and such events, which could be injurious to the harmonious relationship of the association, must be borne with good will and the time-honored ethic of the medical profession. In a true legal partnership, the patients are considered to be patients of the partnership, and again, the partnership documents indicate how a practice division will take place on dissolution.

The reason for this emphasis on patients and their records is the way practices are valued by lending institutions, by the court in the case of legal action such as a professional liability suit or a divorce action against one of the partners, and by medical brokerage companies, which can facilitate the sale of the practice upon death, disability, or retirement. Whose patient is it? It is important to clarify this question at the start of your professional association.

In partnerships and associations, compatibility is perhaps even more important than monetary considerations. Are you and your associate like minded? Do you share the same medical philosophy toward patients? If not, will you be able to fit in with the other person's manner of practice? Do you know this person very well? Are you able to tolerate the other person's idiosyncracies and personality quirks? Are you able to discuss your differences and come to satisfactory resolutions?

Frequently, as your training period is concluding, an offer will come from an established attending physician you have met. At first you may be flattered and gratified, and sensing the security of a ready-made practice, you may be quick to accept the offer. Before you accept, spend some time with this physician in the office. Talk to the people who work there. How are they treated? Does this doctor treat them as you would wish to be treated? Look at the medical records. Are they of high quality? Talk to this physician's friends and associates. What is the physician's reputation? Do not be overawed by the fact that this individual is a practicing doctor and you are still in training. If you work there, you may stay there for a lifetime. Such an association constitutes a marriage of sorts; if you come to disagreement and have to leave, anticipate a divorce with all its attendant financial consequences. Occasionally, the younger physician who joins the older remains the "junior partner" and patients, especially when they are in great difficulty, gravitate to the more senior physician. You must consider the possibility that joining a senior physician may leave you, for many years, in his or her shadow. Even more unfortunate is when the senior physician takes advantage of the junior, requiring more on-call time and more weekends. In the first year or so, the junior doctor may have to "pay dues," but after a reasonable period of time, both physicians in an association or partnership should be coequal. If there is to be an exception to this rule, it should be clearly spelled out, either in a contractual document or in the basic partnership agreement. Failure to establish this difference in seniority, perks, remuneration, and on-call time from the beginning of the association can lead to resentment and eventual separation.

The worst scenario you could face as a young physician after separation from such a partnership may be when you realize that your patients and their records continue to belong to the senior doctor, and the time and effort you have put in have not established a practice of your own.

Mixed-specialty associations and partnerships can be fraught with difficulties. The graduating physician may not appreciate the significance of the choice of associates or partners. For example, if you, as an internist, joined a highly visible and successful surgeon, you could be paid extremely well to work up patients and do postoperative care, but in fact you may be dependent on the surgeon and have little chance of establishing your own internal medicine practice.

The converse can also be true. For instance, suppose a group of family practitioners takes in a surgeon. The surgeon's referrals will tend to come only from the partners. Physicians outside the partnership may well perceive the surgeon as a competitor rather than as a consulting surgical specialist to whom they can refer their patients. When partnerships cross specialty lines, they are usually sufficiently large to generate their own referral base.

The association and the partnership offer the emerging physician a good way to get started, preserving many of the advantages enjoyed by the solo practitioner with the security of one or more others to share expenses and responsibilities.

The coming years will see many complex forms of physician associations that have not existed before. Linkage of physicians through IPAs and PPOs will sharply increase. Health planners are formulating health maintenance organizations (HMOs) "without walls"—an HMO in your office. You can expect in the future to practice medicine with physicians you scarcely know, the medical team caring for the patient having been assembled by an insurance company or a practice association. You will be steadily bombarded with brochures and contracts to join PPOs and HMOs. The caveat issued when selecting a partner or associate or joining a group holds true here. Carefully read the description of the program and read beyond the page where they describe your compensation. If possible, talk to other physicians who are members of this particular plan and try to ascertain if the plan subscribers are satisfied. You may, for example, find yourself with a patient enrolled in such a plan who is desperately sick and urgently needs some form of specialized treatment. The plan may require you to call some long-distance telephone number to get an authorization for such treatment, and you may find yourself on the telephone for a long time, being shuffled from one department to another, each requiring that you explain carefully what it is that you want. This may be a burden that all doctors must bear in the future, but some health plans are more notorious for their bureaucracy than others. You should attempt, when possible, to be selective.

To cut expenses, physicians are beginning to share space such as waiting rooms, treatment rooms, and laboratories. To increase revenues, physicians are creating limited partnerships and joint ventures, purchasing and operating medical diagnostic and treatment equipment, medical office buildings, and clinical laboratories. Physicians are now sharing billing services and transcription services, and most large urban centers have doctor-owned professional liability insurance companies. Despite legislation proposed both at the federal and state levels, physicians are increasingly huddling together under the onslaught of government regulation, attempting to preserve revenues and lower costs. Associations and partnerships in the year 2000 will probably be the second most common form of practice for physicians.

Group Practice

Medicine is an occupation for slaves.
                                                    (Benjamin Rush)

Group practice, in reality, is a partnership sharing both income and expenses. In the preceding section, partnerships and associations were discusssed together, suggesting that the emerging physician would join with one or two other physicians. The usual implication of the term "group" is that three or more physicians are involved; large groups may include hundreds of doctors and paraprofessionals. Groups can be either one speciality (usually the smaller groups) or multispecialty (generally larger groups). A group is formed to maximize professional and economic benefits and, in the same fashion, share professional and economic liability. Typically the young graduating physician will respond to a group's advertisement in a professional journal or through a medical society. For the young physician, there is immediate security, stability, and the knowledge that he or she is needed and will have a steady flow of patients. From the start, the new physician will benefit from the business acumen of the group which has already been established and will share in the group's reputation and ongoing success. The new physician will, in effect, surrender some of the independence that the solo physician enjoys for the many immediate benefits offered by the group.

Many established physicians, particularly in primary care specialties, who see their incomes dwindle and responsibilities and risks exponentially increase, have opted for employment in large group practices. It is rare today to see a number of practicing or new physicians coalesce into a small group; economically and philosophically, it is extremely difficult. The trend appears to be the financially battered physician joining a large, established group or HMO: in effect, getting a job.

As with other commodities, salary ranges have been developed for most physician specialties. You will be paid more to join a group in an urban setting than to do so in the countryside, more in the West than in the East. In some highly competitive markets (e.g., Minneapolis, Minnesota) with aggressively competing HMOs, physicians' salaries are among the lowest in the nation. Still, these ensured salaries may look very attractive to the beleaguered solo practitioner faced with relentless overhead and uncertain reimbursement. It is important for the beginning doctor to appreciate the subtler aspects of group practice compensation. The salary offered by the group carries with it the expectation that you will render a certain number of hours or units of service; these will be carefully monitored. If the group does well, there may be year-end bonuses, and in some groups there are complex formulae to offer further incentives to the members. Your view may be that the salary is paid to you because of who you are and your credentials. From the group's perspective, you are paid according to cost-benefit analysis and your performance within the group must meet certain expectations. The guaranteed minimum provided by the group is comforting, but the income cap is often not carefully considered by the doctor joining the group.

Health-care educators who regularly contribute articles to hospital management magazines suggest that group practice is the method by which most medical care will be delivered in the future. Certainly the group practice, if well managed, can develop great business strength. Professional business managers can fine-tune the more mundane aspects of practice and achieve economies and efficiencies that the individual clinician cannot. The group can enter into contracts with insurers and payors and, if large enough, can exert leverage and drive discounts for services. Large groups can influence hospital, laboratory, and x-ray charges by virtue of the volume they control.

Some sages are predicting that the hospital of the future will contract with a single, large-group practice to be its medical staff. Such ideas at first may seem revolutionary, but the economies of cost achieved by group practice are undeniable. Hospitals, as public institutions, are ecumenical when credentialing a medical staff, and the resultant mix of primary care-givers and specialists is usually grossly out of balance. Currently, a medical staff of 1000 doctors, for example, may include 100 nephrologists or 100 orthopedists. There will be hardship for the doctors in the oversubscribed specialities as they compete for patients in the hospital's limited catchment area. Group practices carefully select the type and number of specialists needed to service a given primary-care base. It is anticipated that if, as predicted, physicians are rearranged into increasingly larger group practices, there will be considerable disruption and rearrangement in existing medical communities. The emerging physician who is prepared to understand these changes and who is able to make informed and wise choices will be the successful physician of tomorrow.

A successful group practice depends on everyone fitting in and, in the metaphor of the row boat, pulling their respective oars in the same direction. It is important for you to be able to fit in. As you would with a partnership or association, examine the members of the group. What is this group's reputation? Examine the medical charts. Talk to the employees. Remember, you will have much less autonomy in a group. You must avoid group situations where you might become a "doc in a box," an undistinguished "plain-vanilla" doctor confined in an undistinguished, plain-vanilla office, wading through an endless sea of dissatisfied patients. You will probably have to attend group meetings. Will there be protracted arguments over who jammed the copier machine? Will your group, as some do, go over every item on the phone bill? Compatibility is still the key. Obviously, in a larger group it is unlikely that everyone will become life-long friends. Keep a sharp eye out for problems. Is there a doctor in the group who is especially troublesome? Is the group in financial difficulty? A friendly visit with the group's manager or bookkeeper may give you valuable information on which to base decisions. Do not feel intimidated. Because you are the potential new physician, you may hesitate to ask questions and investigate possible problems. Remember that you are, in fact, a desirable person; otherwise, the group would not be considering you.

In most group practices, there is a trial period during which the new physician serves a probation to test compatibility. At this time you should consider the group, rather than yourself, as on probation. Read carefully the contractual material the group presents to you. Having an attorney go over the contract may be the best money you ever spent, but not every attorney will be appropriate: you should select a lawyer well versed in health-care matters and in group practice contracts. As physicians, we too often allow our egos to get in our way, and we assume that because we have had many years of postgraduate medical training, we can fully understand a legal contract. What is not in the contract may, in fact, be more important than what is. An experienced health-care lawyer can tell you if the group's contract is usual and customary or whether there are extraordinary and draconian features applied to you. The lawyer may be able to negotiate removal of some of the more objectionable features from the contract.

In very large groups, which may have hundreds or even thousands of doctors, the contract you will be offered will have few areas of flexibility. Established health plans such as Kaiser Permanente have developed mechanisms by which new physicians join their group. As the years pass and seniority increases, the physician acquires greater financial participation and increasing benefits. Be extremely careful when joining the large group, especially if you are considering relocating to another city and are not familiar with the group's reputation. In a city where group health plans are competing, it is not uncommon for one HMO to be identified as the "expensive one," another as the "bare-bones outfit," and another as the one with "too many patients," or where "you don't want to go if you are really sick." The medical philosophy of the group may be contrary to your own; remember, you will have to pull your oar in the same direction or you will not fit into the group and will not be successful.

The trend in health care seems to be toward increasing corporatization. The perceptive Mayo brothers, who founded their clinic a century ago, are replaced today by business-school graduates with M.B.A.s in health management. Buzz words like *health-care marketing, indirect costs, risk pooling, payor mix, cost-benefit ratio,* and *profit center* seem irrelevant to an elderly patient with congestive heart failure. However, a two-tier medical care system that serves both those who can pay and those who cannot is today a reality, and this economic stratification is likely to become more pronounced in the 1990s. Many states have laws preventing the corporate practice of medicine, but these laws are currently under fierce assault. As government funding is withdrawn, the corporate sector is steadily infiltrating the health-care business to answer increasing demand. Will medicine be dispensed in the future by large corporations, bought and sold by conglomerates whose primary interest is shareholder return? Regrettably, this appears to be the trend. However, as Starr concluded in his Pulitzer-prize-winning book, *The Social Transformation of American Medicine:* "A trend is not necessarily fate. Images of the future are usually only carica-tures of the present. Perhaps this picture of the future of medical care will also prove to be a caricature. Whether it does depends on choices that Americans have still to make."

Many physicians graduating today can be heard to say repeatedly that their main interest is in taking care of patients and that they will leave financial matters to others. This is naive thinking; in fact, financial matters have a direct bearing on how you take care of your patients and the quality of medical care that your patients receive. You have finished your medical training. You are an expert clinician. You are now faced with learning a new body of information—the complex and rapidly changing world of medical economics. If you turn your head and look away, considering all of this as irrelevant and unimportant to the practice of medicine, you will be making a grievous error and you and your patients will suffer for it.

Suggested Reading

Battler, W. S., in *The Doctor's Dream*. Leeuwordon, Holland: Miedema and Co., 1877.

Fischer, M. H., in Fabing, H. and Marr, R. *Fischerisms*. New York: Little Brown and Co., 1978.

Gabel, J. Cohen, H., and Fink, S., "Americans' Views on Health Care: Foolish Inconsisten-cies?" *Health Affairs* 8:103–118, 1989.

Holmes, O. W., in *Medical Essays: Currents and Countercurrents in Medical Science*. London: Boosey, 1984.

Inglehart, J. K., "Moment of Truth for the Teaching Hospitals." *New England Journal of Medicine* 307:132–136, 1982, p. 132.

Jolly, P., "Medical Education in the United States, 1960-1987." *Health Affairs* Vol 16 (suppl.):144–157, 1988.

McCue, J. D., *Private Practice: Surviving the First Year*. Lexington, MA: Collamore Press, 1982, p. 262.

Osler, W., in Strauss, Maurice B. (Ed.). *Familiar Medical Quotations*. Boston: Little Brown and Co., 1968, p. 153.

Owens, A., "Who Will Be Your Patients?" *Medical Economics* March:35–53, 1986.

Relman, A. S., "Assessment and Accountability: The Third Revolution in Medical Care." *New England Journal of Medicine* 319:1220–1222, 1977.

Ringel, S. P., "The Future of Academic Neurology: A Colorado Perspective." *Annals of Neurology* 27:100–102, 1990.

Rush, B., in Strauss, Maurice B. (Ed.) *Familiar Medical Quotations*. Boston: Little Brown and Co., 1968, p. 296.

Starr, Paul, *The Social Transformation of American Medicine*. New York: Basic Books, 1982, p. 449.

12 An Overview of the Principal Characteristics of Different Legal Entities

RICK L. GROSSMAN, ESQ., JD, LLM AND ROBERT D. GIRARD, ESQ., LLB

Physicians and other health-care providers have available a number of options as the legal structures for the ownership, development, and operation of a professional practice or other business venture. Each choice presents distinct advantages and disadvantages, and the selection of the appropriate organizational format will vary depending upon the character of a particular commerical or professional enterprise. If one or more physicians wish to organize a group medical practice, a professional corporation may be the preferred choice. A partnership may represent a more suitable structure than would a corporation when a group of investors desire to purchase a medical office building. As a result, prior to the formation of any business venture, regardless of its size or scope, consideration must be given to the legal and tax consequences associated with alternative organizational structures.

This chapter provides a topical overview based upon California and federal law of the principal legal and tax characteristics of a general corporation, professional corporation, nonprofit corporation, general partnership and limited partnership. It is not intended to be an exhaustive treatment of all aspects of each form of organization or the differences in the applicable law of other states. Rather, it provides an introduction to the fundamental attributes of each option, and will serve as a foundation for further investigation and research on relevant tax and legal issues and as a guide for the coordination of the development of a new business venture with legal, accounting, tax, and other professional advisors.

Formation

General Corporation

One or more persons or legal entities may organize a corporation for any legitimate purpose by preparing and filing articles of incorporation with the state governmental authority designated with the responsibility for corporate public record maintenance. Articles of incorporation generally contain (1) the formal name of the corporation, (2) either a general statement regarding or a detailed list of the business purposes of the corporation, (3) the name and address of the corporation's agent for service of process, who is the individual initially designated to be the recipient of legal process in the event the corporation is named as a party to a judicial or other proceeding, and (4) a designation of the classes and the number of shares of each class of capital stock that the corporation will be authorized to issue, including a description of the rights, privileges, preferences, and restrictions associated with each class of stock. In addition, the articles of incorporation may include the names and addresses of the initial directors of the corporation, an authorization for the directors to levy assessments against the shares of the corporation's capital stock, a grant of preemptive rights to the corporation's shareholders, special qualifications for persons to become shareholders, a requirement that more than a majority of the shareholders approve certain corporate actions, a condition that shareholders approve certain corporate actions not otherwise subject to shareholder approval, restrictions on the transferability of shares, and any other provision for the management or conduct of the affairs of the corporation that is not in conflict with general corporate law.

The other principal organizational document of a corporation is the bylaws. The bylaws specify rules and procedures for the direction of a corporation's business affairs, such as (1) the number of directors, (2) the time, place and manner of calling, conducting, and giving notice of shareholders', directors' and committee meetings, (3) quorum requirements for shareholders' and directors' meetings, (4) the manner of execution, revocation, and use of proxies, (5) the qualifications, duties, and compensation of directors and officers, (6) the tenure and appointment procedures for corporate officers, and (7) the preparation and distribution of annual reports and financial statements. The applicable provisions of a state's general corporate law will govern administration of a corporation when the bylaws do not specify a particular rule or procedure. Bylaws may be amended, modified, or supplemented by directors or shareholders and are required to be available during normal business hours at the principal executive office of a corporation for inspection by directors and shareholders.

Professional Corporation

Most state licensing statutes governing the practice of medicine and other allied health professions prohibit a corporation or other legal entity from holding professional rights, privileges, and powers. In some jurisdictions, the foregoing restriction also limits the employment of a physician or other licensed professional by a general corporation, on the theory that when a corporation employs a professional, a nonlicensed person in a supervisory position over an organization's employees may have the power to direct the licensed individual and influence his or her professional judgment and decision-making. These traditional legal constraints on the relationship between a general corporation and a license holder resulted in the inability to incorporate a professional practice. However, during the 1960s, as a response to the significant tax incentives created under the federal income tax law for corporations that were not available to individuals, trusts, or partnerships, a number of states enacted legislation permitting the formation of professional corporations.

A professional corporation is organized in the same manner as is a general corporation, through the filing of articles of incorporation with the applicable governmental authority. The articles of incorporation of a professional corporation must state that its purpose is to engage in a designated profession. In all other respects, the articles of incorporation and by-laws are similar to those of a general corporation. The submission of a certificate of registration or the receipt of a permit from the governmental body regulating a profession also may be necessary in order for a professional corporation to conduct business activities and provide professional services.

Nonprofit Corporations

There are three classifications of nonprofit corporations: public benefit corporations, mutual benefit corporations, and religious corporations. The major distinction among the different types of nonprofit organizations is the purpose for which each is formed. A public benefit corporation may be formed for any public or charitable purpose, and its assets must be used exclusively for and irrevocably dedicated to such purpose. A mutual benefit corporation may be created for any lawful purpose, and its assets are held and used for the collective benefit of those persons who are members or otherwise associated with the organization. Finally, a religious corporation must be organized for a religious purpose and its assets dedicated to such purpose.

Nonprofit corporations are organized in the same manner as are general corporations. Articles of incorporation are filed with the applicable governmental authority and contain (1) the name of the corporation, (2) the name and address of the corporation's initial agent for service of process, and (3) a statement of the corporation's purposes. The articles of incorporation of a nonprofit organization that wishes to qualify for an exemption from federal and state income tax also must stipulate that no substantial part of the corporation's activities will consist of carrying on propaganda or otherwise attempting to influence legislation, that the corporation will not intervene or participate in any political campaign on behalf of a candidate for public office, that no part of the net earnings of the corporation will inure to the benefit of any officer, director, member, or other private person, and that upon dissolution the assets of the corporation will be distributed to another tax-exempt entity organized for similar charitable or public purposes. The bylaws of a nonprofit corporation fulfill the same purposes and are similar in form and substance to those of a general corporation.

General Partnership

A general partnership is formed upon the association of two or more persons as co-owners to carry on a business for profit. Because of the breadth of this definition of a general partnership, the law specifies certain co-ownership and business arrangements that will not be classified as partnerships, such as corporations, associations, joint tenancies, tenancies in common, employers and employees, debtors and creditors, landlords and tenants, annuities, and other similar relationships that may be based upon the sharing of business revenues or profits. However, absent sufficient facts to justify that an affiliation or revenue-sharing arrangement is not a partnership, the formation of an enterprise by two or more persons to pursue a business or professional venture will be presumed to be a partnership.

Neither the preparation and execution of a partnership agreement nor the filing of a charter, articles, or other organizational document with a governmental authority is necessary in order to formally organize a general partnership. Good business practice, however, dictates that partners enter into a partnership agreement in order to formally establish the roles and relationships of the partners and to take advantage of the flexible profit-sharing and business management arrangements available in the general partnership format. Absent a written partnership agreement, the Uniform Partnership Act (UPA), as adopted by virtually all of the jurisdictions in the United States, governs the management of the partnership, intrapartner rights and remedies, the legal relationship of the partnership and its partners with third parties, and the rights of partners with respect to the property of the partnership.

Limited Partnership

A limited partnership is a partnership formed by two or more persons having as members one or more general partners and one or more limited partners. In contrast to a general partnership, a written certificate must be prepared and executed by the partners in order to effectively organize a limited partnership. The Uniform Limited Partnership Act (ULPA), the limited partnership law adopted by a majority of the states, establishes a number of components that must be contained within a certificate of limited partnership, including the identification of the name and principal place of business of the partnership, the character of the partnership's business, the name and place of residence of each partner, the term for which the partnership will exist, the amount and nature of the capital contributions and the additional capital contributions to be made by each partner, the share of profits that each partner will receive in exchange for a capital contribution, the voting rights of the limited partners, and other matters relating to the management and operation of the enterprise. The ULPA will govern all aspects of the limited partnership's activities that are not specified within the certificate. The certificate, executed and acknowledged by all partners, must be recorded in the county where the limited partnership maintains its principal place of business.

Several jurisdictions, including California, have adopted the Revised Uniform Limited Partnership Act (RULPA), which simplifies the procedures for organization of a limited partnership. In order to form a limited partnership under RULPA, (1) a certificate of limited partnership containing the name and principal business location of the partnership, the names and addresses of the general partners, and the name and address of the partnership's agent for service of process must be filed with the governmental authority with responsibility for the maintenance of public records regarding limited partnerships, and (2) the partners must enter into a partnership agreement. The RULPA does not mandate any specific requirements for a limited partnership agreement, and the statutory provisions of the RULPA will govern the activities of a limited partnership to the extent that a partnership agreement does not enunciate any rights, powers, or privileges of the partners.

Equity Holders

General Corporation

There are no specific limitations on the classes of persons or legal entities that may be shareholders of a general corporation. A general corporation's stock may be held by individuals, revocable or irrevocable trusts, employee benefit plans (such as pension and profit-sharing plans), general or limited partnerships, professional or nonprofit corporations, and other general corporations. However, as further described below, if a general corporation elects to be treated as an "S corporation" for federal or state income tax purposes only individuals and certain trusts may become shareholders.

A general corporation's shares may be issued for money paid, for labor or other services performed for or on behalf of the corporation, for tangible or intangible property actually received by the corporation, or for the cancellation of indebtedness. Under California law, shares may not be issued in exchange for a promissory note unless the note is adequately secured by collateral other than the shares to be acquired, or in exchange for the promise to perform future services for or on behalf of the corporation.

Professional Corporation

Individuals licensed to practice a specific profession and certain related professionals are permitted to be shareholders of various types of professional corporations. For example, podiatrists, psychologists, registered nurses, optometrists, marriage, family and child counselors, clinical social workers, and physician's assistants may, in addition to physicians, be shareholders of a professional medical corporation organized under California law, provided that the allied health professionals hold no more than 49% of the total outstanding shares of the professional corporation and that the remaining shares are held by physicians. Further, a shareholder of a professional corporation is prohibited from entering into a voting trust, a proxy, or any other arrangement vesting another person (other than a licensed individual otherwise qualified to hold and vote such shares) with the authority to exercise the voting power of any or all of the shares. Shares of a professional corporation may be issued for the same types of consideration as for a general corporation's shares.

Nonprofit Corporations

Nonprofit corporations generally are not authorized to issue shares of capital stock; instead, a nonprofit corporation may—but is not required to—admit persons as members. If a nonprofit corporation does not authorize the issuance of memberships, the corporation will be controlled by its board of directors, and the rights, powers, and privileges normally granted to members of a nonprofit organization will be held by the board. Any person or legal entity may become a member of a corporation that permits members, subject to any rights, privileges, conditions, or restrictions imposed on the qualifications for membership. A membership in a nonprofit corporation may be issued for any form of consideration, including those prohibited in the case of a general or professional corporation.

General Partnership

Any person may become a partner of a general partnership. Thus, as with a general corporation, partners may include individuals, revocable or irrevocable trusts, employee benefit plans (such as pension and profit-sharing plans), general and limited partnerships, and professional, nonprofit, and general corporations. However, employee benefit plans and tax exempt nonprofit corporations may suffer adverse federal income tax consequences as a result of participation in a partnership. Further, there are no restrictions on the categories of consideration that may be paid for a partnership interest. As a result, partnership interests may be issued in return for a promissory note or the agreement to perform future services to or for the benefit of the partnership, as well as for money paid, labor performed, or the contribution of tangible or intangible property.

Limited Partnership

The eligibility criteria of persons who wish to become partners in a limited partnership are the same as those governing participation in a general partnership. Also, the types of consideration that may be transferred in exchange for a limited partnership interest are identical to those permitted in a general partnership, except that a limited partner may not receive a partnership interest in return for an agreement to perform future services to or for the benefit of the partnership.

Limited Liability

Avoiding exposure to personal liability for a business's debts and obligations is a crucial factor that influences the selection of the form of legal organization for a new enterprise. Participants in an endeavor may make significant economic contributions or devote substantial personal efforts for an activity to succeed; however, absent extenuating circumstances, most individuals will not risk their personal wealth to satisfy a business's obligations.

General Corporation

Shareholders of a general corporation are not personally responsible for the company's debts and liabilities. A corporation is treated as a legal entity separate and apart from its shareholders, and in most instances, its assets are the sole source of funds for the satisfaction of an obligation. Thus, as a general rule, the maximum financial loss that a shareholder may suffer as a result of participation in a corporation is his or her economic investment.

There are several exceptions to the liability protection accorded to shareholders of a general corporation.

Purchase price obligation. Every person to whom shares are originally issued by a corporation is obligated to pay the entire sum agreed to be paid for the shares. If a shareholder fails to pay the amount due, a creditor of a corporation may enforce the payment obligation against the shareholder and use the funds in satisfaction of a corporate debt.

Return of corporate distributions. A corporation may not distribute cash or other property to its shareholders when the corporation's liabilities exceed its assets or if the corporation, as a result of a distribution, would be unable to meet its liabilities as they mature. If a shareholder receives a corporate distribution knowing that it violates one of these prohibitions, a creditor of the corporation may retrieve the distributed funds from the shareholder and use the funds to liquidate a corporate debt.

Witholding tax liability. A corporation is required to withhold certain federal, state, and local taxes from the wages paid to its employees. A shareholder who exercises operational control over a corporation that fails to deposit or pay withheld taxes when due may be personally responsible to the applicable taxing authorities for 100% of the nonpayment.

Personal guarantees. As a practical matter, most financial institutions, landlords, and other parties extending significant credit to a new or closely held professional or business venture require that the owners of the enterprise personally guarantee the entity's debts and obligations. The provision of personal guarantee defeats the immunity otherwise available to the shareholders of a corporation.

Alter-ego liability. When a corporation is a "shell," without a meaningful identity separate and apart from its shareholders (i.e., a mere alter ego of the shareholders), and a court determines that it is inequitable to permit a corporation's shareholders to benefit from limited liability to the detriment of a creditor, the shareholders may be held personally accountable for a corporate liability. Factors that the courts have relied upon to establish personal liability under the alter-ego theory include (1) the failure to observe corporate formalities, such as the maintenance of adequate corporate minutes and records, the regular election of officers and directors, the proper issuance of capital stock, and the maintenance of separate corporate accounting records; (2) the disregard of separate corporate existence through the use of business assets for personal motives or the commingling of corporate and personal funds; and (3) the failure to adequately capitalize a corporation, resulting in the lack of sufficient assets to fulfill the corporation's liabilities as and when due.

Professional Corporation

The rules governing the liability of a general corporation's shareholders apply to the shareholders of a professional corporation. A shareholder of a professional corporation also may be held responsible when he or she negligently renders professional services on behalf of a professional corporation. Normally, one shareholder of a professional corporation will not be personally liable for the professional negligence of another shareholder. However, the courts in several jurisdictions do not permit the use of a professional corporation to limit liability and have concluded that all shareholders are personally responsible for the professional negligence committed by one shareholder.

Nonprofit Corporations

Generally a member is not personally liable for the debts, liabilities, or obligations of a nonprofit corporation. However, a creditor will have the right to enforce the member's obligation to pay the purchase price for or any dues or assessments levied against a membership and to require a member to return any amount received from the corporation in violation of the prohibition on corporate distributions.

General Partnership

A partner of a general partnership is not accorded any protection against the liabilities of the partnership or the liabilities of the other partners. Partners are jointly and severally liable for the negligent or wrongful acts or omissions of any partner acting in the ordinary course of the partnership's business and for the misappropriation of funds by a partner. As a result, one partner may be held fully responsible for the payment of any losses or damages caused by another partner, subject only to each non-negligent partner's right to require (1) the negligent partner to reimburse the non-negligent partners for losses or damages, and (2) the other non-negligent partners to contribute toward a pro-rata share of the obligation. Each partner of a general partnership is also jointly liable for a pro-rata share of all other debts and obligations of the partnership.

Limited Partnership

Limited partners are ordinarily protected against personal liability for the debts and obligations of a limited partnership. Responsibility for the partnership's liabilities rests with the general partner. Thus, as in the case of a shareholder of a corporation, the maximum financial risk usually faced by a limited partner is the amount of his or her economic investment in a limited partnership. There are certain exceptions to this rule.

Control. A limited partner may become obligated for the debts of a limited partnership if he or she actively participates in the control of the business. Neither acting as a contractor for or an employee of a limited partnership nor the exercise of the voting rights granted to limited partners will constitute sufficient active participation in a partnership to expose a limited partner to liability.

Representation. If a limited partner represents the partnership in transactions with a third party, the limited partner may become liable for any debts or obligations owed to the third party if such person reasonably believed that the limited partner was a general partner of the partnership.

Use of name. If a limited partner allows his or her name to be used in the limited partnership's name, the partner may be held liable for all liabilities of the partnership to persons who reasonably believed that such limited partner was a general partner.

Return of distributions. A limited partner is obligated to return a distribution of cash or property received from a limited partnership if the partnership's liabilities exceed the fair market value of its assets as of the date of the distribution. A creditor of the limited partnership may retrieve the distributed funds from the partner on behalf of the partnership and use the funds to discharge the partnership's obligation to the creditor.

Capital contribution obligation. Every limited partner is obligated to make a capital contribution to the partnership in exchange for his or her interest. If a limited partner fails to pay all or any portion of the amount due, a creditor of a partnership may enforce the payment obligation against the limited partner and use the funds in satisfaction of a debt of the partnership.

Management and Control

Another important factor that may affect the choice of a particular form of organization for a new business venture is the ability of the owners to participate in its management and control.

General Corporation

Shareholders normally do not actively participate in the management and control of a general corporation. Instead, shareholders determine who will administer the operations of a general corporation through the election of a board of directors. They may also affect the general direction of the corporation through the exercise of approval rights over significant corporate issues, such as amendment of the articles of incorporation, the sale of substantially all of the corporation's assets, the merger of the corporation with another entity, or its dissolution.

Generally, the business and affairs of a corporation are managed and all corporate powers are exercised by or under the direction of a board of directors. The board may delegate its responsibilities to a committee, an independent person, or a management company; however, the ultimate accountability for the corporation's affairs rests with the board. A board of directors must comprise a minimum of three members; however, a corporation with only one shareholder may have only one director and a corporation with two shareholders may have only two directors. There is no limit on the maximum number of persons who may serve on a board of directors. Decisions of a board of directors normally require the approval of a majority of directors attending a meeting at which a quorum (a majority of the authorized number of directors) is present, unless the articles of incorporation, bylaws, or applicable corporate laws dictate a greater number.

A director owes a duty of loyalty to a corporation and is obligated to perform his or her duties in good faith, in a manner believed to be in the best interests of the corporation and its shareholders, and with such care, including reasonable inquiry, as a reasonably prudent person in a like position would use under similar circumstances. If a director executes his or her duties in compliance with the foregoing standard, the director will not be liable for any alleged failure to discharge obligations.

When a director intentionally or negligently fails to perform his or her corporate responsibilities, participates in the making of a loan to—or a guarantee of the obligation of—any director by the corporation without the requisite approval of the shareholders, approves a distribution to shareholders in violation of statutory limitations, or violates any of the other responsibilities owed to the corporation and its shareholders, the director may be held personally responsible for any loss suffered by the corporation's shareholders and creditors. A director or officer also may be liable for any negligent or intentional acts or omissions committed while in the scope of fulfilling his or her corporate duties. Personal liability exposure may be reduced and, in some instances, eliminated through the power of a corporation to indemnify its officers and directors. Directors' and officers' liability insurance may likewise be available to help insulate those individuals serving in a corporate capacity from personal liability; however, such insurance is often not available for start-up enterprises and frequently excludes coverage for the professional negligence of a corporation's officers and directors.

A general corporation is required to have a chair of the board or president, a secretary, and a chief financial officer in addition to a board of directors. Other corporate officers are permitted if their duties and titles are stated in the corporation's bylaws or otherwise determined by the board. The officers serve at the pleasure and direction of the board of directors and are generally responsible for the daily operation of the corporation.

Professional Corporations

The management and control of a professional corporation is regulated by the same rules and limitations applied to a general corporation, subject to the following exceptions:

Directors and officers. The directors or officers of a professional corporation must be licensed individuals and are limited to those persons who may be shareholders of a professional corporation. This rule is modified in the case of a professional corporation with only one shareholder, where an unlicensed individual may serve as the corporate secretary of the organization.

Term of office. In contrast to general corporations where directors of nonpublicly traded companies are allowed to serve for only one year, directors of professional medical corporations may serve for terms of three years. If a medical corporation has more than 200 shareholders, the term of a director's office may be extended to six years as long as no more than 50% of the members of the board plus one additional member have six-year terms.

As noted in connection with general corporations, it is essential for a professional corporation to adhere to the formalities imposed upon corporations, such as the maintenance of corporate minutes and records, the regular election of officers and directors, the proper issuance of capital stock, and the preparation and execution of employment agreements between the corporation and its shareholder-employees, in order to prevent the loss of the separate identity existing between a corporation and shareholders. Failure to comply with these requirements may result in the loss of corporate status and the risk of significant personal liability for the corporation's shareholders.

Nonprofit Corporation

The rules governing the management and control of nonprofit corporations also are similar to those of a general corporation. The members of a corporation participate in the supervision of the corporation through the election of members to the corporation's board of directors and the approval of significant corporate issues, such as the amendment of the articles of incorporation, the dissolution of the corporation, and the sale of substantially all of the corporation's assets. The board of directors is charged with the responsibility for administration and direction of the organization. Some of the principal differences between the governance of a nonprofit corporation and that of a general corporation include the following.

Corporation without members. As noted above, a nonprofit corporation may be organized without members, in which event all corporate powers, including the election of directors, rest with the board of directors.

Term of office. Directors of a nonprofit corporation may serve for a term of three years if permitted in the articles of incorporation or bylaws. Directors may serve for up to six years in a nonprofit corporation without members.

Interested directors. No more than 49% of the directors of a nonprofit public benefit corporation may be persons who are compensated for full- or part-time services rendered to the corporation during the 12-month period prior to election, other than compensation paid for services as a director of the organization.

Limited liability for volunteer directors. Directors and officers of a nonprofit public benefit corporation who are not compensated for their services may be immune from liability for monetary damages resulting from an alleged failure to discharge their duties as officers or directors if their corporate responsibilities are performed in good faith, in a manner believed to be in the best interests of the corporation, and with such care, including reasonable inquiry, as a reasonably prudent person in a like position would use under similar circumstances. Personal liability is also eliminated for any damages to third parties resulting from the negligent acts or omissions of volunteer directors and officers.

General Partnerships

Each partner of a general partnership maintains an equal right to participate in the management and control of the enterprise. Every partner is deemed an agent of the partnership for purposes of its business operations, and the act of a partner in furtherance of such operations binds the partnership, unless the partner had no authority to act and the person with whom he or she was dealing knew that the partner had no such authority.

Partnership decisions require the approval of a majority of the partners. Certain actions—such as an assignment of partnership property to creditors, the disposition of a partnership's goodwill, the confession of a judgment against the partnership, the submission of a partnership claim to arbitration, or the commission of an act that makes it impossible for the partnership to carry on its business activities—require the approval of all partners. Normally, each partner is granted one vote on all issues, regardless of any differences in the partners' profit-sharing ratios. The Uniform Partnership Act (UPA), however, permits the partners of a general partnership to agree upon a modification of most management powers granted to the partners. Thus, for example, partners may designate one individual as a managing general partner and limit the authority of other partners to act on behalf of the partnership or mandate unanimous consent for the approval of all partnership decisions. The partners also may modify the partners' voting rights so that the number of votes held by each partner corresponds to his or her share of the partnership's profits.

Limited Partnerships

Limited partners have a limited right to participate in the management and control of a limited partnership. They may vote on significant issues affecting the limited partnership, such as an amendment to the partnership agreement, the dissolution and winding up of the partnership, the sale of substantially all of a partnership's assets, the incurrence of indebtedness other than in the ordinary course of business, the removal of a general partner, and an election to continue the buisness of a partnership after a general partner ceases to act in such capacity. However, without risking the loss of limited liability, they are not otherwise authorized to participate in the management and control of the partnership's business.

The authority of a limited partnership rests with the general partner, who assumes a duty of loyalty and the responsibility to act in good faith and in a manner believed to be in the best interests of the limited partners and the partnership. Similar to the members of the board of directors of a corporation, a general partner of a limited partnership may be held personally liable to the partnership and its partners for any losses or damages resulting from the failure to discharge duties in compliance with this standard.

Continuity of Existence

General Corporations

A general corporation exists indefinitely absent a contrary intention expressed within the organization's articles of incorporation. Thus neither the death of a shareholder nor the retirement of a member of the board of directors, nor any other event affecting the corporation or its directors or shareholders, will automatically cause a dissolution or termination of a general corporation.

Professional Corporation

A professional corporation also exists indefinitely; however, as further discussed later in this chapter, the death of the sole or remaining shareholder of the corporation may lead to the dissolution of the organization if no licensed professional succeeds to the ownership of the entity.

Nonprofit Corporation

The existence of a nonprofit corporation is governed by the same rules that apply to a general corporation.

General Partnership

In contrast to corporations, the life of a general partnership is not indefinite and is contingent upon the occurrence of certain events. Generally the death, bankruptcy, withdrawal, or expulsion of an existing partner or the admission of a new partner will cause the dissolution of a general partnership and obligate the partners to terminate and wind up the partnership's business affairs. However, the partners may agree in writing to eliminate one or more of the listed events and to continue the existence of the partnership upon the occurrence thereof. Further, the partners may agree upon a specific term for the existence of a partnership, in which case the partnership will automatically terminate and dissolve at the end of the term.

Limited Partnership

The existence of a limited partnership is dependent upon the occurrence of certain events affecting the general partner. When a general partner ceases to act in such capacity as a result of a withdrawal from the partnership, removal as general partner, the bankruptcy of the general partner, the death or dissolution of the general partner (if the general partner is other than a person), a limited partnership will dissolve unless there is a remaining general partner to continue the partnership's business affairs or all of the limited partners agree to continue the partnership and appoint a new general partner. As with a general partnership, the partners may agree upon a specific term for the partnership's existence, in which event the limited partnership will automatically terminate and dissolve on the appointed date. The death, bankruptcy, or withdrawal of a limited partner does not adversely affect the existence of a limited partnership.

Transferability of Ownership Interests

General Corporation

The shares of a general corporation are not subject to any corporate limitations on transferability. Thus a shareholder may convey shares of a corporation's stock to any person at any time.

Other rules, however, may affect the transferability of corporate shares. For example, the issuance of securities, whether by a corporation or a limited partnership, is subject to the application of federal and state securities laws. These laws are designed to protect the public against fraud through the dissemination of accurate and current information concerning a company and its securities. The applicable rules and regulations governing securities require (1) the disclosure of sufficient information regarding a corporation or other issuer coincident with the offer and sale of securities, through a prospectus or other mechanism, in order for a prospective investor to make an informed and reasoned decision regarding the purchase of securities; (2) the registration and qualification of securities with federal and state governmental agencies prior to the sale of the securities, which includes a review of and opportunity to comment on the information to be distributed to prospective investors; and (3) depending upon the number of investors and the value of the assets of an organization, the annual filing of financial statements and other information regarding the entity's business operations and securities ownership.

In order to ease the process for sales of securities in connection with start-up business ventures and for sales that are limited in scope, both federal and state laws contain a number of exemptions to the presale registration requirements. For example, under federal securities law, a corporation will not be required to register the sale of its stock with the Securities and Exchange Commission if the shares of stock will be sold only to residents of one state. Further, under federal securities law and the securities law of most states, a corporation will not be obligated to register the sale of stock with the applicable governmental authorities when the shares of stock will be sold only to a limited number of unsophisticated investors (eg, usually 35) who have the capability to evaluate the merits and risks associated with the investment. Qualification for one of these registration exemptions does not remove the obligation to comply with the information disclosure requirement associated with the sale of securities.

Most new business or professional enterprises rely upon an exemption from registration in connection with the initial sale of equity securities. When securities are sold in reliance upon a registration exemption, the securities are considered restricted and may be resold only if subsequently registered or if a registration exemption for the resale of the securities is available under federal or state law. As a result, although general corporate law may not impose any restrictions on the transfer of shares, applicable federal and state securities law usually limit the free assignability of corporate stock.

Shareholders of a closely held general corporation also may wish to voluntarily impose restrictions on the transferability of shares. The success of a business enterprise is often tied to the identity and compatibility of the entity's owners. If one shareholder of a corporation transfers his or her shares to another party, the new shareholder may break up the harmony that existed among the former owners of the corporation and business operations may suffer. To prevent the possible disruption of an enterprise, shareholders of a corporation frequently enter into a buy/sell agreement that imposes restrictions on the transfer of shares. For example, a buy/sell agreement may provide that shares may not be conveyed without the prior written consent of a corporation's board of directors or the other shareholders of the enterprise. The agreement may grant a right of first refusal to the corporation or to the other shareholders if a shareholder receives an offer to buy his or her shares from a third party. Further, the agreement may provide for the repurchase of shares by the corporation or by the other shareholders upon the occurrence of certain events, such as the death, disability, or divorce of a shareholder.

Professional Corporation

The transferability of the shares of a professional corporation is subject to several limitations. First, shares may be assigned only to individuals who fall within the specific classifications of licensed persons who are permitted to be shareholders of a professional corporation. Thus, for example, a shareholder of a professional medical corporation may transfer shares to another physician or to a licensed podiatrist, but may not transfer the shares to a dentist. Second, within six months of the death of a shareholder of a professional corporation, or within 90 days of the date a shareholder becomes legally disqualified to practice his or her profession, the shares of a professional corporation must be transferred to another licensed person or back to the corporation. A corporation's charter or governmental registration may be revoked for failure to comply with the repurchase obligations. Shareholders of a professional corporation also use a buy/sell agreement to voluntarily regulate the transfer of ownership interests, including the repurchase of shares when a shareholder ceases to be associated with a professional group practice.

Nonprofit Corporations

Generally memberships in a nonprofit corporation are not transferable unless expressly permitted within the articles of incorporation or bylaws of the organization. Thus, absent express approval within the entity's governing documents, all rights of a member cease upon the member's death or dissolution.

General Partnership

A partner's interest in a general partnership is freely transferable absent a written agreement of the partners to the contrary. In the event of an assignment of a partnership interest, the assignee only acquires the share of profits to be received by the assigning partner and does not obtain any rights to participate in the management and affairs of the general partnership until formally admitted as a partner by the other general partners. As noted above, unless the partners expressly agree otherwise, the admission of a new partner to a general partnership results in the dissolution of a general partnership and the reconstitution of the entity as a new partnership that includes the new partner as one of its members. Provisions similar to those contained in a corporate buy/sell agreement are often included in a general partnership agreement to control the transfer of ownership interests by the partners.

Limited Partnership

All or any portion of a limited partnership interest is assignable by a limited partner, subject to the application of any restrictions imposed by federal and state securities laws in the manner described above. Assignment may be restricted through appropriate provisions in the limited partnership agreement. Transfer of a limited partnership interest does not dissolve the partnership, nor does it entitle the assignee to become or to exercise any rights accorded to a limited partner. Instead, the assignment entitles the assignee to receive the distributions and allocations of income, loss, deduction, credit, or similar items to which the assigning limited partner would be entitled. The admission of the assignee of a limited partnership interest as a limited partner requires the consent of all partners, unless the limited partnership agreement specifies otherwise.

Distributions

General Corporation

Distributions of cash or property by a general corporation with respect to its capital stock are paid proportionately based upon the number of outstanding shares of stock held by each shareholder. If a corporation is authorized to issue more than one class of stock, the priorities and preferences conferred upon each class of stock in the organization's articles of incorporation will govern the receipt of distributions from the corporation.

Distributions by a corporation to its shareholders may be made only (1) when the amount of the corporation's retained earnings prior to the distribution exceeds the amount of the distribution, or (2) when, after taking the distribution into account, (a) the sum of the corporation's assets is at least 125% of the sum of its liabilities, and (b) the corporation's current assets are at least equal to its current liabilities. Distributions are also prohibited when a corporation is insolvent or insolvency would occur as a result of the distribution.

Professional Corporation

Distributions by professional corporations are governed by the same rules and restrictions that apply to general corporations.

Nonprofit Corporations

Nonprofit corporations are prohibited from making distributions of any kind or nature to their members.

General Partnership

Distributions of cash or property by a general partner to his or her partners will be allocated first to repayment of each partner's contributions of capital or advances to the partnership and then equally among the partners based upon the partnership's net profits. There are no restrictions or limitations on the time when a distribution may be made by a partnership to its partners.

The partners may modify the general statutory formula for partnership allocations and agree in writing upon any other method for the allocation of partnership profits or distributions. Thus, for example, as opposed to an equal distribution of the partnership's profits, the partners may agree that certain partners will receive a share of net profits based upon their original capital contributions, even after such contributions are repaid. The partners also may agree that certain partners will receive a specific amount of money from the partnership regardless of the overall net profits of the entity. This flexibility, which is not available in the corporate form, makes the general partnership a preferable vehicle for many business ventures.

Limited Partnership

A limited partnership's profits and losses will be allocated among its partners, and cash or property will be distributed by a partnership to its partners, proportionately based upon the capital contribution of each partner. As with a general partnership, the partners may agree upon any other formula for the allocation of a partnership's profits or losses and for distributions of cash or property. There are no limitations or restrictions on the time when a limited partnership may make a distribution to its partners; however, as noted earlier, a partner may be required to return a distribution if, after the distribution, the partnership's liabilities exceed the fair market value of its assets.

Federal Income Tax Liability

A dominant factor in the determination of the type of organization to be adopted for a new business venture is the potential federal income tax liability that may be incurred by the enterprise and its owners. Significant differences exist between the taxation of a corporation and that of a partnership, and the economic effect of these differences must be considered along with the other issues discussed in this chapter.

General Corporation

A general corporation is treated as a taxable entity separate and apart from its shareholders for federal income tax purposes. As a result, each fiscal year a corporation is required to account for and pay a federal income tax based upon its income, gains, losses, deductions, and tax credits. Current federal income tax rates imposed on the net taxable income of a corporation are 15% on all income up to $50,000, 25% on all income between $50,000 and $75,000, and 34% on all income in excess of $75,000. The highest corporate rate exceeds the maximum federal income tax rate of 31% imposed upon individuals.

A corporation may not claim a deduction for dividends paid to its shareholders. Therefore the distribution of a corporation's after-tax earnings is potentially subject to a second level of taxation upon receipt by a shareholder. For example, if a corporation earns $100 of net taxable income, a corporate income tax of $34 will be assessed on the income. If the corporation distributes the remaining $66 to its shareholders, assuming application of the maximum individual income tax rate, the shareholders must pay an individual income tax of $20.46 on the amount received in the distribution. The result is a combined corporate and individual federal income tax of 54.46%.

Another consequence of the separate tax treatment of a corporation is that the character of income earned at the corporate level does not flow through to the shareholders. For example, if a corporation recognizes $100 of long-term capital gain and distributes the same amount to its shareholders, the shareholders will be treated as receiving ordinary income and not long-term capital gain. Any benefit that the shareholders may realize from characterization of the income as long-term capital gain is eliminated.

The adverse effect of "double-taxation" may be ameliorated through the use of alternative means for the distribution of income to shareholders in such a manner that it is deductible at the corporate level. This may be accomplished through payment of interest by the corporation on loans from its shareholders, payment of reasonable compensation (either in the form of a salary or bonus) by the corporation for services rendered by its shareholders, or payment of rent or other similar consideration for the use of a shareholder's property by the corporation. Although permissible under current federal tax law, both the substance and form of these techniques are carefully scrutinized when the Internal Revenue Service audits a corporation's income tax return. If the IRS finds that a situation is abusive, it may exercise the authority to reallocate or recharacterize items of income, gain, loss, or deduction, which may result in the loss of a favorable tax result. Therefore, taxpayers should carefully document all transactions between a corporation and its shareholders to prevent disallowance of a beneficial tax consequence.

Another mechanism to avoid the imposition of a federal income tax at the corporate level is for the shareholders of a corporation to elect treatment as an "S corporation." When an S corporation election is properly filed, no federal income tax will be assessed on the corporation's net taxable income. Instead, the character and amount of all income, gain, loss, deduction, and tax credits will be allocated among the shareholders of the corporation and includable on the shareholders' individual income tax returns. The effect of the S corporation election in most circumstances will be to reduce the maximum potential federal income tax to 31%.

The following criteria must be satisfied in order to initially qualify as an S corporation and to continue to qualify after an election is made:

Status. The corporation must be a United States domestic corporation and may not be a member of an affiliated group. This latter requirement means that an S corporation cannot own 80% or more of the stock of another corporation.

Number of shareholders. An S corporation may not have more than 35 shareholders. For this purpose, a husband and wife are treated as one shareholder.

Type of shareholders. Individuals and certain categories of trusts are permitted to be shareholders of an S corporation. Foreign and domestic corporations, partnerships, nonresident aliens, and foreign trusts are not eligible to be S corporation shareholders.

Classes of stock. An S corporation may have only one class of stock. Differences in voting rights will not, in and of itself, create more than one class of stock for this purpose.

Election. An election to be taxed as an S corporation must be signed by all shareholders and other persons who have interests in the stock of the corporation, such as a spouse with a community property interest. The election will be effective as of the first day of a taxable year if it is filed with the Internal Revenue Service on or before the 15th day of the third month of the corporation's taxable year. If it is filed any time thereafter, the election will be effective as of the first day of the immediately succeeding taxable year.

Professional Corporation

A professional corporation will be treated in the same manner as a general corporation for federal income tax purposes; however, all of its income will be subject to tax at the maximum federal rate of 34%, as opposed to the graduated rate schedule available to general corporations. The federal income tax can be averted through an election to be treated as an S corporation, which is available on the same terms as for a general corporation.

Nonprofit Corporations

The fact that an organization is formed as a nonprofit corporation does not necessarily result in exemption from the imposition of a federal income tax on its taxable income. Regardless of the purposes for which a nonprofit corporation is created, a nonprofit corporation will be subject to taxation under the same rules that apply to a general corporation unless it applies for and receives tax-exempt status from the Internal Revenue Service.

There are a number of categories of tax-exempt organizations, including charitable organizations, trade or business associations, business leagues, social clubs, voluntary employee benefit associations, fraternal beneficiary societies, and credit unions. The requirements for qualification for exempt status vary for each class of organization. However, there are certain opportunities that may be pursued through a tax-exempt organization, such as the operation of a hospital, the conduct of medical or scientific research, or the publication of a professional journal, and if one is interested in the use of a tax-exempt organization to pursue one of these endeavors, the appropriate professional advisors should be consulted.

General Partnership

A general partnership is not treated as a separate taxable entity for federal income tax purposes. Instead, the amount of its income, gains, losses, deductions, and tax credits flows through to its partners, who include on their individual income tax returns their respective distributive share of the partnership's tax attributes. In certain instances, the character of an item realized at the partnership level retains its tax character at the individual level and may be netted against or included with other similar items realized by a partner. Unlike a general or professional corporation that does not elect S corporation status, there is no double taxation of a partnership's net taxable income.

It is important to note that a partner recognizes income or loss from the receipt of a distributive share of a partnership's tax items regardless of whether any distributions are made by the partnership to its partners. As a result, if a partnership recognizes significant profit but fails to distribute any cash or property to its partners, the partners will be obligated to pay individual income tax on their allocable shares of the income, yet will not have any additional cash to make the payment. Conversely, if a partnership makes a cash or property distribution to its partners during a taxable year when the partnership recognizes a net loss, no tax will be levied against the distribution unless the distribution exceeds a partner's adjusted basis for his or her partnership interest, in which case the partner will recognize a capital gain. Finally, subject to certain limitations and restrictions, a partner may be able to offset his or her allocable share of a partnership's net loss against income recognized by the partner from other sources.

Limited Partnership

A limited partnership generally will be treated in the same manner as a general partnership for federal income tax purposes.

Income Tax Incentives and Attributes

The following discussion highlights several categories of tax incentives and benefits that are available to the owners/employees of partnerships and corporations. For purposes of this discussion, "C corporation" refers to a corporation that has not elected to be treated as an S corporation.

Health Insurance Premiums

Health insurance premiums paid by a C corporation for the benefit of a shareholder/employee are deductible by the corporation and excludable from the income of the shareholder/employee. For taxable years commencing prior to January 1992, 25% of the health insurance premiums paid by a partnership for the benefit of a partner/employee is excludable from income. No similar exclusion is available for a shareholder/employee of an S corporation.

Medical Reimbursement Plans

Medical expenses of a shareholder/employee paid under a reimbursement plan adopted by a C corporation are deductible by the corporation and are excludable from the income of the recipient of the benefit. No similar benefit is available to partners or shareholders of an S corporation.

Disability Insurance Premiums

A C corporation may deduct disability insurance premiums paid for the benefit of its shareholder/employees and the premium payments will be excludable from the income of the shareholder/employees. No similar benefit is available for partners or shareholders of an S corporation. However, if a shareholder/employee excludes the premium costs from his or her income, any payments received by the employee under the insurance policy upon disability will be subject to federal income tax.

Term Life Insurance

A C corporation may deduct the premium cost of up to $50,000 of term life insurance purchased on the life of a shareholder/employee, and the premium payment is excludable from the income of the shareholder/employee. No similar benefit is available to partners or shareholders/employees of an S corporation.

Dependent Care Assistance

C corporations, S corporations, and partnerships may deduct the costs of dependent care assistance benefits provided to shareholder/employees or partners. Any benefits received are excludable from income by the shareholder/employees or partners.

Educational Expense Assistance Plans

C corporations, S corporations, and partnerships may deduct the costs of educational expenses incurred under employee assistance plans developed by an employer. Any benefits received are excludable from income by the shareholder/employees or partners.

Cafeteria Plans

A cafeteria plan permits an employee to choose among two or more qualified fringe benefits available under the plan, one of which may be the payment of cash compensation. Benefits paid under a cafeteria plan are deductible by the employer as long as there is no discrimination in favor of highly paid employees. Only C corporations may establish cafeteria plans.

Pension and Profit Sharing Plans

The significant differences that formerly existed among C corporations, S corporations, and partnerships in the deductions available for contributions to and for the benefits payable from qualified pension or profit-sharing plans have been effectively eliminated. As a result, regardless of the organizational form selected for a business enterprise, the entity will be able to establish and make deductible contributions to a qualified employee benefit plan.

Several differences remain between qualified employee benefit plans of

C corporations and plans maintained by partnerships or S corporations. A shareholder/employee of a C corporation may borrow money from a qualified plan, whereas a partner or shareholder/employee of an S corporation generally is prohibited from borrowing from a plan. The rules governing the aggregation of qualified employee benefit plans of related employers for eligibility, discrimination, and other purposes treat a C corporation in a more favorable manner than a partnership or S corporation. An employee benefit plan maintained by a C corporation may invest its assets in life insurance policies for the benefit of the plan's participants. Plans maintained by partnerships and S corporations may not make similar investments. A participant in the qualified employee benefit plan of a C corporation may be entitled to income averaging in connection with a lump sum distribution made to the employee upon the separation of service (whether by death, retirement or any other reason). Participants in a partnership or S corporation plan will not receive this favorable tax treatment.

Death Benefit

A C corporation may pay and deduct up to $5000 of additional compensation on the death of a shareholder/employee, which will not be taxable to the shareholder's estate or any other recipient. A similar benefit is not available to partnerships and S corporations.

Dividends-Received Deduction

A C corporation that owns the stock of another corporation is entitled to deduct 70% of any dividends received with respect to such stock. The effect of this deduction is to reduce the maximum federal income tax payable on dividends received by a C corporation to approximately 10.2%. No similar benefit is available to partnerships and S corporations.

Fiscal Year

A C corporation may adopt a taxable year other than the calendar year for federal income tax purposes. The taxable year of a partnership is determined by reference to the taxable year of its partners, which usually results in the use of a calendar year by a partnership. An S corporation is required to use the calendar year as its taxable year. The principal advantages of adoption of a noncalendar year are an initial deferral of tax for the shareholder/employee on income that otherwise may have been taxed in the first year of incorporation, and a continuing ability to allocate the individual income of shareholder/employees between two calendar years by the timing of salary payments.

A professional services corporation is denied the right to have a taxable year other than the calendar year, unless the entity is willing to elect to make certain minimum distributions to its owners/employees prior to the end of each calendar year. The effect of this election is to eliminate any advantage available through the use of a noncalendar fiscal year. As a result, for all practical purposes, a professional corporation will be required to adopt the calendar year as its taxable year.

Method of Accounting

A C corporation is required to report its taxable income under a method of accounting other than the cash receipts and disbursements method. Normally, C corporations will adopt the accrual method of accounting. This presents a potential disadvantage to a C corporation because it will be required to report and pay taxes on its outstanding accounts receivable, although it may be able to deduct all or a significant portion of its outstanding accounts payable. A professional C corporation may be able to use the cash method of accounting if its annual gross receipts are less than $5 million. If a partnership has a C corporation as a partner or is considered a "tax shelter," then it must use the accrual method of accounting. Otherwise, a partnership and an S corporation may use the cash method of accounting.

Worthless Stock Loss

Generally, any loss recognized by a shareholder on the sale or disposition of corporate stock is treated as a long-term or short-term capital loss depending upon the period of time that the stock is owned. However, if the stock of a small business corporation is deemed worthless, a shareholder may treat the loss as an ordinary loss rather than a capital loss. For this purpose, a "small business corporation" is any corporation that received less than $1 million as capital contributions and paid-in surplus of its stock and, during the five-year period prior to the determination that its stock is worthless, more than 50% of its revenues were received from sources other than rent, royalties, dividends, interest, and other passive types of income. The maximum amount a shareholder may claim as an ordinary loss is $50,000, or $100,000 in the case of a husband and wife filing a joint return.

Planning Ideas

The selection of a legal structure for a particular professional or business endeavor will depend both upon the objective factors outlined in this chapter and upon the subjective concerns of the participants in the enterprise, such as risk aversion, prior business experiences, and the recommendations made by professional advisors. Because of the variety of and relative importance often placed upon the subjective factors, it is impractical in this context to suggest that a specific business activity must conform to one organizational format. However, certain structures are recommended for distinct categories of professional or business ventures.

Professional Practice Groups

The prevalent formats for the ownership and operation of a professional practice are either a professional corporation or a general partnership.

Personal liability. A professional corporation offers several distinct advantages over a partnership, including (1) the ability in most states to shield the shareholders of the organization against personal liability for the professional negligence of one shareholder, (2) limited personal liability of the shareholders for the general debts and obligations of a practice, and (3) the opportunity to take advantage of the tax incentives and fringe benefits available to corporate shareholder/employees that are unavailable to partners of a partnership. A general partnership presents a greater risk of personal liability for its partners; however, exposure to certain liabilities may be reduced or effectively eliminated through the acquisition of adequate professional liability (malpractice) and general liability insurance.

Governance. A professional corporation requires a greater degree of procedural formality than does a partnership, such as the regular election of a board of directors and corporate officers, the maintenance of corporate minutes and other records, and the documentation of the employer/employee relationship between a shareholder and the corporation. Depending upon the size of a professional practice group, the existence of corporate formalities forces the members of a professional corporation to deal on a periodic basis with the issues faced by the enterprise, such as compensation, growth, practice development, and other similar matters. Corporate law also establishes the structure for the governance of a professional corporation, which in a large practice group may avert the need for discussions and decisions that must occur in the partnership context regarding the framework for professional practice management.

Profit sharing. The general partnership allows for greater flexibility in the structuring of the allocations and distributions of a professional practice's net profits than does a corporation. In a partnership, profits are not required to be allocated on a pro rata basis. As a result, some partners may receive a greater share of the net profits and other partners may receive a lesser share. Partnership allocations also may be arranged in such a manner that certain partners receive a predetermined dollar amount each fiscal year regardless of the entity's net profits, whereas other partners receive a specified percentage of net profits and are subject to any increases or decreases in profitability. A professional corporation is not as versatile. Net profits of a professional corporation, when distributed, must be allocated proportionately based upon the number of shares held by each shareholder. Some of this rigidity may be eliminated through creative compensation arrangements between the corporation and its shareholder/employees and variations in the number of shares held by each shareholder; however, the tax and other financial effects of such arrangements in results in the professional corporation context are often less favorable.

Other Business Arrangements

The preferred legal structure for other types of business arrangements will depend upon the factual circumstances surrounding the development, ownership, and operation of the venture. Several general issues to be taken into account are as follows:

Double taxation. Use of a general corporation (that does not elect S corporation status) presents potential adverse federal income tax consequences when a business is organized to own and hold real estate or any other appreciating tangible or intangible asset. Upon the sale of an appreciated asset, a corporation will recognize a gain and incur a federal income tax liability on the transaction. A distribution of the after-tax sale proceeds to the corporation's shareholders will result in the imposition of a tax at the shareholder level and further reduce the net sale proceeds received by a shareholder. Further, if an appreciated asset is held by a corporation, double taxation cannot be avoided through a distribution of the asset to the shareholders in connection with a dissolution of the entity or a redemption of its shares because a tax will be levied against the corporation on the appreciation existing at the time of the distribution. As a result, the preferred format for this type of business venture is one that avoids a tax at the entity level, such as a general partnership, a limited partnership, or an S corporation.

S corporation limitations. An S corporation appears to be an ideal format for most business enterprises because it receives the nontax benefits of a general or professional corporation, yet no federal income tax is assessed at the corporate level. However, there are certain restrictions associated with an S corporation which limit its utility. An S corporation is unavailable to a widely held enterprise because it may have only 35 shareholders. It may also be impractical when a business wishes to obtain equity capital from sources other than individuals and the few permitted categories of trusts, because professional corporations, general corporations, and employee benefit plans are prohibited from becoming shareholders of an S corporation. A limited partnership is often preferred to an S corporation by reason of its liability protection for limited partners and lack of restrictions on the categories of persons who may become investors in the business enterprise.

Loss limitations. The discussion of the federal income tax consequences associated with an S corporation, limited partnership, and general
partnership indicates that a shareholder or partner of one of these organizations is allocated a distributive share of the tax items recognized at the
entity level and is required to include these items on his or her individual
income tax returns. If a net loss is recognized at the entity level, a shareholder or partner may be able to apply this loss against income from other
sources and reduce his or her overall tax liability. However, there are
certain statutory limitations on the ability of a partner or shareholder to use
a distributive share of losses against income from other sources, and these
rules must be taken into account in determining the effect that a particular
legal structure may have on an individual's income tax situation.

A shareholder of an S corporation is prohibited from using his or her
distributive share of losses from the corporation in excess of (1) the shareholder's adjusted basis in corporate stock (generally determined as the
amount of a shareholder's initial and additional capital contributions to the
corporation, which is adjusted annually based upon a shareholder's allocable share of net profits or net loss and cash or property distributions from
the corporation), and (2) the amount of any loans made by the shareholder
to the corporation. When a shareholder's share of losses exceeds this
amount, use of the losses is suspended and is available for use by the
shareholder in subsequent years. To ensure that a shareholder has sufficient basis to use losses, when a corporation needs capital, it is beneficial
for a shareholder to borrow the money from a third party and contribute or
loan the funds to the corporation, thereby increasing the shareholder's
basis.

A partner may use his or her distributive share of losses from a partnership to offset income from other sources only to the extent that the losses
are not greater than the (1) adjusted basis of a partner in his or her partnership interest (which is initially determined and adjusted annually in the
same manner as the adjusted basis of the shares of an S corporation shareholder), and (2) the partner's allocable share of partnership liabilities. When
a partner's distributive share of the partnership's losses exceeds this
amount, the losses are carried forward and may be applied by the partner in
future taxable years. In contrast to a shareholder in an S corporation, a
partner of a partnership does not receive any additional benefit for loans
made by the partner to the partnership, but does increase his or her basis by
a share of partnership liabilities. Thus, when a partnership requires additional capital, it is advisable for the funds to be borrowed by the partnership.

The *at-risk rule* also limits the deductibility of losses by a partner or
shareholder of an S corporation to the amount that the person is at risk with
respect to a particular activity. Amounts at risk are generally defined as the
sum of the money and adjusted basis of any property contributed by a
person to a particular activity as well as the amount of any funds borrowed
for use in the activity if the borrower is personally liable for repayment of

the loan. A taxpayer will not be considered at risk when he or she is protected against loss by virtue of a third-party guarantee of an indebtedness, a stop-loss agreement, or other similar arrangement. All business activities, including real estate, are subject to the application of the at-risk rule.

A third limitation on the ability of a partner or shareholder of an S corporation to deduct his or her distributive share of an entity's losses is the passive loss limitation added by the Tax Reform Act of 1986. This rule is designed to prevent the use of losses from passive investments, such as tax shelters, to offset income recognized from active sources, such as compensation or other fees paid for personal services. For purposes of the passive loss limitation, there are three types of income: passive, active, and portfolio. Portfolio income generally includes income from royalties, dividends and interest. Active income generally includes income earned for personal services, and passive income is income earned from participation in a passive activity. A passive activity is defined as an activity that involves the conduct of a trade or business and in which a person does not materially participate. *Material participation* is defined as the involvement in an activity on a regular, continuous, and substantial basis. Ownership of a limited partnership interest is presumed to be a passive activity.

Generally, the passive loss limit permits losses recognized from passive activities to only offset income recognized from passive activities. As a result, otherwise deductible losses from a limited partnership may be useless if a limited partner has no other passive income to apply against the loss. Losses that are not used in one taxable year may be carried forward and applied in subsequent taxable years when a taxpayer may have passive income.

The passive loss limitation applies to individuals, estates, trusts, S corporations, partnerships, personal service corporations, and closely held C corporations. The many rules that govern the application of this limitation are beyond the scope of this chapter; however, two matters should be noted. A closely held C corporation that is not a personal services corporation will be permitted to deduct its passive losses against earned income but not against portfolio income. Further, even though rental activities are generally considered passive activities, certain taxpayers may be able to deduct up to $25,000 of losses from rental real estate activities against active and portfolio income.

Suggested Reading

B. Bittker, and J. Eustice, *Federal Income Taxation of Corporations and Shareholders* (5th Ed.), Boston, MA: Warren, Gorham & Lamont, 1990.

Blazek, J., *Tax and Financial Planning for Tax-Exempt Organizations.* New York: John Wiley & Sons, Inc., 1989.

Grant, I. M. and W. R. Christian, *Subchapter S Corporations* (2nd Ed.), Shephard's/ McGraw-Hill, Inc., Colorado Springs, CO, 1990.

Hargrove, J. O., (Ed.), *Attorneys' Guide to California Professional Corporations.* Berkeley, CA. Continuing Education of the Bar, 1989.

Harroch, R. D. (Ed.), *Start-Up Companies: Planning, Financing, and Operating the Successful Business.* New York: John Wiley & Sons, Inc., 1987.

Hopkins, B. R., *The Law of Tax-Exempt Organizations.* Boston, MA: Warren, Gorham & Lamont, 1989.

W. McKee, W. Nelson, and R. Whitmore, *Federal Taxation of Partnership and Partners* (2nd Ed.), Law Journal Seminars-Press, New York, N.Y., 1990.

13 | Choosing Your Practice Location

JUDITH E. BERGER

As you are probably aware, it is going to be more difficult for physicians to locate practices during the next decade—especially in the Sunbelt and in urban areas—because of the predicted surplus or maldistribution of physicians already in these areas. Over 50% of young physicians grow dissatisfied with their practices and choose to leave within the first two years. Limited practice growth, inadequate earnings, lack of coverage and support from the medical community, and disappointments in the quality of life for themselves and their families are often cited as primary factors motivating their decisions to relocate. Many of the problems contributing to practice dissatisfaction and decisions to relocate are avoidable and often are a result of incomplete preparation and faulty decision-making during the practice selection process. Residents and fellows do not have enough knowledge or experience to select a practice opportunity, evaluate the different financial arrangements, and set up a comprehensive interview. In addition, the average resident has approximately $35,000 to $80,000 in loans or indebtedness. These circumstances can force new physicians to compromise their ideals in order to obtain a position that will allow them to pay off their debts. All of these factors, in addition to other, personal ones, affect selection of the practice location.

This chapter addresses the different types of practice opportunities available, how to evaluate different arrangements, and the importance of ensuring a successful interview and visit. Included at the end of this chapter is a practice selection timetable and a practice rating guide to help you through the evaluation process.

The first step in selecting a practice location after you have determined the type of practice is to decide in what part of the country you want to live. Most physicians choose a location that is somewhat familiar to them: perhaps they or their spouse was born or educated in that community or part of the country, or they know someone in a specific community.

Once your location is selected (East, West, Midwest, South, etc), you need to choose the size of the community in which to practice: rural (up to 5000 population); semirural (5000–10,000); urban (50,000 and up); or suburban (up to 50,000). Many people have no concept of size of cities and sometimes go to a rural community, thinking it has about 50,000 residents.

It is important to find out the cost of living in the community. Learn the population of the town and its surrounding areas. What type of recreation is available? Does it meet the needs of your family? Are there parks and city-sponsored programs like soccer, Little League, swimming, and summer programs for children? What types of cultural activities are available (eg, theater, summer stock, dances, concerts)? To some people, this is very important. Also, if these activities are not available in the community, how long must one drive to find them?

When physicians and their spouses move to a community away from their families, public transportation and access is very important. It is vital to investigate airline, bus, and train schedules and major highways. Are there major roadways that make the town easily accessible?

Another factor to investigate is the growth potential of the area and what the major industries are. Have there been any major layoffs or closings of industries? Who are the major employers and how many people do they employ? Is there an economic development council that is soliciting new business and industry for the community? It is important, also, to consider opportunities for youth after graduation from high school and college: without these opportunities there is little or no incentive for young people to return. What places of worship are available, and are there adequate shopping facilities to meet all of your family's needs?

When visiting any community, have a real estate agent take you around to look at residential areas. Take into consideration the prices, taxes, location, and types of homes. Find out how prices have varied over the past five years and how easy it would be to sell a home there. Also, look at loan and mortgage rates.

Make sure employment is available for your spouse. If your spouse is also a physician and you are looking at a group practice, make sure the group hires married couples—some do not.

A final consideration in evaluating a community for your practice location is the school system. For example, how many students are there? What is the student-teacher ratio? What are the education requirements of teachers? What is the basic curriculum? How well have the students scored on standardized, statewide tests? What percentage of students go on to college?

It is very important to focus on the practice opportunities available, not solely the position's financial compensation and benefits.

In selecting a practice, the first important question to ask is why the opportunity is available. Is there a need attributable to retirement, death, or replacement of someone leaving, or just a need for additional physicians? Once you have determined that there is a need, you must look at the practice volume, patient composition, and payor-physician mix.

Find out how many doctors have left the community in the past five years and why. Speak to them if possible. Where did other physicians in the community train? Are they board certified? Why did they choose to practice in that community? What are the current referral patterns? Do referrals come from other physicians or self-referrals? Does the hospital have a referral service? Speak with the physicians who would be referring patients to you.

If you are going into a solo practice, is cross coverage available? If it is a group practice, are there other physicians in your specialty? What is the future of the practice three to ten years down the road?

What type of hospital would you be using? Where is it in relation to the office practice? Is the hospital a for-profit or not-for-profit institution? How many beds does it maintain? What major services and facilities does it offer? What specialties are represented on the medical staff and what is the quality of the nursing staff? What is the attitude of the administration and the board of directors toward physicians' involvement in the hospital? Are there teaching opportunities available? And finally, what is the long-term viability of the hospital?

If you are looking into a group practice opportunity, find out what the group's overhead or department overhead is.

What are the average earnings by specialty? Is there a production formula, buy-in and/or prepayment component to the practice, and if so, what is the percentage? What does the benefit package include—malpractice, health insurance, relocation expenses, interview expenses, rent, medical society dues, vacation, education time, medical books, and so on?

Keep an open mind when choosing your practice location. No situation is perfect; sometimes an ideal practice is not realistic in today's health-care environment. Before choosing your practice location give priority to the aspects that are most important to you, both professional and personal, and then focus your attention on those areas.

Remember also to consider the nature of your specialty and your type of patients when choosing your location. Finding a new, developing community with young families is ideal for a family practitioner or pediatrician, but locating in such a community could prove to be a financial disaster for a rheumatologist, urologist, or geriatrician. Conversely, a retirement community is an excellent site for a cardiologist or a geriatrician but a poor choice for an obstetrician. These examples, although extreme and obvious, nevertheless convey a key point—that is, know the demographics and referral base of each location you are considering.

Practice Selection Timetable

Much information in this chapter has focused on selecting your practice location, but keep in mind that the timing is also crucial. Residents and fellows should plan to select a location early in their last year of training. Table 13.1 is a checklist for you to use in your practice search.

Many of the items in Table 13.1 can be condensed if the pace of your final year of residency prohibits you from starting to look until later in the year. However, it is not wise to omit any items. All are equally important in making your first day pleasant and in making the last weeks leading up to that day much less harried and frantic. Also important are the support systems that will carry you through these times; your family, friends, and colleagues can provide you with valuable information, advice, and feedback. They can also be an invaluable source of reassurance. In any case, use

Table 13.1 Practice Selection Timetable

Activity	Time before target date	Date completed
1. Choose desired general or specific locations(s).	9–12 mos.	_____
2. Consider type of practice to establish or join, comparing solo opportunities, single-specialty and multispecialty group settings, HMO or other corporate settings, and academic positions.	9–12 mos.	_____
3. Discover what opportunities are available in the areas you have chosen that fit your desired practice style. Discuss opportunities with your program director, review advertisements in specialty journals, consult recruiting firms to see what they are representing, and contact state or specialty associations to review their listings.	8–11 mos.	_____
4. Through telephone interviews, narrow choices to no more than five opportunities that would suit your needs, based on practice style, location, and other important factors.	8–9 mos.	_____
5. Arrange visits and conduct interviews in person for the opportunities you have chosen as your most suitable alternatives, including all facets of a visit previously discussed.	7–8 mos.	_____
6. Visit prospective employers for a second visit.	6–7 mos.	_____
7. Make final decision about practice choice and politely decline other offers.	5–6 mos.	_____
8. Apply for hospital privileges, tour the community for housing options, and apply for necessary loans.	4–5 mos.	_____
9. With the assistance of the group you are joining, order announcement cards and advertisements, stationery, business cards, and any patient information packets you especially like.		_____
10. With the assistance of the group you are joining, apply for life, health, disability, and malpractice insurances and provider numbers.	3 mos.	_____
11. If you are going solo, in addition to doing #9 and #10, plan how you will market yourself, order signs and furniture, plan staff, and set fees.	3 mos.	_____
12. Meet community leaders and physicians.	1–2 mos.	_____
13. Take a short vacation to relax.	1–2 mos.	_____
14. Move.	2–4 wks.	_____

Table 13.2 Practice Rating Guide: Community

Factor	Score*: (1 2 3 4 5)
Social/cultural amenities (theaters, shopping, other social/athletic/ cultural items)	_____
Natural attractions (seashore, lake, mountains, etc.)	_____
Special attributes (historical or other significant points)	_____
Facilities (parks, country clubs, golf, tennis, swimming opportunities, preschools, gyms, etc.)	_____
Schools (rating of local schools compared with state average; access to colleges and universities)	_____
Accessibility of activities missing from this community	_____
Career/social opportunities for spouse	_____
Living arrangements (housing availability, desirability, and affordability)	_____
Proximity to family and friends	_____
Economic climate	_____

*Scoring: 1 = poor; 2 = fair; 3 = good; 4 = very good; 5 = excellent.

the information as needed, allowing it to guide you through a paced final year of residency.

Practice Rating Guide

The purpose of the practice rating guide (Tables 13.2–13.5) is to help physicians identify the strengths and weaknesses of practice opportunities as they relate to their professional and personal needs over time. The instrument was developed with the recognition that factors that increase attraction to practice opportunities (such as income or location) may not

Table 13.3 Practice Rating Guide: Pay and Benefits

Factor	Score*: (1 2 3 4 5)
Salary (comparability with similar positions)	_____
Appropriateness to level of clinical activities; recognition for extra-clinical responsibilities; incentives for productivity	_____
Income guarantee (are the payback provisions fair and reasonable?)	_____
Competitiveness of net income guarantee	_____
Benefits (competitive with the market; incentives for remaining; life, health, disability, and malpractice insurance; retirement provisions; deferred income; vacation and educational leave)	_____
Projected income potential in two, five, and ten years	_____
Partnership potential (buy-in provisions for professional corporation, building, and equipment)	_____

*Scoring: 1 = poor; 2 = fair; 3 = good; 4 = very good; 5 = excellent.

Table 13.4 Practice Rating Guide: Scope of the Practice

Factor	Score*: (1 2 3 4 5)
Services provided and their compatibility with training, interest, and medical philosophy	_____
Patient volume and patient/payor mix	_____
Peer participation (quality in number of physicians in practice, provisions for backup, and relations to other providers)	_____
Extra-clinical activities	_____
Off-duty separation from the practice (ie, reasonableness of call schedule, does the community tend to intrude on the physician's private time)	_____
Administrative/management expectations (nonmedical clinic activities and other community activities)	_____
Clinic operations (clinic hours and adequacy of staff in quantity, quality, and training)	_____
Clinic facilities (physical plant, location, size, layout, and physical condition)	_____
Clinic equipment (adequacy for patient load and services, provisions for updating, and how well maintained)	_____
Continuing education (availability, appropriateness, quality, and reimbursement for cost)	_____
Opportunity to combine academics and research with clinical practice	_____

* Scoring: 1 = poor; 2 = fair; 3 = good; 4 = very good; 5 = excellent.

Table 13.5 Practice Rating Guide: Medical Community

Factor	Score*: (1 2 3 4 5)
Hospital practice (proximity to office, ER call arrangements, adequate specialty referral sources, and participation in hospital staff)	_____
Competition for patients and competitive climate	_____
Participation in local/regional medical affairs (medical society, hospital staff, CME, and informal peer contacts)	_____
Continuing medical education (accessibility, funding, provided on-site in the clinic, provision for backup)	_____
Referral sources (availability of referral network and ability to enter)	_____
Contact with peers (other physicians in clinic, in community, and in referral chain)	_____
General Comments: _____
_____
_____
_____

* Scoring: 1 = poor; 2 = fair; 3 = good; 4 = very good; 5 = excellent.

provide sufficient motivation to remain in the practice if other factors are not present, such as support in the medical community. As such, it provides a method to evaluate a variety of factors related to selection and retention, including geographic location, community life, scope of practice, medical community, and compensation and benefits.

Numerical scoring is strongly recommended in order to establish a reasonable baseline. There are not provisions, however, for totaling the score, given that there is no way to equate the values in one section with those in another (eg, compensation and benefits vs. community life). Physicians are encouraged to discuss their impressions with family, peers, colleagues, and prospective employers to aid in the success of practice selection.

Summary

Some of the major points to consider when looking for practice locations are as follows. First—and most important—what type of clinical practice opportunity are you looking at: are you interested in a group, solo, or hospital-based practice or an HMO? When making this decision, consider the location; for example, in small, rural communities, there are not many large group practices.

First, look at the clinical practice, second find out what you and your family are looking for from a personal viewpoint, be it recreational facilities, housing, access to large cities, and so on. It would be wise to make a list of all these different items in order of priority, and in doing so, make sure the community offers at least a majority of these factors.

The other important consideration is the attitude of the administration and the board in the area and in the practice at which you are looking. Make sure that they can provide you with detailed information as to the need for a new physician.

The important issue is not geographic location, but the practice opportunity, the need for physicians, and the opportunity for continued success in the community. There is a place for everyone. However, if a community has a high unemployment rate and little industry, or if it is losing whatever industry it has, that will have a great effect on the future of your practice, so consider it carefully.

14 | Finding Practice Opportunities

MICHAEL J. BENENSON, MPS
AND LESLIE C. YOUNG, MS

For the young physician entering practice or the physician opting to alter an established career path, a range of basic practice modes are possible. Once the physician has made some choices about the type(s) of practice of interest, the practical aspects of seeking out and securing opportunites must be considered. This chapter begins by defining and differentiating the major types of medical practice. General criteria for selection from among the options are offered, including a method for applying the individual physician's personal weighted value to each criterion.

For each of the major practice options, we offer a number of approaches to uncovering the real opportunities available within a given community. These approaches range from undertaking the research required to establish a brand-new solo practice to applying for employment with a targeted organization. The interview process should include the physician's own evaluation of the working environment and compatibility of medical philosophy, often assessed by obtaining introductions to other physicians already in the organization. Evaluation of employment contracts, fringe benefits, partnership agreements, and the details of establishing a new practice are addressed by other chapters of this book.

Although many view the practice of medicine as more restrictive than ever before, it is also true that an unprecedented variety of possibilities exists. It is not necessary for newly trained physicians to accept only those opportunities that present themselves. It is advisable, however, that they narrow their focus to those few practice modes and locales of greatest interest and concentrate their efforts to secure a position within these parameters.

Types of Practice: Basic Options

The types of practice opportunities available and of interest to an individual physician will, of course, be heavily influenced by the clinical specialty and credentials of the doctor in question. Many physicians have even combined some of these options over the course of a career or at a given time. Moreover, as will be discussed later, many of these classifications are not mutually exclusive. They are offered as a general taxonomy of practice settings in order to help organize the physician's own personal choices.

There are literally hundreds of specific practice opportunities, most of which fall into one of the following broad categories:

private practice (solo)

private practice (single-specialty group)

private practice (multispecialty group)

hospital-based or clinic employee

HMO staff model

Public/federal/military medicine

Academic medical practice (including research)

Administrative medicine

A multiplicity of variables will influence the specific characteristics of any given option. For example, the geographic region, group practice size, payor mix, special populations served, and terms of the employment contract or partnership structure will all affect the descriptions provided here as well as the benefits and disadvantages of each option.

Private Practice: Solo

Solo practice is the traditional model of the self-employed single doctor, and it still represents the majority of private practice physicians in the United States. The solo practitioner is his or her own boss and is responsible for all clinical as well as business aspects of the practice. Solo practice physicians retain independence and control over their professional lives. There are no conflicts with associates, dilution of authority, compromised medical values, arguments over work schedule, responsibility for colleagues' actions or reputation, or sharing of profits. On the other hand, the solo physician is burdened with total responsibility for supervision of staff, business decisions and financial performance, and 24-hour coverage of patient care.

In spite of working longer hours, the solo physician generally sees fewer patients and earns less than his or her group practice counterpart. This is typically a function of both practice overhead costs and non-revenue-producing demands on the physician's time. Another factor may be that solo practitioners are often in specialties that earn less money, such as general/family practice, pediatrics, or internal medicine. The ability to support state-of-the-art equipment and generate ancillary revenues related to such equipment also places the solo practitioner at a disadvantage compared with a group practice. Additionally, the solo practitioner may experience greater personal and professional isolation. With the growth in group practice demonstrated over the past two decades, there are some who predict the demise of the solo practice physician. The start-up cost for a new medical practice is the key reason that most young physicians entering private practice are not going solo. Nonetheless, solo practice is generally more lucrative than is practice as an employee of a group or clinic and academic or administrative medicine. Again, the location, specialty, and entrepreneurship of the physician, among other factors, will affect these general patterns regarding compensation as well as the viability of the solo practice mode in the larger marketplace.

Finding opportunities. The decision to establish a new solo or small associated practice is more ominous than the acceptance of a "job." This is not only a function of the initial capital investment, lease commitments, and other financial risks, but also a matter of the basic non-transferability of one's patient base. The practitioner pursuing this option (especially in primary care specialties) should have a high level of commitment to living in the community selected. This is not a good option for the nomadic personality.

In order to find opportunities for entry into a new solo practice, it will be necessary to research various aspects of the local marketplace. In particular, you must acquire information on the economic and demographic characteristics of the areas, population growth forecasts, the number and geographic distribution of specialists of your type, and whether or not these numbers support the addition of another physician to the area. Primary source demographic information is available from local governmental and planning agencies as well as chambers of commerce. Because not all physicians join local medical societies, the best source of inventories of physicians by specialty is the local yellow pages. Large group practices serving mainly HMO patients often do not list there, yet their doctor count figures into the doctor-to-population ratios for the area. You should first target your likely hospital affiliation(s) and locate the medical staff development specialists on their staff. Many hospitals provide the following types of assistance:

Rule-of-thumb doctor/population ratios for your specialty (Also available from the American Medical Association)

Inventories of local medical office space

Inventories/maps of competing local specialists

Introductions to solo or two-doctor practices looking to bring in a junior partner

Introductions to current staff members

Assistance with practice start-up, including loans and assistance with purchasing equipment and subsidizing the cost of space

Practices available for sale

Information on moonlighting opportunities (such as in the emergency room or in hospital-sponsored clinics) in order to create an income source while building a new practice

Other practice-building opportunties such as HMO/PPO contracts

Income guarantee programs

Attempt to meet other practitioners, both within your specialty and in specialties that are natural referral sources for your specialty, to assess the degree to which you will be welcomed into the medical community. If you are a specialist targeting a populous area, consider joining more than one hospital's medical staff in order to broaden your initial referral base. If you are an established physician relocating from another area and you have special expertise of some kind, investigate opportunities to enhance visibility by speaking at medical staff conferences and continuing education programs. Planning your entry into a community from a long distance will require a number of well-organized trips to the locale. Make contacts, plan meetings, and schedule appointments by corresponding with your targets before the trip.

Consider engaging a professional practice consultant, financial advisor, and specialized attorney for advice on starting a private practice. Among other things, this should include assistance with locating the practice, equipping and staffing the office, and setting up administrative procedures and policies as well as developing initial income streams. In addition, the relative costs and advantages of purchasing an existing practice (be sure to seek professional advice on practice valuation) should be weighed against the capital costs, initial income, and cash flow forecasts for starting a new practice.

Private Practice: Single Specialty Group

A group practice, defined as three or more physicians practicing in association, may take many forms (partnership, stock corporation, professional corporation, association agreement, expense-sharing only, or employer-employee contract). A single-specialty group may consist of primary care physicians (general or family practice and internists) or specialists of a like type. A single specialty group is afforded the usual advantages of group practice: easy consultation with colleagues, sharing of coverage, sharing of overhead expenses (economies of scale), and ability to support a business manager or designate the managing physician, thereby relieving those interested in only clinical practice from these responsibilities.

The single-specialty group can often support the purchase of expensive specialty-related diagnostic equipment or the offering of technical services ancillary to the specialty. Examples of these include ophthalmic lasers for in-office eye surgery, physical therapy and diagnostic radiology as adjuncts to orthopedics, a hematology laboratory to support an oncology practice, or cardiac stress testing equipment. Diversification of practice revenues generally increases group income. In addition, such service offerings reflect a level of sophistication that enhances the group's reputation and generally provides for patient convenience. When these services are provided through the doctor's office at a lower cost than when offered institutionally, they improve the physician's competitive position in the marketplace. Given the many forces that are currently reducing income derived from direct physician labor, alternate sources of revenue are increasingly important. In 1988, the median total compensation for physicians in single-specialty groups exceeded that for like specialists practicing in multispecialty groups for all specialties except family practice (see Table 14.1). This may correlate with differences in fee structure and/or level of participation in "discount medicine" (Medicaid, Medicare, PPOs, and HMOs) when comparing single-specialty groups with multispecialty groups.

Finding opportunities. Approaches to finding practice opportunities with single-specialty groups are similar to those used for multispecialty groups and are discussed in the following section.

Private Practice: Multispecialty Group

A multispecialty group generally combines primary care physicians with a number of specialty physicians. Within a small multispecialty group the specialties represented may be limited to pediatrics, obstetrics, gynecology, and subspecialties of internal medicine (e.g., cardiology, neurology, gastroenterology, pulmonology) and also, perhaps, a general surgeon or dermatologist. In very large multispecialty groups, virtually all specialties (with exceptions among the tertiary specialties) may be represented.

The compensation levels experienced by group practice members vary greatly depending upon the individual physician's status in the group: for instance, shareholder or partner versus salaried physician, equity position, longevity with the group, specialty, production level, and other factors. Upon formation of a new group, whether single- or multispecialty, the associated physicians may have equal ownership position and yet may have different income levels depending upon the income distribution scheme utilized by the group. A young physician brings no established patient clientele and is most likely to begin as an employee of the group, with partner or ownership status to be available after a time.

Finding opportunities. In order to identify specific opportunities within single- or multispecialty groups, one might begin with an inventory of the established groups in the area of choice. Such an inventory is best developed with the assistance of the yellow pages, the local hospital, health plans with whom they might contract, a few local doctor contacts, and the local medical society. Larger groups may also be listed as members of the Medical Group Management Association or the Group Practice Association of America. Having identified these groups, you should attempt to make personal contact with the group manager or senior partner to determine whether the group is recruiting for your specialty. Practice opportunities within smaller groups are typically known to the medical staff development officers of the local hospitals and are sometimes advertised.

Additionally, you may utilize physician search firms or medical employment agencies to aid in finding opportunities to join group practices,

Table 14.1 Median Physician Total Compensation by Specialty and Group Type

Specialty	Group Type					
	Single specialty		Multispecialty		All Groups	
	Number of Responses	Total Compensation	Number of Responses	Total Compensation	Number of Responses	Total Compensation
Allergy/immunology	5	*	106	$124,663	111	$124,000
Anesthesiology	93	$192,188	171	$174,934	264	$182,470
Cardiology: invasive	119	$265,000	222	$185,923	341	$228,500
Cardiology: noninvasive	43	$185,000	156	$136,625	199	$145,187
Dermatology	18	$186,940	177	$128,398	195	$130,398
Emergency medicine	26	$130,519	156	$100,708	182	$104,000
Endocrinology/metabolism	13	$147,532	109	$110,352	122	$112,665
Family practice	368	$88,542	1,765	$90,414	2,133	$90,000
Gastroenterology	36	$178,089	268	$161,318	304	$162,576
Gynecology	3	*	35	$148,093	38	$148,547
Hematology/oncology	53	$160,407	218	$124,005	271	$130,900
Infectious disease	2	*	64	$112,473	66	$114,114
Internal medicine	148	$127,064	1,287	$100,000	1,435	$100,850
Neonatology	12	$324,000	26	$139,502	38	$154,289
Nephrology	6	*	96	$121,878	102	$124,603
Neurology	81	$156,070	196	$118,536	277	$126,126
Obstetrics/gynecology	116	$230,112	670	$152,731	786	$159,329
Occupational medicine	*	*	52	$95,445	52	$95,445

Specialty	N	Median	N	Median	N	Median
Ophthalmology	68	$272,218	260	$149,868	328	$168,990
Otclaryngology	46	$207,863	218	$149,714	264	$155,299
Pathology	6	*	85	$140,600	91	$139,000
Pediatrics	69	$117,244	787	$93,552	856	$94,704
Physical medicine	18	$123,000	24	$121,300	42	$123,000
Psychiatry	31	$104,000	143	$96,340	174	$96,870
Pulmonary disease	48	$176,719	192	$130,067	240	$134,980
Radiology	218	$277,714	228	$175,450	446	$220,072
Radiology: therapeutic	26	$225,307	30	$149,169	56	$193,068
Rheumatology	24	$154,388	126	$105,014	150	$108,131
Surgery: cardiovascular	22	$427,513	63	$285,688	85	$316,837
Surgery: general	44	$187,177	588	$151,201	632	$151,587
Surgery: hand	18	$330,858	6	*	24	$272,458
Surgery: head and neck	1	*	9		10	$207,358
Surgery: neurological	45	$370,000	62	$224,589	107	$316,765
Surgery: oral	4	*	17	$129,050	21	$131,045
Surgery: orthopedic	331	$287,845	421	$188,112	752	$231,611
Surgery: plastic	5	*	33	$165,300	38	$173,983
Surgery: vascular	21	$307,776	82	$206,420	103	$216,803
Urology	34	$218,737	227	$159,507	261	$165,354

* An asterisk indicates that a median value is suppressed when the number of individual responses is less than 10. An asterisk in the "Number of Responses" column should be interpreted as a zero. Excluded from this table are data for university- and government-affiliated medical groups, physicians earning less than $20,000 per year, and all professionals born before 1923. This table includes data for both single-specialty and multispecialty groups.

Source: MGMA Physician Compensation Survey Report, 1989 Based on 1988 Data, Table 3, p. 12, reproduced with special permission from the Medical Group Management Association, 1355 South Colorado Bl., Suite 900, Denver, CO 80222.

generally under an employment contract. The placement fees of the search firms are typically paid by the employer. It behooves the physician to submit résumés to as many such firms as possible.

Similarly, the local medical society and your national specialty board may have information exchanges for practice and employment opportunities. These may be job banks in addition to paid advertisements in the classified sections of their affiliated journals. For easy access to the classified sections of the many medical journals now published, use your local university's, hospital's, or other medical library's periodicals section. You may also access the classified sections of general circulation newspapers from around the country at a good university library.

Hospital-Based or Clinic Employee

Some specialties, such as anesthesiology, pathology, and radiology, by their nature lend themselves to hospital-based practice and hence involve either a contracted or salaried relationship to the institution. Although the hospital-based physician often pays certain expenses, such as malpractice insurance premiums, he or she does not incur the expense of starting up and operating an office.

Many institutions now operate hospital-based or satellite ambulatory care clinics in primary care or other specialties, including occupational and industrial medicine and urgent and emergency care. These are no longer limited to teaching hospitals or inner-city charity clinics. Limitations on the corporate practice of medicine in most states prohibit the employment of physicians by other than physician-owned professional corporations. Whether an employee of the hospital/clinic or an employee of the medical corporation contracted to it, physicians in nearly all specialties will find opportunities to take jobs with such organizations. A trend in which hospitals are purchasing has evolved established physician practices as a means for hospitals to increase their patient bases. More and more young physicians are opting for this route, if not for a lifetime, at least until training debts are paid and resources are developed with which to open a practice.

A physician's own experience with this type of practice may vary significantly depending upon the patient population served, type and location of the facilities, and the service or teaching goals of the organization. In general, physicians practicing in this mode will generate lower average incomes than will those in private practice. To a degree greater than in group practice, these physicians experience regular schedules, time off, freedom from 24-hour call, and the ability to pursue other personal and professional interests. The physician has virtually no involvement with administrative or financial performance issues for the practice and may or may not have staff supervision responsibility. It is often possible to practice office-based medicine only, if desired, with hospitalizations attended by other colleagues. Such positions are often associated with a great deal of financial security, little or no practice-related expense, and substantial fringe benefits, which can include health and disability insurance and holiday, vacation, and sick pay as well as a retirement plan. Some institutions may even provide assistance with establishment of a private practice in the area, after a period of service with the clinic.

Finding opportunities. For hospital-based opportunities, direct contact with the hospital administration or medical director is the appropriate avenue. If private practice is your eventual goal, initiate frank discussion about assistance with this before accepting the position. The hospital may be aware of still other opportunities in non-hospital-sponsored clinics as well. However, do not expect the hospital to provide leads to clinics that do not use that hospital. Urgent-care centers can generally be found in the yellow page listings. The state or county health departments that provide licensure to some ambulatory clinics may also be able to provide inventories of their licensees. Remember, however, that physician-sponsored clinics conceived as "doctors' offices" may not need such licensure and may not, therefore, be found in these inventories.

These kinds of facilities are likely to use medical recruitment firms and classified advertising so, again, the classified ads in your professional journals are important.

HMO Staff Model

Also known as Prepaid Group Practice, the HMO staff model is nothing more than a medical group or clinic organization devoted exclusively (or almost exclusively) to servicing patients of a health maintenance organization (also called a prepaid health plan). The income levels, benefits, and drawbacks of this type of practice are similar to those of a physician-employee of a fee-for-service clinic or group. Prepaid group practice physicians do derive average incomes that are slightly below those of their counterparts in fee-for-service groups and solo practitioners in private practice. However, the differences are not great except for the highest earners within fee-for-service medicine. The very definition of *staff model HMO* implies physicians are employees of the health plan. Technically speaking, many staff model plans (such as Kaiser Foundation Health Plan) actually contract with the medical group (in this case Permanente Medical Group). Hence some physicians may hold ownership in the group whereas others are employees. Profit distribution (bonuses) to the partners is even possible under this model.

The distinction between fee-for-service and pre-paid groups becomes more blurred in regions where HMOs network with independent multispecialty groups on a nonexclusive basis. This produces group practices whose revenues are a blend of prepaid contracts (under which the group assumes some insurance risk for professional and outpatient ancillary services) and fee-for-service income from cash-paying and indemnity-insured patients. The percentage of the group's revenue from prepaid sources may range from a very small proportion to 100%, with literally dozens of contracted HMOs. Even solo-practice physicians may participate in HMOs to a small or a great degree, through independent practice associations or as direct contractors.

Finding opportunities. Direct contact with and application to the plan of interest and use of search firms and classifieds are appropriate. In order to inventory staff model HMOs and their locations, the best source will be the Group Health Association of America, your state-level HMO trade association, if any, and medical management journals in the university library. Additional search tools are the various guides to periodical hospital and medical literature. The local medical society or hospital trade association may also be of assistance.

Public/Federal/Military Medicine

The many branches of the U.S. military, the U.S. Public Health Service, the Veterans Administration, and state and local public health organizations offer a plethora of professional opportunities to physicians. The variety makes it nearly impossible to compare characteristics of work environment and job demands among these options. Although pay ranges within this broad category are among the lowest, the fringe benefits are among the most substantial. The prospects for travel to unusual places and involvement in important government-sponsored research and training programs are extensive, as are opportunities to combine medical practice with medical administrative challenges and even public policy development, if desired. Through such programs as the National Health Service Corps (NHSC) a diversified practice in areas of great human need is possible. In addition, the NHSC offers a private practice option that assists physicians in setting up a private practice in underserved areas.

Finding opportunities. Make direct application to any organization of interest, whether or not jobs are advertised. Direct application can be made to the various branches of the military, U.S. government, and state and local health departments. In some cases, taking a civil service examination may be required. Government positions are not typically advertised in periodicals, nor do they typically use search firms. However, postings of all specific openings are generally available via direct visits to the personnel offices of these agencies. More convenient information may be available at the student placement service of your university medical school or that affiliated with your residency program.

Academic Medical Practice

Involvement in academic medicine suggests a combination of teaching, research, administration, and clinical practice. This can be a very exciting and stimulating life. The satisfaction derived from being on the cutting edge of new technological or scientific developments as well as in the training of new medical minds may offer great fulfillment. Academic advancement may be very much dependent upon a capacity for and productivity in the area of research because research grants and other "soft money," meaning nonrecurring revenue, provide the funding for approximately 80% of the medical education system. Advancement within academia may mean appointments that expand administrative responsibilities, which may or may not be viewed as a plus depending upon the proclivities of the individual. Certainly, academic physicians may experience a greater share of competition among faculty and administrative complexities than does the self-employed private practitioner.

The income possible in academic medicine varies greatly from institution to institution. It depends not only on the specialty and tenure of the professor, but also on the resources of the institution and its policy regarding fee-for-service private practice. Since the income potential is significantly lower than for a specialist in private practice, more than half of the medical schools in the United States now permit faculty to engage in private practice in order to supplement their salaries. In fact, some schools now arrange for the facilities in which the faculty can conduct practice. Supplemental income may also be derived from publications, speaking honoraria, and specialty consultations. Fringe benefits are typically very liberal. It should be noted, of course, that many physicians engaged primarily in private practice also hold part-time faculty appointments as a means to satisfy their desire for the academic experience.

Finding opportunities. The inroad to academia is likely to be based primarily on one's specialty area, the prestigiousness of training and academic rank from medical school, and previous performance on research projects. Involvement with senior faculty on research with long-term funding, combined with display of leadership— for example, as senior resident — is the most likely route to opportunity here. Application directly to medical schools and teaching hospitals of interest is possible. Presentation of one's qualifications will require detailed information on research, papers, previous appointments, and academic honors. Faculty recommendations out of the residency program will be paramount.

Administrative Medicine

This is a very broad, nonspecific category inasmuch as many modes of medical practice offer the opportunity for administrative or managerial responsibility. Its inclusion here is intended to highlight the expanding numbers and types of opportunities for physicians in administrative roles. This is especially true within the burgeoning field of managed care. The 1980s witnessed an explosion in the demand for medical direction over programs of utilization review and management and quality assurance driven by the advent of the Medicare prospective (based on diagnostic-related groups [DRGs]) payment system, PPOs and, in particular, HMO enterprises. Independent medical review companies have sprung up in great numbers and utilization management/quality assurance departments within health plans have expanded.

Many community hospitals that previously had no paid medical director have created such posts in response to changes in the Medicare program and the HMO industry. Even some large employers that are self-insuring their employee health plan have found a need to hire physicians as medical administrators. All of these developments reflect the evolution of interest on the part of all third-party payors in controlling the cost of care by having a much more direct influence on physician practices than ever before. In order to do an adequate job of this while still addressing the concern over ensuring that quality of care is upheld, the skills of lay administrators must be supplemented by those available only from trained physicians. Physician presence in corporate board rooms and committees of upper management is increasingly common.

Since this is a relatively new arena, the average salaries of administrative physicians, which tend to be very low compared with practicing physicians', may be changing. For the physician who may not prefer hands-on clinical medicine and who may enjoy the development of practice criteria and review procedures, new options are on the horizon.

Finding opportunities. The physicians found in administrative roles typically have paid their dues in clinical practice and gained a certain level of maturity before making the switch. Without this hands-on clinical background and exposure to the real world of the medical industry in practice, the physician is unlikely to command the respect necessary from other physicians and lay administrators for such a role as medical director in a community hospital or even in a health plan or medical corporation. For the physician interested in diversifying his or her workload into the administrative arena while still participating in patient care, many part-time opportunities may be available. An administrative role within a medical group, clinic, or staff model HMO typically evolves out of an established relationship with the organization. Part-time positions as medical directors of small clinics or in medical criteria development with health insurance plans or utilization management companies are more likely opportunities in the short term. To access these opportunities, classifieds in periodicals, professional journals, and, for full-time positions, the medical search firms are the best route. It is advisable to contact target employers directly, based on an inventory process to identify the firms. Hospital administrators and health plan representatives can be very helpful if made aware of your interests.

Criteria for Evaluating Practice Options

The practice options available to most physicians are significant enough in number that a process of criteria development and application should be devised. This may help the individual doctor focus in on the mode(s) holding the greatest appeal so that very specific opportunities can then be considered. Criteria that may be used are discussed in the following sections.

Compensation Level

Some general patterns we have noted after reviewing data from multiple sources, including the American Medical Association's surveys on physician incomes, include the following:

The 1988 median net income for all physicians nationwide was $120,000 per year; the mean was $144,700.

Private practice physicians earn approximately 27% more than do salaried physicians.

Group practice physicians earn more than do solo practitioners.

Single-specialty group practitioners earn more than their multispecialty group counterparts.

Pediatricians, general and family practitioners, psychiatrists, and occupational medicine doctors are among the lowest-paid physicians.

Anesthesiologists, radiologists, and pathologists are among the highest earners, along with the surgical specialties (especially cardiovascular, orthopedic, hand, and neurosurgery), obstetricians/gynecologists, neonatologists, radiation oncologists, and invasive cardiologists.

Physicians in metropolitan areas with populations under 1 million earn slightly more than do physicians in larger metropolitan areas and even more than do those in nonmetropolitan areas.

Female physicians earn less than do male physicians in all specialties (this may correlate to status as employed vs. self-employed and to age differences between the genders).

Generally speaking, group practice physicians in medium-sized multispecialty groups (16–100 doctors) have better earnings than do those in smaller or larger groups. Among the primary care specialties, however, the larger the group the better. This pattern may relate to the economies of scale (including the ability to generate income from alternate sources) attainable in medium-sized groups, offset by the correlation between very large groups (with more than 100 doctors) and participation in managed care programs.

The degree of participation in managed care is a very inconsistent predictor of earnings. Generally, primary care physicians fare better under full fee-for-service medicine, whereas some specialists (especially psychiatrists) actually earn more with moderate participation (less than 40% of patient volume) in managed care. This may be attributable to the channeling of patients to the specialists participating in such programs.

Two additional trends are important to consider: "real," that is, inflation-adjusted, historical earnings increase over time and the potential that exists for greater regulation of physician fees in the future. Although increases in physician net income (before taxes) have occurred in all specialties at an average annual rate of 7.3% (nominal income), the annual growth rate in real net income, when adjusted for changes in the consumer price index, was only 0.5% for the period from 1975 to 1986. For pediatricians, general and family practitioners, and internists, real income actually declined over this period.

To some degree, regulation of physician fees has already occurred in the sense that many government and private insurance programs set maximum allowable fees based on "usual, customary, and reasonable" fee standards. The physician, however, is free to accept the maximum or charge his or her patient the difference. A long-awaited study produced by a team at the Harvard University School of Public Health was delivered to the Health Care Financing Administration in 1988. This study, which sets a scale of relative values for the various physician services and procedures, is expected to be used widely in the 1990s to set national price controls on physician fees. Of significance is that the scale attempts to adjust for previous biases that favored the surgical specialties and places higher values on the "cognitive" medicine of family practitioners and internists. This could lead to a narrowing of the differential currently seen between medical and surgical specialty incomes.

Financial Security

As discussed previously, self-employed private practice physicians experience greater concerns over financial security than do salaried physicians. In private practice, whether solo or as a group partner, there are no income guarantees or other fringe benefits except those arranged by the physicians for themselves. The self-employed, nonsalaried physician may be more vulnerable to changes in the medical marketplace, both nationally and locally, which can negatively affect his or her financial standing.

Quality of Life

Practice within a group, an HMO staff model, or as an employee physician may provide for fewer financial worries, a greater amount of discretionary time, and greater freedom from production pressures and administrative headaches. For the purposes of this exercise we rate these factors high on the quality of life scale (see Table 14.2). However, this scale is of such a subjective and personal nature that the individual physician may choose to make adjustments.

Retirement Benefits

The private practice solo physician will have to undertake self-imposed retirement planning. A component of this plan will include possible sale of

Table 14.2 Practice type criteria scoring.

CRITERIA/TYPE	Solo	S Sp Grp.	M sp Grp.	Clnic Emp	HMO Staff	Publ/ Milit	Acad emic	Adm. Med.
Compensation % Weight:	60	90	70	45	60	30	50	50
Fin. Security % Weight:	40	70	70	80	70	80	60	60
Quality/Life % Weight:	50	80	80	90	90	60	70	80
Retirement % Weight:	50	60	60	70	70	90	80	60
Satisfaction % Weight:								
Control % Weight:	90	80	70	60	50	60	60	30
Patient Cont. % Weight:	70	80	80	90	80	50	20	10
Adm/Clerical % Weight:	90	60	60	10	60	20	70	95
TOTAL WEIGHTED SCORES								

the practice upon retirement. It will be difficult to know the value of a practice much in advance of the retirement date. Furthermore, a process of transition to part-time practice as retirement approaches causes the trade-off of reducing the practice value. At the other extreme, government service generally offers substantial retirement benefits (although based on a lower income base) after 20 or 30 years of service and a chance for a second-phase career.

Ego Satisfaction

Such qualities as prestige, intellectual challenge, interpersonal relationships, sense of achievement, self-image, and opportunity for variety are all factors that contribute to professional ego satisfaction. Although we commonly think of academia and/or research roles as being associated with most of these factors, such may not be the case for a given individual. A great sense of achievement and self-image may be connected with entrepreneurial success for one individual and with helping underserved populations for another. Valuation of this criterion will be highly individual.

Control of Medical Decision-Making

Generally speaking, private, self-employed, solo practice with no involvement in managed care offers the highest degree of discretion in medical decision-making, though concern over cost to the patient does influence medical decisions. The interjection of utilization management programs associated with many prepaid and other health plans subjects the physician's decisions to the greatest degree of scrutiny. Between these two extremes, typically, is the employee physician. Similarly, academic medicine is based very much on group conferencing of diagnostic and treatment choices. Also, quality assurance and utilization programs in the inpatient setting do affect all physicians practicing in that arena. The relative weight of this control criterion (Figure 14.1) depends greatly on the temperament of the individual doctor.

Patient Contact

Administrative and academic medicine as well as some segments of government practice (such as research or policy administration) generally offer the least direct patient contact. A component of the patient contact criterion that may be important to the practitioner is continuity of contact. In urgent and emergency care, continuity is at its lowest. It may also be low in government-sponsored clinics, military medicine, and, to some degree, an HMO staff model, though this can vary dramatically depending on the organizational policies relating to case management. Clearly, some specialties lend themselves to more or less patient contact, ranging from virtually none in radiology and pathology to high levels of involvement in family practice, pediatrics, and psychiatry.

Administrative/Clerical Demands

Solo practitioners are free to allocate their time as they see fit, but administrative and clerical demands often create a diversion. Typically, salaried clinical positions and group practice offer the lowest demand for administrative and clerical involvement as well as the least degree of influence over administrative procedures and policies. Interestingly, these same settings offer the greatest potential to combine patient care with administrative duties, should this be one of the proclivities of the practitioner. Such opportunity tends to expand with age and experience and, in all but solo practice, may be limited by judgments about the practitioner's qualifications for the administrative responsibilty. The administrative demands of practice are an important issue primarily because medical education typically offers no specific training in these matters.

Applying Criteria to Practice Type Options

Table 14.2 is a blank matrix into which the physician may insert his or her own rating score for each practice type option, specific to each criterion using a scale of 1 (lowest) to 100 (highest). The rating score should be inserted into the upper left segment of each cell. We have inserted a suggested rating for each based upon the foregoing general discussion, with the exception of the satisfaction criterion. Next, applying the doctor's own highly individual value system and personal preferences, a weight (expressed as a percentage of 100) should be given to each criterion. The weights should be inserted after "% weight:" in the left-hand column under each criterion. Multiply the weight percentage by the score for each option, and insert each weighted score into the lower right segment of each cell. Add the weighted scores for each option and insert the total at the bottom of each column. Do not make critical career choices based upon the bottom line scores. Rather, use these scores to examine your subjective instincts about your preferred options. This may help you narrow your range of choices and focus your energies on pursuing specific opportunities.

Conclusion

Because of the incredible variety of medical practice modes available to today's physician, finding practice opportunities begins with an appreciation of the wide range of possibilities and the relative advantages and disadvantages of each; one should be mindful of the many variables, such as specialty, geography, payor mix, and status of the particular doctor, that affect the truisms of each option. This is necessarily followed by some application of the individual physician's personal goals and preferences in order to narrow the field of choices to something manageable. Each physician should develop, and periodically reassess, his or her personal strategy for a career progression over time. Finally, seeking out specific opportunities is a matter of organizing one's research, taking advantage of the variety of outside resources available, and structuring the initiative.

Suggested Reading

American Medical Association, *Socioeconomic Characteristics of Medical Practice, 1989.*Chicago, IL: AMA.

Coile, Russell C., Jr., *The New Medicine: Reshaping Medical Practice and Health Care Management.*Rockville, MD: Aspen Publishers, 1990.

Cotter, Patrick, S., "An Analysis of the Changing Patterns in Physician Employment Status 1983 to 1985." In *Socioeconomic Characteristics of Medical Practice.*Chicago, IL: American Medical Association, 1986.

Farber, Lawrence, *Encyclopedia on Practice and Financial Management.*Oradell, NJ: Medical Economics Books, 1985.

Gonzalez, Martin L., "Trends, Variations, and the Distribution of Physician Earnings." In *Socioeconomic Characteristics of Medical Practice, 1987.*Chicago, IL: American Medical Association, 1987.

LaDou, Joseph, and Likens, James, *Medicine and Money: Physicians as Businessmen.* Cambridge, MA: Ballinger Publishing, 1977.

Nelson, Susan "Buying M.D. Practices: The Trend Continues."*Hospitals: Journal of the American Hospital Association*(July 20):63, 1987.

Sandrick, Karen, "Group Practice: What's the Attraction?"*Hospitals: Journal of the American Hospital Association*(April 5):46–50, 1986.

15 | Assessing the Value of a Medical Practice

LESTER J. SCHWARTZ, CPA

This chapter describes an approach to determine the value of a medical practice. It is designed to help the busy practitioner understand the appropriate charges that should be made in determining the total value of a clinical practice. Later in this book, another chapter describes approaches for dissolving or selling a medical practice. Many of the concepts described in this chapter will be repeated at that point, but the purpose of this chapter is to provide greater detail regarding the determination of the value of a practice. This will enable the clinician not only to determine how to increase the value of his or her practice for possible future sale, but more importantly, to assess those elements that should be considered in making the decision to purchase a practice.

A group practice of three orthopedic surgeons came to me with a problem. A personality dispute had polluted their working environment and one of the partners had walked out in a huff. The remaining partners continued their arrangement and, believing they were acting in good faith, paid their former colleague for his share of patients' billings collected and their other assets.

Still miffed, the former partner sued his ex-associates claiming, he was also due compensation for his portion of the goodwill—that highly intangible factor viewed as crucial to generating future earnings—that he had helped accrue to the practice. A lengthy court battle ensued that was complicated enormously by the fact that the partners had failed to obtain a partnership agreement with a clear formula for determining the value of the practice.

The two remaining partners eventually won this case when the judge determined that the plaintiff was not entitled to any compensation for the group's goodwill because of the manner in which he had departed the partnership. Still, it was a needless exercise that consumed a great deal of time and energy, not to mention money.

Had the partners had the foresight—or, more realistically, had they been advised by a qualified professional—to include a plan for determining everything of value in the original partnership agreement, the legal issues that so complicated this case would have been simpler and far less expensive to sort out. Unfortunately, I come across such oversights all too often.

The above example illustrates just one need for considering the value of a medical practice and the diverse elements that constitute this complex process. Moreover, given the public's current appetite for litigation, pricing a practice and determining in advance how that price will be calculated is more important today than ever.

Practice valuations are required whenever there is a partnership dissolution caused by death, retirement, or, as in the example above, an inability on the part of associates to continue working together. Other circumstances that require valuations include:

Buy/sell agreements

Prenuptial agreements

Divorce

Estate planning

Key man insurance

Professional loans

Establishing a practice's financial health as part of an overall "fiscal checkup"

Rules of Thumb

Ascribing value to a professional practice that is a closely held personal service is difficult because of the intangible nature of goodwill.

Unfortunately, there is no rule of thumb here that can be trusted for a quick and reliable estimate of valuation, because medical practices are extremely difficult to compare. Income figures alone are not a trustworthy barometer: for example, the length of time required to generate the income is equally important. A practice that takes 40 hours of work to generate a given level of income is far more valuable than one that requires twice the time to generate the same income.

Because rules of thumb are coarse oversimplifications, they can in some cases lead to grossly incorrect conclusions. The importance of individual expertise, location, referral sources, board specializations, and licensing barriers make it impossible to readily substitute one practice for another. Therefore, the only rule of thumb I subscribe to is never to rely on a rule of thumb to determine value.

The Internal Revenue Service recommends the same cautious approach. Revenue Ruling 59-60, the agency's primary guideline for valuing all businesses, notes that the circumstances of each valuation need to be considered and that rules of thumb, though not specifically ruled against, are best avoided.

Consequently, placing a value on a medical practice is more an art than it is a science. The knowledge and experience of the appraiser are paramount, as is sensitivity to the purpose of the valuation. For example, a valuation for a buy-sell agreement could be more conservative so as not to burden the remaining partners. A practice that liberally could be valued at $450,000 might be set at $300,000 to minimize life insurance costs. For federal estate tax purposes, the beneficiaries of the physician usually want to keep the lowest possible value on the practice to minimize the tax bite. However, in a divorce proceeding the attorney for the physician's spouse is likely to value that same practice in a far more liberal light to maximize his or her client's claim.

Fixed elements set by statute or case law, which vary widely from state to state, must also be taken into account. But even when every element is considered, in the end it all comes down to a professional judgment.

Another reason it is dangerous to rely on rules of thumb is that methodology for arriving at valuation often is subjected to close scrutiny when proceedings turn adversarial. If methodology is to withstand hostile attack, it must be complete and supportable. Rules of thumb are inadequate on either score.

The Elements of Value

Eight basic categories listed in Revenue Ruling 59-60 must be considered in determining valuation.

1. The nature of the practice and its history. Among the questions to be considered is whether patients are of long standing or recent additions and the age and health of the practitioner. Another important factor is whether the practice is dependent upon one group of referrals for a disproportionately large percentage of its income.

2. The general economic outlook as well as that for the practice's specific economic environment. Factors to be considered in this category include whether there is any possibility of an economic downswing and what impact such a downswing might have on medical demand. For example, plastic surgeons, psychiatrists, and other medical disciplines viewed by the public as performing services of a more elective nature tend to be more vulnerable to an economic downswing than are critical care and emergency physicians. Then there is the question as to increased competition on the horizon, represented today, in part, by health maintenance organizations and preferred providers.

3. Book value of stock, if applicable, and the company's financial condition. The organizational form of a medical practice can vary widely; they can be proprietorships, partnerships, or corporations. Many practices are organized in some combination of these three options for tax and other business considerations. Because financial statements are normally prepared at cost, they must be interpreted differently to determine fair market value.

Most professional practices keep their financial statements on the cash basis of accounting and do not give effect to accounts receivable or accounts payable. Further analysis is required to adjust for these and other items not reflected on the financial statements. A practice may have an obligation to repay excess charges made to Medicare, Medicaid, or insurance companies. Deferred tax liabilities may also exist.

In a corporate setup it is important to note that loans to shareholders may represent disguised dividends, just as loans from shareholders may be equity and not debt.

4. Earning capacity. The issue here is prospective income, or potential. Have salaries, travel, entertainment, auto use, and other owner perks been considered? One way to anticipate potential is to scrutinize past performance with an eye on anticipated changes in circumstance.

5. Dividend-paying capacity. Here again, the emphasis is on capacity, not actual payout. With corporately structured medical practices, the focus needs to be on cash-flow projections, with dividend capacity related to earning capacity. Also, has due consideration been given to the need to reinvest in the practice?

6. Sales of stock or any other interest and the size of the stock or interest to be valued. This is applicable only if the practice has a corporate or partnership structure, but if so, recent sales are most important. Also, has an interest been sold to insiders, and what percentage of the practice has been sold? Consider whether any recent events have significantly affected the value of the practice.

7. Market price of stocks of corporations engaged in a same or similar business. This is almost impossible to apply to any professional practice, medical or otherwise, because of how rare it is to encounter a practice structured as a corporation that sells stock. There is literally almost no opportunity for comparison.

8. Goodwill or other intangible value. In most instances, goodwill and accounts receivable will be the major assets of a medical practice. Actually, the same might be said for any personal service practice. In a professional practice, business-oriented goodwill is attributable to the same elements found in any business—location, staff, patient base, and operating systems—and can have significant and readily transferable value; however, professional goodwill depends upon the unique characteristics of the medical provider. Substitution, or transferability, of such goodwill may be difficult.

Tangible Assets

The tangible, or hard, assets of a practice are easier to value than are the intangibles. Medical equipment, office furniture and fixtures, supplies, and real property constitute the tangible assets of a medical practice.

Compared with most businesses, a medical practice's tangible assets often account for a relatively small portion of its value, because only a nominal investment in equipment may be required to generate income. Of course, this is not the case with specialists such as radiologists, who may spend large sums on state-of-the-art equipment.

Two approaches exist for valuing tangible assets: the *cost method* and the *market method*.

The cost method values tangible assets by using the net book value, which is the original cost minus the accumulated depreciation. The market method defines the value of an asset by its replacement cost based on like assets currently available in the marketplace. The market method is commonly applied to real estate, equipment, and furnishings.

With both methods, it is important to pay close attention to the date the valuation is to be determined, because this becomes the benchmark used to measure all value, regardless of later changes in the worth of assets. That benchmark remains the standard until a new valuation is established. Therefore it is important that the parties to the valuation know when to reassess value.

Valuations obtained for prenuptial agreements or when divorce or death has taken place do not require reevaluation because they are point-in-time valuations that are not commonly affected by later changes in circumstances. However, valuations for purposes of buy/sell agreements, for example, do require reevaluation because changing circumstances will make the practice more or less valuable as time goes by.

Accounts Receivable

The valuation of the accounts receivable also requires special attention. Account balances by themselves can be very misleading; what needs to be determined is the level at which actual payment can be expected. Do the books reflect stated charges, or the figure that Medicaid or private insurance is likely to cover? The proper amount may be much less than the practitioner's stated rate, because he or she has agreed that the latter amount will retire the full patient debt.

Bills outstanding for one year or more are likely to be uncollectible. Likewise, those that have been turned over to a collection agency would have limited, if any, value. Accounts receivable within 30 days of billing are generally considered more likely to be collected than are those over 120 days. After a reasonable period of time, which varies according to the experience of the practice, accounts receivable are deemed to be of little worth unless payment is to come from a government agency or insurance company.

With reasonable billing and collection procedures, 70% to 90% of all physicians' charges are collected.

Pricing the Value of Goodwill

The goodwill of a practice is constantly searching for a definition. That most often cited comes from Justice Story in *Commentaries on the Law of Partnerships:*

> Good-will may be properly enough described to be the advantage or benefit, which is acquired by an establishment, beyond the mere value of the capital, stock, funds or property employed there-in, in consequence of the general public patronage and encouragement, which it receives from constant or habitual customers, on account of its local position, or common celebrity, or reputation for skill or affluence, or punctuality, or from other accidental circumstances or necessities, or even from ancient partialities or prejudices.

The California Business and Professions Code puts it more succinctly, simply noting that "the good will of a business is the expectation of continued public patronage."

Traditionally, goodwill has been described as a preference by patients which arises from the reputation, skill, and manner of the physician.

One accounting measurement of goodwill is calculated by applying a factor to the amount of the physician's earnings in excess of a normal rate of return. Again, that factor would vary depending upon judgment and circumstance.

An accounting method for calculating the factor is a straight-line method in which the average net profits are multiplied by a rate based on judgment. This results in the total value of the practice, including the book value and the goodwill.

Another method provides for a specified rate of return on the book value, or capital, of the practice other than goodwill, which is deducted from the average profits. Depending upon a purchase plan of three to five years, these excess profits are then multiplied.

Yet another method calculates a percentage return on the tangible assets of the practice prior to the date of valuation, which is then deducted from the average earnings for the same period. The value of that remainder is normally capitalized at a rate of 15% to 20%, and the figure is considered the value of goodwill.

In a practice, one should always consider a reasonable amount for the services to be performed by the doctor, which should be deducted from earnings.

Also, one should always look at the market value approach to determining goodwill. Have there been any arms-length transactions between physicians that would help to gauge this amount? For taxes and other reasons, the components of a practice that has been sold are sometimes clearly defined. The source of such information can be obtained from brokers who facilitate the buying and selling of professional practices.

Courts have noted the importance of goodwill in establishing valuation. The California Court of Appeals in Golden v. Golden held that the community property of the parties included a value for goodwill of the husband's medical practice for purposes of dividing the property in a divorce.

Conclusion

Placing a value on a medical practice requires the assistance of a qualified certified public accountant, professional appraiser, or specialized broker. Even equally skilled and experienced persons can and do come up with widely varying estimates of valuation because of the inexact nature of the process and the existence of conflicting methodologies.

In most instances, valuation is a result of good judgment and agreement, but in the marketplace for medical practices, perhaps the truest measure of the value of a medical practice is what a buyer is willing to pay and what a seller is willing to accept.

16 | Negotiating Employment Opportunities: Terms And Conditions

SHERWIN L. MEMEL, ESQ., JD

A reality of today's health-care market is that there is a growing number of physicians who are employees of other physicians, medical groups, hospitals, health maintenance organizations, or other health-care entities. The growth of physician employment relationships can be traced from changing practice patterns, increased competition, more mobility, and the broad expansion of alternative delivery systems such as health maintenance organizations. Consequently, it is likely that today's physician at some time will come into contact with a physician employment contract, either as an employee or as an employer.

This chapter will address the basic terms and conditions that should be included in a physician employment contract; it is designed to be useful to both the physician-employee and the employer in defining and maintaining the employment relationship. The basic elements of a physician employment contract will be the same regardless of whether the employer is a medical group, hospital, or other entity, but employment agreements will need to be tailored to reflect the special needs of each specific employment relationship. Additionally, although this chapter does not address independent contractor, partnership, or other nonemployment arrangements, the general topics discussed should be useful in identifying issues to be reviewed in any physician service relationship.

General Guidelines

An employment contract should be drafted according to the principle that "it is easier to do a good job now than to fix it later." The employment relationship between the physician and the employer potentially can last for years. Given the significance of the relationship, both financially and professionally, it is incumbent upon the parties to fully discuss and mutually understand the rights and obligations that are contemplated under the employment contract.

After the parties' agreement is put into writing, it will be difficult to argue that the contract is not an accurate reflection of their intent. It is critical to give careful consideration to the terms and conditions of the employment arrangement and to give specific attention to ensuring that the written contract is an accurate reflection of the agreement. If the physician and his or her employer take the time at the outset to satisfy themselves that the contract meets their needs and accurately reflects their agreements and enabling the termination of the relationship to be handled in an amicable and businesslike manner.

Another reality in today's health-care market is that very few physicians now stay with one practice for their entire career. Accordingly, the physician employment contract should be drafted with the realization that the employment relationship may be severed and the parties may go their separate ways at some future time. When this occurs, it is almost equally likely that there will be some disagreement over the respective rights and obligations of the parties. Referring to a well-structured physician employment contract at this time can provide a means for resolving such disagreements and enabling the termination of the relationship to be handled in an amicable and businesslike manner.

Finally, the legal environment surrounding physician relationships, particularly relationships involving referrals, has become substantially more complex in recent years. Corporate practice of medicine, antitrust, Medicare fraud and abuse, state anti-kickback and fee-splitting prohibitions, and other similar issues generally arise in conjunction with physician joint ventures and independent contractor relationships, rather than with the bona fide physician employment arrangements that are contemplated in this chapter. Nevertheless, because these areas of law are changing rapidly, whenever possible a physician employment contract should be drafted or reviewed by an attorney who specializes in health-care law.

Basis Elements of the Physician Employment Contract

Recitals

The *recitals* are general statements describing the reasons for and the parties involved in the proposed employment relationship. The names of the parties, a description of their legal capacity (individual, corporation, partnership), and a general statement of the work to be performed are set forth in the recitals. The recitals should state that the written contract is a full statement of the respective rights, obligations, and responsibilities of the parties in connection with the employee's provision of services on behalf of the employer.

The recitals also should contain a statement describing the qualifications of the physician employee. For instance, the recitals may indicate that the physician employee is duly licensed to practice medicine in the state where the contract is to be performed. Any specialties of the physician employee also should be mentioned, as should any board certifications or other special qualifications. Because of the importance of the descriptions set forth in the recitals, the contract should incorporate the recitals by reference or otherwise clearly state that the language in the recitals is binding on the parties.

Duties and Responsibilities

The contract should contain a provision that specifically describes the medical and administrative services the physician employee is expected to perform on behalf of the employer. These clauses also often provide that the physician employee will faithfully serve the employer and will devote such time as may be necessary to fulfill the listed duties. The contract should require the physician employee to conduct his or her professional activities in accordance with any and all applicable laws, regulations,and ethical and professional standards, as well as any rules, policies, and procedures of the employer. Additionally, this provision should state that the physician employee will maintain his or her license to practice medicine in good standing throughout the term of the contract.

If the physician employee's services are not to be performed only at specific locations, the contract should so state. Similarly, the number of hours the physician employee is expected to work should be described. The fact that the physician employee may be required to provide care to the employer's patients during nonbusiness hours, or pursuant to on-call scheduling, also should be discussed. The physician employee should agree to abide by the employer's on-call schedule and/or the on-call schedule of other related health-care entities, and to fulfill all the duties of an on-call physician.

The contract usually will provide that the employer has the duty to provide all office space and equipment necessary for the physician employee's activities under the contract and to undertake billing, collection, and other management functions. The contract should state that the employer has the right to establish all fees and to hire and fire all personnel. Also, in order to maintain clear lines of authority, the contract generally will provide that the employer alone has authority to determine space and equipment needs, billing and collection practices, and other issues related to administering the business of the employer.

Outside Activities

As indicated above, an employment contract usually will provide that during its term the physician employee must devote his or her full energies, interests, abilities, and productive time to performance of the contract. Often, language is included in this section which allows the physician employee to expend reasonable time for participation in teaching, research, civic or charitable activities, seminars, conferences, other continuing education, and other activities related to the physician employee's professional development. If such language is adopted, the employer may include an additional provision requiring the physician employee to refrain from such outside activities if they materially interfere with the services the employee is required to render to the employer.

The contract also can address whether the physician employee will be allowed to maintain private medical offices or otherwise treat patients outside the scope of the contract. Most physician employment agreements will contain a provision that the physician employee shall not, without the written permission of the employer, directly or indirectly engage in any activity that competes within a specified area with the employer's activities during the term of the agreement.

Term of Agreement

The contract should specify how long the employment will last. The contract can be for a specific term, such as one year. Alternatively, the employment need not be for a specific length of time, but rather can last as long as neither party terminates.

In general the physician employee benefits more from having a longer-term contract. If a physician employee is subject to a long-term contract but wants to leave, it is very difficult, and usually politically undesirable, for the employer to try to force the employee to stay. However, if an employer terminates an employee without cause before the end of the contract term (for instance, in the first year of a three-year contract), then the employer may be required to pay the contracted-for compensation to the employee for the remainder of the contract term. Thus, even though the physician employee will be obligated to mitigate damages (ie, seek other employment to lessen the amount the employer would have to pay), the longer-term agreement provides the physician employee with greater security.

The employer, on the other hand, would be better served to have an unspecified term or a short term. In fact, employers often adopt language stating that the physician employee is not employed for any specific length of time and that no provision of the contract is intended to be construed as a promise or guarantee of continuing permanent employment. A reference to the fact that the employment is *at-will*—that is, the employment can be terminated at any time for any reason that does not violate public policy— is desirable for the employer. Such at-will language may protect the employer from future contract damages in the event the employer needs to release a physician employee on short notice.

Compensation

A primary concern and motivation for entering into an employment contract is to specifically detail the terms of the employee's compensation. The physician employment contract should state the amount of compensation and how it will be calculated. In determining the methodology for paying the physician employee, the employer should consider carefully the sources of its revenue and the effect contracts with third parties may have on the employer's cash flow. An employer may wish to compensate its physician employees differently depending on whether the employer participates in a substantial number of capitated contracts now prevalent in the prepaid health sector.

Taking these issues into account, physician employment contracts vary widely in setting forth compensation provisions. For instance, compensation may be based upon a flat salary, production, or a combination of the two. The efficiency of the physician's practice (for instance, proper use of ancillary services) also can be used to determine compensation. Minimum guarantees and bonuses may be considered. The employer may wish to retain flexibility to modify compensation in the event of changes in the employer's finances, whereas the physician employee will prefer certainty throughout the term of the contract. The contract also may contain a provision permitting the parties to review the compensation terms at specified intervals.

Benefits

Employees generally will have the right to receive a variety of fringe benefits. It is usually sufficient in the contract to refer to the fact that the physician employee will receive the vacation, disability, retirement, and other benefits that are provided under the employer's standard personnel policies. The contract should state that these benefits can change from time to time and that the physician employee is entitled to only those benefits then existing.

Fringe benefits that will be provided in addition to those set forth in the employer's personnel policies should be listed in the employment contract. These may include pay for attending conferences, professional meetings, or other continuing education. Any additional benefits not available to the employer's other employees, such as additional life insurance or stock option plans, also should be included in the physician employment agreement to avoid future misunderstandings.

Professional Liability and Other Insurance

The physician employment agreement should contain a provision regarding the physician employee's professional liability insurance. It is common for the employer to promise to provide and keep in force professional liability insurance on behalf of the physician employee and also to set the limits of liability coverage. The provision should require maintenance of such professional liability insurance during the life of the contract. The employer may insist on a provision that such insurance will be maintained only as long as it is commercially available at reasonable rates, as determined by the employer.

A provision concerning automobile insurance may also be appropriate in some instances. If a physician employee uses his or her car in the course of employment and an accident occurs, the employer may face liability if the employee does not have insurance or the insurance is not sufficient to cover the damages. Consequently, an employer may wish to include a contractual provision obligating the physician employee to carry appropriate levels of automobile insurance.

Ownership and Confidentiality of Records

Another provision that should be included in the physician employment agreement pertains to patient-related information. The contract should provide that all patient records, histories, and other files concerning patients of the employer shall belong to and remain the property of the employer. Moreover, the agreement should include a provision requiring that all such records, reports, and information be kept in strictest confidence.

The contract also should cover all business records of the employer. Business records would include fee schedules, accounts receivable records, patient lists, employer lists, and other materials or information regarding the business methods and operations of the employer. The contract should state that these business records are confidential and shall belong to and remain the property of the employer.

The physician employee should be required to keep accurate records of all professional work he or she performs. Additionally, the physician employee should be required to assist in preparing any documentation that is required under public and private reimbursement programs, such as Medicare and private insurance.

Termination

An important provision in any physician employment contract addresses when and under what circumstances the employment can be terminated prior to the expiration date set forth in the contract. As stated above, unless otherwise specified in the agreement, the term of employment will be indefinite or at-will—that is, terminable by either party simply by notice to the other. In such instances, it is common for the contract to state that a specific number of days' prior notice must be given by the terminating party.

As in negotiating the overall term of the contract, it is advantageous for the physician employee to seek as long a notice period as possible when at-will termination will be permitted. If the employer desires to retain the ability to terminate the physician employee immediately or on short notice, a severance package for the physician employee may be considered.

When the physician employment agreement is for a specific term, such as a year, the parties may nevertheless wish to acquire the ability to terminate the agreement immediately upon certain occurrences. Many physician employment contracts permit either party to terminate the agreement upon a *material breach* by the other party. A material breach generally means a failure by one party to fulfill its obligations under the contract. This type of contract provision can lead to disputes regarding whether a party's actions or omissions actually constituted a material breach. Consequently, in addition to or in lieu of such provision, the employment contract also should list any specific events that will be grounds for immediately terminating the agreement.

The most common grounds for immediate termination of a physician employment contract include the death of the physician employee, the suspension or revocation of the physician employee's license to practice medicine, and suspension or revocation of the physician employee's medical staff membership or clinical privileges at specified facilities. If the physician employee will provide services to health maintenance organizations or other entities that credential physicians, the physician employment contract also could be terminable based upon loss of any such credentials.

The employer's failure to pay salary or fringe benefits often will be a reason for early termination. Additionally, the employer's inability to obtain or maintain professional liability insurance on behalf of the physician employee at reasonable rates, and the conviction of the physician employee of a felony or any other crime involving moral turpitude, also may be grounds for termination. Additional grounds for "for-cause" termination by the employer could include failure of the physician employee to comply with the employer's policies and procedures, chronic absenteeism, alcoholism, or drug addiction.

If the physician employee is hired to perform services under a specific contract between the employer and a third party (e.g., an HMO), then the employer may wish to have the ability to terminate the physician employment contract in the event the underlying third party contract is terminated. Again, in such instances, a severance package for the physician employee may be considered.

If the employer is a hospital or other entity that has a medical staff, then the relationship between the employment contract and applicable medical staff membership or clinical privileges should be addressed in the employment contract. Generally, termination of such membership or privileges will result in immediate termination of the employment contract, and termination of the employment contract likewise will result in termination of the employee's medical staff membership or clinical privileges. However, some states may have laws that prohibit employers from undertaking such a mutual termination or that otherwise require the employer to provide certain hearing rights.

The termination provisions of the contract also should discuss any continuing relationship of the parties after termination. The following are examples of posttermination rights and obligations that may need to be addressed: the status of the physician employee as a shareholder in the employer; any obligation of the physician employee to resell ownership in real property of the employer; any obligations of the employer to continue any of the physician employee's compensation, medical insurance, malpractice insurance, expense allowance, or other benefits beyond the date of the physician employee's termination of employment; any limitations on the physician employee's right to solicit patients of the employer; and any obligation of the physician employee to assist in the transition of patients to their new physician to ensure the continuity of the patients' medical care.

Other Agreements

The physician employment contract should incorporate by reference any other agreements containing obligations that will be fulfilled by the physician employee. One example would be an agreement between the employer and a referring health maintenance organization. The physician employee should be required to read and agree to act in accordance with—and be bound by the terms, conditions, requirements, and guiding principles set forth in—such related and incorporated agreements.

Amendments and Notices

After the contract is executed, changes in the practice and employment relationship may necessitate changes and amendments to the physician employment agreement. Accordingly, employers and physician employees should consider including a provision that provides for amendment of the contract. The contract should require that all amendments be in writing and signed by all the parties. Likewise, all notices, demands, requests, and other communications required or permitted by the contract should be required to be in writing.

Assignment

Because of the unique qualifications of the physician employee, the contract should provide that the physician employee not have the right to assign any rights or delegate any duties under the contract without the prior written consent of the employer. Likewise, because of the unique nature of the employer, the physician employee may request that the employer be prohibited from assigning its rights under the contract to a third party without the prior written consent of the physician employee.

Restrictive Practice Covenant

Frequently, physician employment contracts contain a restrictive covenant clause or a "promise not to compete." Such a clause holds that if the physician employment relationship is terminated, then the physician employee is prohibited from establishing a practice competing with that of the employer. Restrictive practice covenants must be drafted carefully to take into consideration the reasonable expectations and needs of the parties. For instance, a physician employee who brings a substantial number of patients into the employment relationship may desire to have the right to also take these patients with him or her when the employment agreement terminates.

Generally, restrictive covenants are disfavored legally because they discourage competition. Only a carefully drafted restrictive covenant will be permitted by law. An enforceable restrictive practice covenant must be reasonable in terms of geographic scope, time frame, and scope of activities prohibited. Physician employees and employers should be aware that the statutes and judicial decisions in individual states may differ regarding the enforceability of restrictive practice covenants.

Informal Dispute Resolution and Arbitration

The parties should consider the need for a clause requiring informal dispute resolution and/or arbitration in the event of a dispute over the terms of the contract. Informal dispute resolution is the least costly way to address contractual disputes. An informal dispute resolution provision may simply obligate the parties to meet and confer in good faith. The process also may be more formalized. For instance, the provision could require the parties to describe their positions in writing and set forth time frames and procedures under which the parties will meet and try to resolve the controversy amicably. If a local medical association or other appropriate trade organization provides informal dispute resolution services, the contract could require the parties to seek the assistance of such an organization when a dispute arises.

If informal dispute resolution is unsuccessful, the parties may litigate or submit the controversy to arbitration. The use of arbitration is a controversial topic. Some say that because arbitration is faster and less costly than litigation, it usually benefits the employee (the party with fewer financial resources). Nevertheless, others argue that arbitration can be as expensive as litigation and that litigation enables both parties to more fully explore all the pertinent issues.

In any event, if arbitration is to be required the contract should so state. Arbitration provisions in contracts vary widely. The contract clause may simply provide that arbitration will be conducted in accordance with the rules of a specified organization, such as the American Arbitration Association. Alternatively, the contract may set forth detailed arbitration procedures. Any arbitration clause should state whether the arbitrator can award costs and expenses, including reasonable attorney's fees, to the prevailing party in the arbitration.

If arbitration is to be used, the parties must decide whether to utilize a *binding arbitration* clause. Under binding arbitration, the decision of the arbitrator is in most cases final and binding on all the parties, and any right to judicial review of the decision is expressly waived. Such a binding arbitration provision may be desirable in that it usually means an end to the dispute and thus should prevent the possibility of expensive litigation.

Miscellaneous Provisions

The typical physician employment contract will contain several other provisions pertaining to the construction and interpretation of the agreement. Specifically, in the event that the contract covers activities in two or more states, a clause should be inserted that specifies which state's laws shall govern the interpretation of the agreement in the event of a dispute. The contract also should contain a provision stating that if any portion of the agreement is or becomes illegal or unenforceable for any reason, the remainder of the agreement will remain in full force and effect. Additionally, an attorney's fees clause should be included in the event any action is necessary to enforce the terms of the agreement.

Finally, the agreement should contain a specific reference to the fact that the agreement supersedes all previous oral and written contracts and agreements and constitutes the entire agreement between the physician employee and the employer regarding the physician employee's employment.

Conclusion

Physician employees and employers constantly experience changes in their practices and the relationships among themselves. For these reasons, physician employment agreements can be a valuable tool in defining the relationship between the physician employee and his or her employer, in ensuring that the parties fully understand their rights and obligations, and in enhancing the likelihood of having an amicable and prosperous relationship.

The author wishes to thank Catherine A. Kay, Esq, and Paul N. Phillips, Esq, for their assistance in preparing this chapter.

17 | Using Advisors Effectively and How Much to Delegate to Them

PETER C. McKENNEY, MBA, JD, CPA, LLM.

Introduction

Unlike very large companies, a small business cannot afford to retain full-time experts for all aspects of its business, but it can assemble a team of part-time advisors and consultants who can be just as powerful a resource. This potential resource can be expensive and hence must be used very wisely. If this resource is used excessively, the marginal costs could exceed marginal benefits and therefore reduce profits. On the other hand, if it is not used enough, the small business can make serious mistakes or, at least, miss profit opportunities.

A medical practice, like many other small businesses, exists in a complex business environment. Although the typical physician is an intelligent, hard-working, and capable person who could master many of these complexities, there often exist impediments to such mastery. The physician often is far too busy practicing medicine to devote the necessary time to learning the details of the business environment; did not receive training or education in very many business areas; may not be very interested in some aspects of the business; and lacks objectivity regarding the practice or its business environment.

The physician, therefore, maximizes his or her chance for achieving practice and personal goals by assembling a team of qualified advisors. Naturally, the physician should be the captain of the team, selecting or changing team members, calling team meetings, controlling and encouraging interaction among members, and setting standards for the team. The team approach works in a large business to achieve goals and is essential to a small business as well.

This chapter will discuss how a team of advisors can be used as a resource to help the physician achieve common business and professional goals, such as delivery of quality medical service, reasonable profits, and reasonable stress levels. It will list commonly used advisors and suggest when to use them, how to select them, what should be expected from them, how much reliance or authority should be given them, and how to control them, and their costs. Futhermore, managing the timeliness of their input and coordinating the work of the various advisors will be discussed.

Practice Goals

The physician needs to keep in mind his or her goals for the practice, and advisors can help physicians develop these specific targets or goals. The physician, of course, has to apply his or her philosophy and personal characteristics to the specific circumstances in arriving at practice goals. Setting goals and developing ways to achieve them is part of a process called *strategic planning.*

The most important goal of all relates to the quality of the medical service to be provided. Most advisors will not have significant knowledge of the technical or substantive medical aspects of the physician's practice. Advisors, nevertheless, can help substantially by periodically encouraging the physician and his or her staff to test the accuracy of their perception of how the patient rates the quality of the service in the practice. If the testing reveals a problem with quality, the physician will have to be coached in the ways of applying his or her medical knowledge in approaching desired standards for quality care.

For example, well-designed patient surveys often can provide significant information about the way health care is provided in the practice. In some instances, the actual quality of the medical care is excellent, but the patients' *perceptions* of the quality is not. In this case, the advisors would suggest ways that the practice can change these unfavorable perceptions.

Another common goal for the practice is to derive reasonable profits that will satisfy the personal needs of the physician. Usually business advisors have more training and experience in ways of improving the profitability of a practice, but the physician needs to decide what changes are acceptable in light of the overall goal of delivery of quality care. For example, some business advisors might suggest that the practice change its patient mix and reduce the number of patients who are Medicare or Medicaid subsidized patients. The physician, on the other hand, may not approve of that type of change and would reject that type of suggestion.

Some ways to increase the quality of medical care and increase the profitability of a practice will have adverse consequences for the physician and his or her employees. Such changes will increase stress levels. For example, forcing the staff to schedule more patients per hour or to process more insurance claims per day may increase short-term profits, but it may also cause tension among the employees in the practice. It may also adversely affect the physician's interaction with patients, staff, and family.

Advisors need to be used from time to time to monitor and improve stress levels in all of these positions. Furthermore, advisors should be mindful of improving quality and profits without unduly increasing stress levels. In other words, the advisor should be able to find ways for the physician and staff to work "smarter" rather than harder.

Commonly Used Advisors for the Medical Practice

Attorney

Many physicians actually have more in common with attorneys than they may think. Physicians like to practice preventive medicine. Similarly, one of the greatest reasons a physician should use an attorney more often is that an attorney knowledgeable about the legal issues common to physicians can help avoid significant legal problems. Attorneys should be consulted periodically in order to review the circumstances of the practice. The attorney can then advise the physician of potential pitfalls before they happen. In other words, like a good patient, the physician should have at least an annual checkup. In addition, he or she should consult with an attorney almost every time a significant transaction in the practice is being considered.

Besides knowing when to use an attorney, it is also important to know how to select an attorney. Like physicians, attorneys can be divided into two broad categories: generalists and specialists. More lawyers are becoming specialists, and it is important to recognize the specialty of each attorney being considered. From time to time a physician is going to need an attorney who is knowledgeable about contracts, employment practices, leases, purchase and sale agreements, corporate law, pension law, collections, real estate law, estate planning, third party reimbursement, litigation, and income taxes.

Very few attorneys have experience and expertise in all of these areas. Even if a physician has an attorney who is strong in several of these categories, occasionally another attorney who has expertise in remaining areas may be needed. Ideally, a physician should select as his or her principal attorney an individual who is associated with a law firm that has specialists in many or all of these areas. When the principal attorney needs help in an area in which he or she is not expert, an associate or partner may be called in to help. Communication within a single firm should be faster and better than among several firms. The physician will always know that the principal attorney is in charge of coordinating all efforts and is accountable for the results.

The actual search for an attorney can start with attorney directories. Martindale-Hubbell lists all practicing attorneys by geographic regions. Local bar associations may have referral programs or lists. Other physicians may also give recommendations. From these various sources, two or more strong candidates should be selected and interviewed. In addition to reviewing the candidate's resume and references, ask about the attorney's areas of practice, number of physician clients, and billing rates. Also ascertain details of the attorney's formal education, such as class standing; whether legal work will be done mainly by associates or by that attorney; and how many hours on average each year are devoted to continuing professional education, what courses are taken, and who sponsors them. By comparing the information from the candidates, a selection can be made.

Attorneys, like physicians, are usually very busy and have difficulty anticipating services that each of their clients/patients will need. It is probably unreasonable to expect attorneys to routinely call their physician clients before a legal issue arises. Thus it is important for the physician and his or her nonattorney advisors to be alert to potential legal issues and to notify the attorney when those issues arise. Once the issue has been handed over to the attorney, the physician should expect a reply within a reasonable period of time. The amount of time needed will depend upon the seriousness of the issue. The best way to manage the timeliness of the response is to request a deadline for the work to be done and then hold the attorney to it.

A physician should expect the attorney to explain the background of the law regarding the particular issue at hand and also give one or more options that might be pursued in dealing with it. Attorneys tend to be conservative in advising clients because of significant risk for claims of professional negligence. Nevertheless, the physician should expect the attorney to be willing to give specific advice when the legal issue is reasonably clear.

Banker

Not all bankers are alike. The physician should search for a banker who knows about professional businesses. The typical banker is trained to look for adequate collateral for asset-based financing, but most professionals have few assets compared with the size of loans that are often needed. For example, when starting a practice, most physicians do not have a substantial net worth complete with ample liquid assets for collateral. In addition, they often have significant educational liabilities that far outweigh the total value of their assets.

A banker unfamiliar with professional service businesses could look at a new physician's balance sheet and conclude that there is no borrowing capacity. Bankers who are aware of the earning capacity of professionals, however, look beyond the balance sheet to the viability of the physician's practice. Even these bankers, who are aware of the potential creditworthiness of physicians, may tend to be conservative, but this conservatism may actually be helpful for those physicians who might otherwise commit themselves to larger start-up costs or personal indebtedness than they should. Physicians can get into trouble if their banker is always a "yes" person.

A physician should also look for a banker associated with a bank that offers a broad range of services because physicians' needs for banking services expand during the course of their professional careers. Obviously, in the beginning of a practice there will be a need for equipment and working capital loans and, perhaps, personal loans to help cover living costs until the practice becomes profitable. A good banker will be able to structure the debt so that the debt will be serviceable. After the practice starts to mature, however, the bank should be able to provide loans for expansion of the practice, capital for outside investments, a retirement plan and trust services, and personal trusts for control of personal assets and estate planning.

Accountant

A good accountant can be one of the most helpful advisors a practitioner can have. Accountants generally offer a wide range of services: tax compliance (preparation of income tax returns), tax planning, business advice, business forecasts, personal financial planning, and audit or "attest" functions. Furthermore, accountants can help compare alternative uses of funds, enabling physicians to improve their chances of reaching goals by making the proper selection among the options at hand. Because accountants provide this wide range of services, they can be a co-captain of the business advisory team, helping the physician coordinate the efforts of the other team members.

Some accountants specialize in particular services. It is common in some of the larger accounting firms for an accountant to be a tax practitioner rather than an auditor. Most physicians need accountants who are good tax practitioners rather than auditors. Nevertheless, an accountant will be most useful if he or she is also aware of ways to help safeguard and control the assets of the practice.

In selecting an accountant it is helpful to know the different levels of professional classification in accounting. The certified public accountant (CPA) is the highest classification of accountant. The CPA has had a number of years of prior experience working for another CPA and has passed a difficult standardized test. Generally, CPAs are the appropriate level of practitioner for a physician practice.

Another classification of accountant found in most states is the public accountant (PA). This is an accountant who has not passed the CPA exam but has met certain other standards of performance. A CPA is able to represent a taxpayer before the Internal Revenue Service but a PA does not have the same standing. A PA would have to become an "enrolled agent" by passing a test in order to represent the taxpayer.

Another classification of accountant does not have either the CPA or PA classification. This person may have had some experience or training but has not yet met the standards for classifications. A physician considering hiring such a person should inquire very carefully into their level of experience and training before hiring them.

The final classification is bookkeeper. Bookkeepers record transactions and summarize the financial information of the practice during the year. Bookkeepers generally have little formal training, or even no training at all, but have learned through experience. Often they do not offer income tax services but rather generate their bookkeeping work product for an accountant who will prepare the tax return from this information.

Professionals who provide accounting and bookkeeping services generally charge for their time based upon the number of hours worked. The rate per hour for each of these classifications usually declines from CPA down through bookkeeper. If a practice has trouble with the record-keeping process, then a CPA may want to utilize the services of a bookkeeper. The bookkeeper could be an employee of the physician or an independent contractor. Utilizing the bookkeeper will reduce the total cost to the practice by reducing the number of hours spent by the CPA.

Selecting an accountant involves a process similar to hiring an attorney: Find candidates through society lists and colleagues, interview them as you would an attorney, and in addition to the questions asked an attorney, ask about the quality (experience, training, stability) of the accountant's staff, how the accountant organizes client services throughout the year, what fraction of clients' returns are extended each year, and how many planning services are available.

Insurance Advisor

Every physician needs a very good insurance advisor. Life insurance, disability income insurance, malpractice insurance, health insurance, business insurance and personal liability insurance must be obtained in order to shift the risk for potential losses. Some insurance advisors are knowledgeable in all of these areas; others have become specialists. Depending on the circumstances, a physician may be able to utilize a generalist. If the situation is particularly complicated, the physician may need to have several insurance advisors who are specialists in each of these areas.

Insurance advisors are mostly *commission driven*—that is, they make money only when they sell a product and receive a commission for the sale. In some states there are provisions for insurance consultants to be paid a fee for work performed, often on an hourly basis. Because most insurance advisors generate their revenue from commissions, consumers are sometimes leery of their motives. Although this attitude is healthy, it should not dissuade the physician from seeking qualified help from an insurance advisor. Most physicians should seek an insurance checkup at least once a year. They also should seek help whenever the practice is being expanded or changed significantly.

A good insurance advisor will tailor a program for the practitioner to reduce premium costs. In order to feel comfortable about the program being offered by the insurance advisor, a physician may want to consult with an attorney or an accountant who is knowledgeable in the physician's business affairs. The attorney or accountant can check the assumptions and conclusions reached by the insurance advisor.

Insurance advisors also have varying degrees of experience. In most states it is not difficult to become an insurance agent; therefore the qualifications of the insurance advisor should be investigated carefully. Those who are chartered life underwriters (CLUs) have passed difficult tests in order to earn their designation. These agents will often have a higher level of awareness about insurance issues than will some of their less trained colleagues. The physician should also seek out agents who are knowledgeable about professional practices.

Many insurance advisors have expanded their knowledge to include estate planning and retirement plans, and some have knowledge about personal financial planning. These agents can be very helpful in working with the physician and the physician's other advisors in handling these important issues. On the other hand, agents who have limited training or experience in these areas but claim to have expertise may lack sufficient knowledge to be helpful. Explore these issues carefully before relying on agents in noninsurance areas.

Investment Advisors

The two most common sources of investment advice are the traditional stockbroker and the registered investment advisor. Brokers earn their living by commissions on the transactions they complete; the registered investment advisor charges a fee usually based on the value of the assets managed. If an investment advisor is used, he or she generally will also have to use a broker to execute the security transactions. Although this appears to be a duplication of costs, generally brokers will charge a discounted rate for that type of trade because they spend less time with the investor.

Selecting a particular investment advisor should follow the pattern for selecting an attorney or accountant. Educational background and experience are important attributes as well as the analytical support available to the advisor. Advisors who have experienced at least two bear markets often have a more realistic and prudent view of the investment world.

In developing an investment portfolio, it is important for investors to find advisors who have a philosophy about investing that matches theirs. For example, risk tolerance needs to be taken into account in selecting an advisor. Once an investment advisor has been selected, the physician and other advisors need to monitor the performance of the investment advisor over a period of time to ensure that established goals are being achieved. Generally it takes about three years for the advisor to fully implement an investment program and have enough time to show the full value of his or her performance. On the other hand, if an investor sees in a short period of time that the advisor is not suitable, a change should be made before too much damage is done or an opportunity is lost.

Other sources of investment advice include banks, insurance companies, and mutual funds. Banks are becoming more aggressive in marketing their investment management services. Insurance companies are also selling investment products through their insurance agent network. Mutual funds are often sold without the involvement of an agent.

Although banks in the past tended to be very conservative in their investments and generally did not perform as well as more established investment firms, recently their performance relative to the others has improved; not all banks have improved equally, however. Each bank under consideration should be carefully scrutinized. If a bank's management service is to be used, the physician should be sure it has an investment mix that is appropriately designed for his or her goals.

When a physician first starts accumulating funds for investment, he or she may not have sufficient funds for a well-diversified security portfolio. The physician can gain instant diversification, however, by using mutual funds. Mutual funds are constantly managed by qualified investment analysts and may be suitable until a sufficiently large portfolio has been accumulated to warrant the use of a stockbroker or registered investment advisor.

Some investment advisors ask for authority to make transactions without the investor's prior approval. This is appropriate for those investors who have had a long-term relationship with their investment advisor and feel comfortable that the advisor's investment philosophy is compatible with their own. In new relationships, granting this type of authority could be risky. In a few situations, unscrupulous brokers have churned the account in order to increase their commission income.

The best way for the physician to objectively monitor the investment advisor is to clearly communicate his or her annual yield expectations to the advisor. The physician should then monitor the overall portfolio to see if those expectations are met after all fees and transaction costs are subtracted. If they are not, the physician and investment advisor should meet to review the performance and determine if changes are needed.

Real Estate Broker

Real estate advice is generally needed when acquiring an office building, home, vacation home, or investment property. Also, advice will be needed when disposing of any of these types of property. Furthermore, real estate advice is helpful in locating space to lease or to find tenants for property already owned.

The real estate world is an aggressive one. Large commissions on potential sales can motivate representatives to be highly competitive and unfortunately, in some situations, to be unethical or dishonest. Couple that with a high turnover rate for agents and the inherent difficulty in regulating their behavior, and it should be clear that selecting a real estate broker is a critical concern.

State laws usually control and classify real estate representatives. Often they have at least three classes: (1) a *salesperson* is a basic trainee, often in the first year of work; (2) a *sales agent* can close a deal independently; and (3) a *broker* can operate an office. In addition, the National Association of Realtors has the *Realtor* designation and requires its members to abide by a set of ethics.

Many people become real estate representatives because most states do not require significant preparation and there is potential for earning large amounts of income. A high percentage of those entering the field fail.

Generally those who have survived five years are likely to have the skills to be helpful. Interview others who have used the candidates and have completed a transaction with them before selecting.

Whenever dealing with brokers, distinguish between those who focus on commercial real estate and those who focus on residential real estate. Residential brokers should be part of a multiple listing service. Also, check the volume of transactions the broker has managed in the past to determine how well they perform and how quickly they may be able to complete your transaction.

General Business Consultant

Often there are very helpful consultants available who do not fit into other categories but, rather, represent themselves as general business consultants. These can include strategic planners or personnel consultants. These advisors can be helpful in assessing the status of the business or in identifying current problems. They should be able to make specific, reasonable recommendations that a physician can readily implement. They should be able to help plan for the future and give ideas on expansion of services, selection of equipment, and resolution of personnel problems among the staff and between the staff and physician.

Consistent with the practices of other professional advisors, general business consultants may seek certification from professional associations. Those with significant experience may have met the qualification requirements of the Society of Professional Business Consultants. The Institute of Certified Professional Business Consultants also has a certification program. The practitioner must pass a test and meet an experience requirement before being designated a certified professional business consultant (CPBC).

Considering that these consultants have a broader scope of experience and expertise than do many other advisors, it usually is critical to interview other physicians who have used their services before hiring them. A physician should be sure to ask whether the consultant gave understandable and usable suggestions. Did the consultant follow up? What were his or her strengths and weaknesses? When a decision to hire is made, prepare a written summary of the work to be performed, when it will be completed, the form of the work product, and the fee arrangement.

Billing Specialist

Small practices often do not have highly trained and knowledgeable billing clerks. Such practices can lose significant amounts of money each year from improper billing. Even worse, the clerk can cause the practice significant legal problems if he or she erroneously overcharges patients and insurance carriers. Medicare, for example, may assess a $2000 per mistake civil penalty. Nationally, several practices have been forced into bankruptcy due to these penalties.

The fee schedule should be reviewed and adjusted regularly. This procedure is necessary to ensure that the practice is generating the appropriate levels of revenue and to reduce the risk of unintentionally overcharging. The staff needs to be instructed from time to time on reimbursement rule changes. Rather than relying on in-house personnel alone, it is usually cost effective to hire an outside billing specialist to review the fee schedules, review the accuracy of claims, and advise on how to code to obtain the maximum revenue without overcharging. Those who do not have in-house expertise should seek the advice of a billing specialist at least once a year.

When selecting a billing specialist, look for those who have had significant years of experience in the area. Many independent billing specialists once worked for Medicare or Blue Cross/Blue Shield and have first-hand knowledge of this highly technical area. It is also important to find someone who is constantly updating his or her knowledge through regular attendance at seminars and training sessions devoted to reimbursement issues.

Retirement Plan Advisor/Specialist/Administrator

Qualified retirement plans and employee benefits are two of the most technically complicated areas of practice management. If the practice has a qualified retirement plan that is not properly administered, the plan may become disqualified, with disastrous results. The employees would have to recognize as current income their entire vested account balance, the employer would lose deductions for current contributions to the extent that they were allocated to unvested accounts, and the trust would no longer have the benefit of tax-free accumulation of earnings.

Considering the potential danger in this area, it is important to have expert advice on retirement plan issues. Generally this begins with having a qualified attorney available to the practice who is knowledgeable about the Employee Retirement Income Security Act. The attorney can advise on drafting the plan document and amendments, antidiscrimination rules, vesting requirements, and other legal issues.

Attorneys, however, usually do not get involved in the day-to-day administration of retirement plans. A physician will need the services of other knowledgeable professionals to assist with plan administration. Some financial institutions, such as banks and insurance companies, have pension experts who can address many of the pertinent issues. Furthermore, banks often act as trustees of retirement plans. There are also professional retirement plan administrators and consultants who specialize in providing these services for retirement plans and other employee benefit plans.

The person engaged to perform these services must be qualified to prepare the annual federal reports (Form 5500), advise on the qualification of the plan and required amendments to the plan, give good plan design ideas that will minimize the cost of administration and maximize the allocation to the owner-physicians, and give annual reports to the participants showing the amount of funds in their accounts or the benefits that they have already earned.

Two common alternatives are to use the plan administrators of large institutions or to find a local plan administrator who deals with various plans for many businesses. The advantage of the former is that such administrators generally have more stability and resources behind them. On the other hand, they may be located in another city and generally will not have personal knowledge of the physician's situation. They may not respond rapidly to some of the physician's needs. Local administrators may not have the same amount of stability and resources, but if they are personally known by the physician they may give better and more personal service.

This is a highly technical area and inquiries should be made regarding educational background, certifications, years of experience, and annual continuing professional education before choosing a plan administrator.

Administrators use two different types of cost structures. Some administrators charge a fixed annual fee, whereas others charge an hourly rate. It is probably wise to find two or three alternative sources of this service and compare the perceived quality of the organization with the projected annual cost and then make a selection from that information.

Practice Administrator

The sophistication of professionals who earn their living managing professional practices has increased dramatically over the last decade. Organizations such as the Medical Group Management Association have raised the level of training, experience opportunities, and management resources available to professionals who manage medical practices. In the past, many physicians promoted nurses or other health-care professionals to bookkeeping roles and then to the position of office manager, regardless of the training and interest of that employee. Some of these individuals have performed well whereas others have not.

A new breed of professional, the *practice administrator*, is available to physicians to fulfill this management role. Such people have had a business education with extensive experience and training in administering a medical practice.

These administrators are usually in-house, full-time employees of the physician. A practice generally must have three or more physicians in order to make this type of position economically feasible. Costs often range between $50,000 and $100,000 per year. Practices that are not large enough to afford a full-time administrator may be able to find administrators working in other practices who are available on a part-time basis for consulting services. In order to have a well-run practice, there should be at least one in-house person who attends to all of the important financial functions on a daily basis. Nevertheless, it is sometimes helpful to have the input of a higher level of management professional. The administrator could be engaged to visit the practice for a day or several hours each week in order to assist the full-time in-house office manager.

Computer Consultant

Most medical practices are already computerized to some extent. The remaining practices will become computerized as the cost for computerization declines and the benefits of the computerized office dramatically increase. Regardless of whether the practice currently has a computer, a computer consultant who is knowledgeable in medical practices is a necessary member of the management team. The consultant can provide input to help the practice choose its first computer, expand the utilization of the present system, or upgrade the present computer system by adding to it or replacing it.

Because of intense competition among computer hardware and software vendors, it is often difficult for physicians and their management team to select among competing proposals. One way to solve this problem is to hire an independent consultant who is not motivated to sell any particular product or system. After considerable analysis and discussion with the physician, the consultant should prepare a request for proposals to send to potential vendors. The consultant should subsequently analyze the competing proposals and make recommendations. A good consultant will be able to prioritize the proposals for the physician's consideration. In order to maintain objectivity, the consultant should be paid a fee, either fixed or based on hours worked. Even if the present system appears to be working well, a consultant should make short visits periodically to help the staff fully utilize the system. They also can warn when the system is approaching capacity.

Selecting a qualified computer consultant is not easy. A successful computer operation requires the selection of a computer consultant who has a significant level of training and experience dealing primarily in medical office financial systems. Many people represent themselves as computer experts without having had formal training or adequate experience. The consultant should have at least three years' full-time experience in medical practice, be knowledgeable about various vendors' hardware and software, and be recommended by other physicians who have used the consultant for some time.

For installed computer systems, the vendor may offer computer consultants who are more familiar than are outsiders with the pitfalls and utilities of the system. Generally they will be cost effective to use, though from time to time an independent consultant may be used to oversee their performance.

Personal Financial Planner

A personal financial planner focuses primarily on the individual physician's family financial situation. The planner must also consider the practice because it is usually the major source of wealth for the physician. The goal of personal financial planning is to maximize family net worth consistent with the primary desires and goals of the family. The personal financial planner will address issues such as adequacy of personal life and disability income insurance; adequacy of homeowner's, auto, and health and accident insurance; development of an appropriate estate plan; planning for college education or caring for other dependents; analysis of an existing retirement plan in light of retirement goals; review of investment performance in relation to personal goals; and closely held business issues such as valuing and arranging for the future sale of the physician's interest in the practice.

Many people call themselves personal financial planners, but few have significant experience or training. Organizations exist that certify personal financial planners after they have passed examinations and met certain education and experience requirements. The American Institute of Certified Public Accountants (AICPA) has an *accredited personal financial specialist* planner designation (APFS). The International Board of Standards and Practices for Certified Planners of Englewood, Colorado, awards the designation of *certified financial planner* (CFP). The American College of Bryn Mawr, Pennsylvania, confers *chartered financial consultant* (ChFC) designations. Other, similar organizations also rate financial planners.

Personal financial planning is one of the most difficult disciplines to master. The search for a planner should focus on candidates who have substantial education and experience. Ask how many years of experience the planner has and how many plans are done each year. Be sure to check out references and try to see a sample of the planner's work product.

Personal financial planners can be compensated in two ways. Some charge a fee for service, whereas others charge a commission on products they sell during the planning process. Stockbrokers and insurance agents often are compensated by commission but may also have a fee for service. Generally, the trend in personal financial planning has been toward fee-for-service and away from commission-driven planners. This avoids the potential conflict of interest when a planner recommends that the client buy an investment product.

The planning process should be time consuming and thought provoking. During the first phase, the physician should expect to spend a great deal of time collecting personal information and conveying it to the planner. There should be several meetings during which the planner asks questions and helps the family define personal financial goals. Once the planner has this information, a significant amount of time is spent analyzing the information and formulating options for consideration. The options are then presented and the physician is asked to select the most comfortable option. The planner then should work with the physician and other advisory team members, including the attorney, banker, insurance agent, and trust officers in implementing the plan. The physician and the planner will have to meet regularly during the implementation phase and continue to update the plan.

Remember, personal financial planning is not a once-in-a-lifetime event; it should be considered an ongoing process. Unless circumstances change dramatically, however, the future work should be easier than the initial work.

How to Utilize Advisors

Relating to the Advisor: Careful Selection Enhances Future Utility

In selecting advisors, the physician should consider their education and experience and whether they are knowledgeable about health-care professionals. They will be better equipped to relate to questions if they have a broad understanding of the physician's circumstances. Advisors will also be able to provide better services if they have significant resources available to them. In the selection process, the physician should consider the size or depth of the organization to which the advisor belongs, the stability of the personnel in that organization, and their ability to work with others and share information.

Advisors and Their Clients Must Communicate Effectively

In dealing with advisors, as with almost everything else in life, good communication is necessary. The physician should select and hire advisors with whom he or she feels comfortable discussing private and sometimes embarrassing information or questions. It is very important that the advisor have a personality and style that will be conducive to good communication. The advisor must listen well, be willing to advise, and be ready for action.

Whenever the physician is too busy or unable to perform a task relating to the practice, he or she should feel comfortable in calling an advisor. In addition to calling upon them as the physician perceives a need, some of the advisors should be contacted on a regular, frequent basis. The accountant, for example, should be consulted periodically to consider tax planning. He or she should be asked to prepare a tax projection at least once each year. This will enable the physician to set aside in advance the amount of cash necessary to pay tax liabilities on time and avoid unnecessary underpayment penalties. This also gives the accountant an opportunity to point out tax-saving strategies that the physician may want to implement.

The physician may also need to consult with an accountant from time to time regarding practice cash-flow concerns or other business questions. In short, appointments should be scheduled throughout the year with the accountant as well as with the other advisors who are involved in repetitive tasks relating to the practice. These advisors include the investment advisors, pension advisors, lawyers, personal financial planners, and business consultants.

The Role of the Advisor and What to Expect

Simply stated, the advisor's role is to advise, contrasted with the owner's role, which is to decide. Good advisors will give ideas, alternative options, and when possible, make recommendations among conflicting options. Furthermore, good advisors will give timely warnings of impending matters. On the other hand, the owner must make the final judgment regarding which of several conflicting options best suits his or her personal philosophy and practice goals. Therefore, the physician must feel comfortable in making decisions even if those decisions may, in part or in total, conflict with recommendations of the advisors.

Generally it is unwise for an owner of a practice to delegate complete authority to advisors on policy matters. However, it is good use of the advisors to delegate limited authority on matters that are not perceived as critical to the practice. For example, once a decision has been made to acquire a software system or x-ray machine, the advisor could be given authority to select the appropriate option from the available alternatives. The physician should not delegate authority regarding sensitive issues, such as which physician to hire for the practice; that type of decision is too personal to delegate to an advisor.

Controlling Costs

The thought of having a significant number of advisors available to help a small practice may be exciting, but the realities associated with it must be considered. Using a large number of advisors can be costly, though careful use of advisors can have a payback that is far greater than the actual cost. Therefore, when considering engaging an advisor, the physician should compare the potential cost with the ultimate payback from the advice. In some instances, the benefit consists of avoiding a loss. For instance, conferring with an attorney about a Medicare reimbursement issue in advance may avoid a significant loss that would be incurred if the practice were to be penalized.

In order to control costs, the physician should be well prepared for any meeting with advisors. The physician should organize all of the relevant information, make a list of questions and goals regarding the meeting, and if possible, convey this information to the advisor in advance of the meeting. If a task is assigned to an advisor, the physician should describe the form of the work product desired and ask for an estimate of the potential costs in advance. If a flat fee can be quoted for the work, the physician will have a better idea of whether the task will be cost effective. Most advisors, however, will not be able to determine the total amount of time necessary in advance, and therefore will be able to give only an estimate of total hours. At a minimum, they should be asked to give a specific rate per hour for the work, and they should be told that they are authorized to spend up to a specified amount of hours on the project.

To avoid misunderstandings, it is helpful to ask advisors to prepare a letter outlining their understanding of the task, the scope of the work to be performed, and the fee or the way the fee will be determined. The letter should also specify that they are not authorized to exceed the instructions or specified service.

To manage the timeliness of the task, the physician should set specific due dates with the advisors. If the project is a large, complex one, there should be interim checkpoints established by the physician and advisor at which time the physician can review the status and make timely changes in the project. In some instances, preliminary work will indicate that further work is unnecessary, or that further work will be much more expensive than originally thought, and adjustments will need to be made.

Team Meetings

To derive the most value from advisors, it is helpful to have meetings of team members. Some meetings may be regularly scheduled with all members of the team present. Other meetings may include only a few selected advisors when the input of all advisors is unnecessary. An agenda should be distributed prior to the meeting so that all invitees will be as prepared as possible. The agenda should contain a list of possible outcomes.

Minutes of the meeting should be recorded and distributed to interested persons so that those not in attendance will be informed of the discussion. This is important because they may be able to provide input subsequent to the meeting or because the discussion may affect a project they are working on independently. The minutes should contain a list of assignments and due dates of projects derived from the meeting and the date of the next scheduled meeting.

Summary

By assembling a proper team of qualified consultants and advisors, the practice will have access to the same valuable resources available to the largest businesses in the country. The physician should be the captain of the team and should select and control it. The physician may delegate some authority but should maintain control and awareness of assignments. The team should be able to help the physician provide quality health-care services while maintaining reasonable profits and stress levels.

III | ESTABLISHING A PRACTICE

18 | The Physician as Managing Partner

FRANK A. RIDDICK, Jr., MD

The role of the physician as leader of a medical organization is not a new one. Since the 1800s, the great municipal hospitals of the East Coast have had physician leaders, initially called superintendents, but lately termed presidents and chief executive officers. Medical units and medical installations in the armed forces are traditionally commanded by medical officers, and such experience is often a prerequisite for promotion to the higher ranks for military physicians. Medical schools are headed by deans who are physicians, and the evolution of the medical school into the modern academic health center/teaching hospital has been accompanied by the appearance of vice presidents for health affairs as their directors. The large group practices and great clinics of the United States are physician organizations and traditionally have been headed by physicians. Nevertheless, the cadre of well-educated lay administrators has met the general management needs of most hospitals and health-care organizations. Only in recent years has there been a resurgence of the physician as a medical manager and growing perception of his or her role as a general manager.

Issues of leadership apply in physician-directed organizations even when they are not owned by physicians. The large group practices typically grew out of the expanded practices of surgeon founders, who tended to delegate the administrative aspects of the practice to lay managers but who retained the policy-making, planning, and ultimate decision-making authority. As these practices expanded in size and breadth, the multispecialty group practice evolved. Despite variations in ownership forms and organizational arrangements, these organizations typically have a physician at the helm titled chair of the board, chief executive officer, managing partner, or medical director, under the rationale that doctors are more responsive to physician leadership than to that from nonphysicians.

Why should a medical organization select a physician for a leadership role? Physicians, after all, are seldom prepared educationally or by experience for that role and generally deal with individual patients, not a population group. However, a physician will be able to understand and relate to colleagues in the medical profession. A more important reason is that understanding the process of medical care, the clinical imperative, and the physician-patient relationship enhances leadership in defining the goals of a medical organization and in ensuring that its services meet the institution's obligations to its patients.

Group practices are characterized by a fraternal culture and constitute a professional bureaucracy. The physician leader is *primus inter pares* (first among equals), but by only a narrow margin. The leadership is more consensual than hierarchical, and the most successful of its practitioners are those who achieve credibility among the professional staff in a non-threatening manner.

The modern group practice evolved from being the purveyor of individual professionals' services—a model still extant in some communities and academic centers where there is loose professional linkage between the physicians in a single institution or area—to provision of coordinated medical services by a single staff. The emphasis was on provision of services in the most appropriate setting and on effective use of the hospital, with complex technological services and studies available to outpatients and inpatients with equal readiness. We are now moving toward an era in which the physician leader must negotiate with the purchasers of care for the opportunity to provide services to patients who are locked into various medical care systems. This evolution has required leaders to assume roles beyond that of peacemaker and referee among physicians—that is, they must now organize resources for the provision of care as well as acquire the patient stream necessary for the group practice to function.

The stereotypical leader is tall, dynamic, incisive, and inspirational, but many of us do not fit that mold. The effective leader understands the organization and its members, directs planning and strategy, and achieves a balance between the institution's goals and values and those of the professionals within it.

The typical medical executive rarely has the prerogatives or power of a corporate chief executive officer. The organization sees to that, and the professional group provides checks and balances in the form of the governing board or council, which often functions operationally, rather than through establishing policy. Particularly when physicians own the group, the medical executive may have a hierarchical relationship with the operations, finance, and administrative personnel necessary for the organization to function; however, on the professional side, that physician is both the leader and employee of a group, the members of which are simultaneously his or her key workers and the owners of the business.

What is the background of the physician leader? Historically, such a person has been selected from the professional staff of the organization in early or mid-career and matures in lesser management roles and through on-the-job training, complementing the natural leadership skills that brought that person to the fore. The typical activities and responsibilities of the medical executive are discussed in the following sections.

Organizational Planning

Planning, a chief responsibility of the executive, must be based on an assessment of the environment in which the organization functions and its overall mission.

Planning must encompass the decisions necessary for determining optimal staffing, the facilities that will meet the organization's needs, programs that are to be mounted, the equipment required, and the techniques for the financing of all these. The executive must guide the organization through decisions about the desirability of expansion and creation of new ventures. An effective support staff and, often, consultants are helpful in providing the data necessary to evaluate new ventures.

Recruiting Physicians

Intrinsic to the decision to recruit physicians to an organization are the various reasons for addition: replacement of retiring or departed staff physicians or addition of new skills. New physicians may be needed to provide services to the current population served by the organization, or they may be a necessary element in securing an expanded population of patients. When an organization reaches a certain size, the executive must work through the department chair or have an associate to whom much of the recruiting is delegated.

Recruiting begins with identification of suitable candidates. An effective relationship with residency programs will enhance this process. The younger staff members of the institution are often an asset in identifying prospective staff members. Advertisements in medical journals, special society placement agencies, and search firms may all be useful.

The recruitment process begins with an explicit description of the position to be filled. The process flows best when the candidate is given ample information about the institution and community and when information about the candidate is provided to the interviewers who must give an evaluation. The itinerary and list of interviewees must be selected with care.

The candidate's initial visit to the institution should usually be limited to the candidate alone; if there is mutual interest a return visit including the candidate's spouse is arranged. It is helpful to address the candidate's interests and needs during the recruiting process by providing information about and visits to housing, schools, recreational areas, and cultural activities.

One must be sure the candidate understands the nature of the job and is comfortable with those with whom he or she must interact in the same and related departments. Once the selection is made, a formal, written offer should be extended. It should be explicit as to salary, fringe benefits, aspects of partnership and stock ownership, and other attributes of the position.

Developing the Reward System

Among any 100 medical organizations, there are probably 100 different techniques employed in establishing the reward system. The array ranges from group practices with a system that is, essentially, expense sharing—in which the reward is strictly based on collection of professional fees, against which allocation of overhead expenses are made—to purely salaried systems with salaries varying from specialty to specialty, usually with several levels within the same specialty, dependent on seniority and responsibility.

More often, group practices provide an established starting salary that escalates to parity with other physicians of similar specialty and practice volume over a three- to five-year period of time. This usually is augmented by annual bonuses keyed to organizational success and the individual's contribution to that success. The bonus is usually designed to reward performance that the organization wishes to foster, and according to the setting, it is weighted to reward financial productivity, quality of practice, research contributions, involvement in teaching, or achievement and distinction on the national scene.

It is the rare group that still maintains equal distribution of partnership or group proceeds to all the professionals. The wide disparity in earning capacity and marketplace values between the various specialties make this untenable. Most groups have found that they must adjust the reward system to account for the various professional strategies necessary for successful performance in prepayment practice, and that the system must take into account the large volume of discounted professional services and managed care that is provided. The reward system in most group practices has been subject to a great deal of experimentation and fine tuning from year to year. The organization must determine whether it is competing for its staff with hospitals, medical schools, or the general practicing community in adopting the appropriate strategy for attracting and retaining physicians.

A large number of guidelines exist for compensation in the various specialties. The Medical Group Management Association provides not only salary surveys, but also productivity norms for various specialties. The American Group Practice Association provides an annual salary survey, as does the Group Health Association of American for the HMO industry. There is no dearth of consultants eager to assist development of appropriate reward systems, but management must be intimately involved in the establishment of the system for any particular group, as it is the key to recruiting and retaining the professional staff. Any change must have wide support. It is always useful for management to minimize the number of individuals with which it must negotiate in establishing salaries, and it is best to deal with the chairs of the clinical departments rather than with the large array of individual physicians within the departments.

In the final analysis, any system for paying physicians must be perceived by them as having a rational basis, being equitably administered, providing input and redress to the participants, and serving the values of the institution and the needs of the professionals.

Evaluating Physician Performance

Measuring physician performance is an important element in quality assessment, and the value judgments involved are used in decisions on physicians' salaries and bonuses and their promotion and retention, as well as in the process of nomination to partnership or status as stockholder.

Information from department chairs, colleagues, nurses, and—importantly—patients, are valuable in making assessments. Customarily, medical management devises a form listing such attributes as quality and volume of work; relationships with patients, colleagues, and personnel; maintenance of skills and acquisition of new ones; complaints and law suits; and so on. The section or department chair is asked to complete the form, using an explicit rating scale. The evaluations are reviewed by the governing body or by a personnel committee of its members. An important element is sharing the data and judgments from the evaluation with the professional.

The evaluation may be performed annually, if used in bonus calculation, or every two to three years in conjunction with individual or departmental reviews.

Quality Assurance

In the past, group practices have tended to depend on the data generated on physician performance by hospitals for the Joint Commission on Accreditation of Hospitals (JCAH) visits. Although physician performance in the hospital is an important factor, the process of quality assurance cannot be delegated to solely hospital staff mechanisms. An increasing volume of the professional activity of any group is in the outpatient setting.

Quality assurance in the ambulatory setting currently relies on relatively unsophisticated techniques. Important elements include measures of patient satisfaction, effective use of resources, practice efficiency, and patient outcomes. The latter is still used less frequently than are various process measures that professional consensus determines are important elements of quality, but public expectations will demand evaluations reflecting the results of care in the future.

Dealing with Third Parties: Hospitals, Insurance, and Prepayment Groups

The physician chief executive typically represents the organization in various negotiations over services provided by the organization and its physicians.

Discussions with hospitals usually relate to services provided by the group's physicians within hospital departments and the rates the hospital charges patients covered by prepayment who are served by the group. The latter will influence the ultimate amount the group yields from its capitation portion. Because hospitals are increasingly desirous of binding the referring staff to the hospital and ensuring an admission stream, they are increasingly willing to make concessions to large physician groups with respect to the group's expenses. As more patient care shifts from the inpatient to the outpatient area, the physician group must decide whether to use the hospital's outpatient facilities, set up its own facilities and compete with the hospital, or enter into some joint venture with the hospital for provision for these services.

Groups that deal with health maintenance organizations, even those in which they have an ownership position, will find themselves having to negotiate for expected volumes and rates and whether the services will be provided on the basis of capitation or a discounted fee for service. Also subject to negotiation are retention by the HMO of a percentage of fees for year-end adjustment, the relationship of the group's professionals with the HMO—including restrictions on physician behavior—and mandatory authorization for hospitalization.

Increasingly, the executive leadership of the group must represent the group's interests in dealing with various managed care organizations established by hospitals, medical societies, and insurance companies. The latest wrinkle is the expectation by industry and various employer groups for utilization control, discounts, and data on use of facilities by their employees in exchange for an ensured stream of patients; employers are increasingly willing to negotiate for these.

Acquisition of Patients

In the current era, securing a patient base is essential to the medical organization. There are increasing restrictions on the patient's ability to select the institution where he or she will receive care. The choice may be dictated by the employer or strongly influenced by the patient's previous decision to participate in one or another health-care system. Certainly, an important responsibility of the managing partner is to ensure that the organization is not excluded from its traditional source of patients and that it positions itself to secure new patients. The creation of programs to achieve this is the responsibility of management. Negotiations with insurers, employers, and bulk purchasers of care are important.

In this environment it is sometimes easy to forget that retaining current patients is much easier than securing new patients who are not attuned to receiving care from the organization. Particular attention to the techniques for binding and pleasing the current patient population is essential.

Creating and Overseeing an Effective Management Staff

The lay management of the medical organization is essential to its function, and the medical leader must be involved in the selection and empowering of the chief administrator of the organization. In the ideal organization the medical leader relates to one—or at most, two—administrators. The wise physician manager devotes more care to the selection of the chief administrator than to selection of the head of any clinical department in the institution, as the performance of the chief administrator is clearly more important to the physician manager's career. The head of lay management of the organization should be empowered to recruit and oversee the administrative staff and should have an appropriate linkage through reports to the chief executive officer and the governing body. The medical executive provides a conduit for information to the lay staff about the needs and concerns of the professional staff. Often it is the function of medical management to provide some insulation for the lay staff from the demands and expectations of the professionals in the organization.

Future Directions

Some educational institutions have brief courses in management skills targeted to the needs of health-care professionals. These may or may not concentrate on medical topics. In recent years, the educational needs of the physician who enters management have been addressed by professional organizations. The American College of Physician Executives (formerly the Association of American Medical Directors) was founded in 1975 to provide education in management topics to the physician leaders of group practices. This organization broadened its scope when it became apparent that physicians who were assuming such roles in hospitals, the military, HMOs, and the insurance industry had similar needs. Under a grant from the Robert Wood Johnson Foundation, ACPE established the "Physician in Management" courses, intense, short-term exposures taught by the faculty of universities and covering such topics as finance, medical economics, organizational issues, personnel management, medicolegal affairs, labor relations, and marketing.

The American College of Physician Executives has adopted the medical model for physician managers. It offers the trappings of a medical specialty: continuing education, medical conferences, representation of the professional group in varied arenas, accolades such as fellowships, and lately, board certification through an independent American Board of Medical Management. Whether this will be the appropriate model remains to be seen. Some believe that acquisition of management skills through traditional business education and testing these skills in the crucible of the marketplace will be more important.

The physician who enters management in mid-career often must rely on brief courses and continuing medical education to provide a background. The time consumed in directing an organization and attempting to maintain clinical interests often precludes securing formal education. A number of formal educational opportunities are available which minimize the time in residence, and through brief but intense sessions on campus, frequent weekend classes, computer interaction, and teleconferencing, they offer the M.B.A. degree, master of public health, or a master's degree in health care administration. These educational offerings are usually not limited to physicians, but programs specifically targeted to physicians are emerging. More and more physicians are seeking management education early in their careers with the intent of spending a lifetime in medical management.

A question that often arises is how involved the medical executive should be clinically. It is not only reasonable but advisable for the physician who is promoted from within to continue such involvement. It is always wise to keep one's options open if there is the possibility or necessity of a return to practice. Clinical activity, by maintaining the same discipline and obligations to meet patient needs as do one's colleagues, is particularly helpful in maintaining one's credibility with them. In addition, such experience is valuable in providing insights as to how well the institution is functioning from the standpoint of the practitioner. The difficulties of developing a practice, achieving licensure in a new jurisdiction, and qualifying for hospital privileges may make assuming a clinical role impossible for those physicians who are recruited from outside the institution as chief executive officer.

The reward system for one who assumes a management role usually brings some premium above that for a pure clinician. However, as a rule the difference is not marked, and in most instances the institution pegs the rewards for physician managers below those of the more lucrative specialties. For this reason, one finds that endocrinologists, pediatricians, and psychiatrists vastly outnumber orthopedic surgeons and cardiovascular surgeons in the halls of management. Medical management also carries some risks not present in clinical medicine: clinicians rarely lose their jobs, but managers may get fired.

The number of physicians devoting their careers to medical management is increasing. The proliferation of prepayment groups and PPOs, and the expectation that hospitals will have to provide a cohesive product, will continue to create opportunties. More and more physicians will seek formal education earlier in their careers and will plan a career in management from the beginning. The large group practices and the prestigious teaching hospitals will still tend to recruit from within.

The broader issues in establishing medical management as a legitimate pursuit hinge on dissociation of the linkage between the physician executive and a single medical institution that selects and shapes his or her activities. If a career as a physician manager is to be a bona fide professional endeavor, then three key issues must be resolved.

First, if the physician manager of the future is to gain the knowledge and skills necessary for success by a formal educational process and graduated responsibility commensurate with increasing competence, it will require his or her full time and energy. Simply put, he or she will be a physician manager, not an internist/physician manager or a surgeon/physician manager. The burgeoning needs of major medical institutions will not be met by a physician for whom medical management is an avocation rather than a vocation. The by-product of such dedication to a single endeavor is that physicians entering the field may not be able to rely on activities in a clinical medical specialty to earn their living, as they have in the past.

Second, if practice as a physician manager is a full-time, bona fide vocation that does not tolerate falling back to another specialty, then the skills and knowledge of the manager need to be transportable. If those skills and knowledge are applicable to only one organization, then the physician manager faces too high a risk in choosing a managerial career path. Physician managers will require graduated responsibility, but not all organizations will have an opportunity at every tier waiting for their manager at the exact time he or she is ready for advancement, and that includes advancement to the highest position. Health care is a turbulent industry. Good managers will find it necessary, at times, to leave positions and must be able to find other opportunities rather easily.

The last issue is perhaps the most complex of the three and concerns the clinical physician's perceptions of the value added by a physician manager. If physicians are not made cognizant of the physician manager's knowledge and skills and do not see how those talents can improve their lot, then the attraction of the specialty will be lost. It will not be considered a worthwhile field to enter, it will not attract bright individuals, and it will not be able to require formal education and training for entry and advancement.

The task of making physician managers bona fide medical specialists, needed by patients and respected by colleagues, is at hand. It is an exciting task, and as with most exciting tasks, it will prove somewhat risky to those who tackle it.

Resources

Medical Group Management Association, 1355 S. Colorado Blvd., Suite 900, Denver, CO 80222

American Group Practice Association, 1422 Duke Street, Alexandria, VA 22314

Group Health Association of America, 1129 50th St., N.W. Suite 600, Washington, DC 20036

American College of Physician Executives, Two Urban Centre #200, 4890 W. Kennedy Blvd., Tampa, FL 33609

Suggested Reading

Riddick, Frank A., "Quality Assessment in the Group Practice Setting." Group Practice Journal 39: 9–18.

19 | Acquiring Space for Your Medical Practice

HENRY C. KELLEY, JR., MBA, CPM

Space for your medical practice can be acquired in a variety of different ways. Most physicians either lease their space in a building from an unrelated party or own their space individually or through a partnership arrangement. One form of ownership that has proved successful is for a general partner to act as the property manager and the occupants be limited partners. The individual tenant/limited partner pays rent to the general partner/property manager. The tenants are able to deduct their rent as a cost to their practice and receive passive income or losses from their partnership interest. The partner/tenants must pay market rents to make the lease and partnership interests withstand the many trials of partnership administration. An advisory committee or board can be established to assist the general partner with building issues. This assures the limited partner/tenants that their long-term interests are being considered.

Your accountant should help you determine the best form of space use depending on your current financial picture. A lease-versus-buy calculation can be done by your accountant to determine which form of space use would best serve your particular goals

During the early 1980s many financial advisors encouraged their clients to purchase the real estate used in their practice. However, consider the plight of one physician who was encouraged to move from leased space to a new facility in a growing urban area. He became so enthused over the new office project that he found two new partners to share in the project. They acquired the land, constructed the building, and financed it through a local mortgage company for 80% of the appraised value. The loan was almost 100% of the cost. In the mid-1980s it was not unusual for property to be appraised higher than its cost because of escalating land prices and the relatively easy lending practices of that time. Now the owner of the building finds himself without the two partners that were part of the original partnership and is responsible for all of the debt to the mortgage company.

Because his former partners no longer occupy part of the building, he has a specialized medical building with more space than he needs. The building was designed to accommodate three medical professionals with a common lobby and reception area. Unless he can find other medical professionals who can be compatible with his practice he will have to either reconfigure the building or sell the building to another medical group.

A recent appraisal of the building indicates the property has decreased in value by approximately 20% from its construction cost, because of the overbuilt suburban office market in this city, and is worth less than the mortgage balance. The lease-versus-buy analysis this physician did before committing to this type of space apparently did not accurately assess the risk variables he now faces.

To Buy or To Lease

The decision of whether to lease or buy your space cannot be made from a generalized set of rules. The variables that must be considered include the stability of your practice and the predictability of the space needs you will have in the future. Your personal financial picture and your tolerance for risk are primary indicators of whether you should own your property. If you are forced to spend your time looking for tenants for your building, finding qualified repairmen, collecting rents, and other management duties, then this time will be taken away from your practice or personal free time. In either case, few property managers are able to command fees for their management and leasing duties comparable to those of a physician.

The easiest and probably the best route for medical professionals is to simplify their space use by finding leased or owned space in a professionally managed complex. Property management companies handle all types of medical space, including space leased from unrelated parties, condominium space, and where physicians own a part of the partnership and lease space from the partnership. Each type of space is suited for different needs and users.

If you decide to purchase real estate, be sure you understand your obligations with regard to the partnership agreement and any related mortgage arrangements. There is a huge difference between a limited partner and a general partner in a partnership. There is also a tremendous difference between taking part in a project with nonrecourse debt and one with debt that obligates the partners to joint and several liability. Your attorney should review and explain the possible problems of any partnership arrangement you are considering. Learn to ask the question, What happens if this project fails and all the other partners leave?

Standard Units of Measurement

Before you begin shopping for that ideal office, prepare yourself with a basic understanding of terms commonly used in the building management trade.

Full-Floor Net-Rentable Method

This basis includes certain common areas, such as lavatories, hallways, and elevator vestibules.

Multitenant Net-Rentable Floor Method

This measure deletes the common areas, such as corridors, elevators, lobbies, and lavatories. The multitenant net-rentable measure frequently is referred to as the *usable square footage area.*Consistent with this is the so-called BOMA method of measurement adopted by the Building Owners and Managers Association.

The usable square foot measure was prevalent in older buildings; today, however, the majority of office building managers have converted to the full-floor net-rentable basis. On multitenant floors, a load factor generally is applied to the usable area so that the total square footage leased and charged for is equal to the net-rentable area on a full-floor basis.

Gross Building Area

This measure uses outside wall measurements of the entire building and includes the full-floor net-rentable area plus all stairwells, elevator shafts, janitorial closets, and other areas within the exterior walls of the building. As a user of space you should seek an understanding of the common area load factor being applied to your space, if any. Compare as an example two different rental rate quotes from different landlords:

> Landlord A leases on *usable* area (multitenant net-rentable floor method) basis. Landlord A's space is 2000 sq. ft. @ $12.00 per square foot usable area.

> Landlord B leases on the basis of *rentable* area (full floor net rentable area). Landlord B's space is 2000 sq. ft. @ $11.50 per square foot rentable area.

Your first question should be, What is the load factor for the common areas? After you have determined this information you can more accurately compare the two rental rates. If Landlord B has a building with a common area load factor of 15%, then the rental on the two proposals could be as follows:

$$\text{Landlord A} = 2000 \times \$12.00 = \qquad \$24,000 \text{ per year}$$
$$\text{Landlord B} = 2000 \times \$11.50 \times 1.15 = \$26,450 \text{ per year}$$

The purpose of this illustration is to emphasize the importance of comparing the various quotations you receive with a common unit of comparison.

The rental rate you pay should also be considered, keeping in mind services you require and those the landlord includes in the rental rate. If you lease space in a high-rise building you will probably have all utilities, janitorial services, and security included in the rental rate. Most landlords charge for after-hours utility consumption, extra security for after-hours use of the office, and utility consumption in excess of the building standard. You should negotiate a maximum charge for these extra services in your lease, if possible.

Whereas rental rates are often quoted on rentable area (with a load factor), the amount of "tenant finish" is usually quoted on the basis of usable square footage. This technique is utilized because the common areas have been finished—or should be—prior to your occupancy at the building owner's expense.

If, after deciding you like a particular building, the cost estimate of your tenant finish exceeds the landlord's allowance, then you should consider one or more of the following actions. (1) Look for cost-cutting techniques for treatment of wall areas, floor covering finishes, hardware, and number and composition of doors. (2) Ask at least two other contractors to price the job. (3) Ask the landlord to pay all or part of the difference, through either free rent or an increased allowance. (4) Ask the landlord to amortize the excess finish allowance over the term of your lease at a market rate of interest. (5) Write a check!

Whether you are able to improve your position on the tenant finish allowance is directly related to supply and demand. If building contractors are looking for work in your area, then having several contractors bid on the job could save from 5% to 20%. If the landlord needs you as a tenant to meet financial objectives, you may be able to negotiate a favorable rent rate and tenant finish allowance. You should investigate whether the building owner has the financial ability to carry out his or her promise to you. Typically the tenant in a medical space shares with the owner part of the tenant finish cost exceeding a standard allowance.

Building owners establish the building's standard tenant finish allowance in two basic ways. The first technique is to simply state in dollar terms the amount of money the tenant is allowed per square foot of usable area. This technique, along with a complete description of the condition of the space when you start the tenant finish construction, allows for an easily understood construction cost and related overage.

Some building owners provide a *per unit basis* finish allowance. For example, the tenant may be allowed one linear foot of wall area for each 100 square feet of rentable area, one electrical outlet per 150 square feet of rentable area, one telephone outlet per 150 square feet of rentable area, one interior door for each 200 square feet of rentable area, and so forth until all the components of the office are allocated on a square-foot basis.

It is generally believed that landlords can better control their finish costs using this technique through more thorough construction management. A company may prefer to negotiate on dollar allowances per square foot rather than dictating these per unit allowances in order to make their proposal as clear as possible to the prospective tenant. The company will provide a list of approved contractors for their tenants to choose from and will carefully review all plans before approval.

Tenant finish on either a dollar allowance or unit basis is usually based upon the developer's or manager's estimate of the amount required to finish the office for a typical user without extra items in the suite. When space is in oversupply, the developer/manager may become more creative and offer more elaborate finish allowances. Medical space typically costs at least two times more per square foot for tenant finish than space for a general business user. This cost differential is attributable to excess wall areas for the examination rooms, additional electrical and mechanical costs of heating and air conditioning, and extra electrical costs related to the examination room layout in the suite.

Do not enter into a lease in a nonmedical building until you have determined an approximate cost per square foot to finish the space for your needs. Converting nonmedical space to medical space is expensive, and you may find your tenant finish overage amounts to $15 to $20 per square foot over the allowance for a standard business user.

What Should I Ask for in a Lease Negotiation?

A lease is a negotiated contract and you should address the following areas to help provide your practice with the flexibility it may need.

Lease Term

This is the length of term and your related obligation to pay rent. The typical lease term is three to five years.

Option to Expand

This grants the tenant the right to lease a certain amount of space at a certain time and is usually given to larger, key tenants.

Option to Renew

This grants the tenant the right to renew the lease at the expiration of the original term. This is particularly useful when a neighboring tenant desires your space for expansion and is willing to pay a premium for your space. Most landlords will grant an option to renew as long as the rental rate can be set at the market rate at the time you exercise this option. The typical option term will be similar to the primary term of the lease.

Option to Cancel

Sometimes this provision is available to tenants whose business depends on one individual, such as a sole proprietor who is a lawyer or physician.

These points of negotiation are directly dependent on the relationship between the supply of available offices and what the other building owners are offering. Only through research can you accurately determine which of these points you should be able to negotiate into your lease arrangement.

Whether a practitioner or medical group seeks to buy or lease facilities depends on their available capital, their degree of willingness to assume risks in real estate investment, the nature of the real estate market in their community, and their business plan for the future. This section has attempted to familiarize the reader with the questions to consider and terminology he or she will face in making the choice to buy or lease practice facilities. As with every major business decision, take the time to do the research, know what questions to ask, be sure you fully understand all the alternatives, be aware of the pitfalls, and seek your advisors wisely before signing on the dotted line.

Subleasing and Medical Time-Share Arrangements

The previous section discussed conventional alternatives for acquiring medical office space with a lease or purchase. This section explores additional alternatives for locating space through a sublease or assignment from an existing tenant or through a time-share arrangement. The difference between an assignment and a sublease will be explained from a legal perspective. In addition, a discussion of possible solutions for dealing with excess space is included to assist those physicians who find themselves with unwanted office space.

Whenever you enter into a real estate transaction, you should consult an attorney who specializes in real estate matters. Accordingly, this section is intended to provide you with enough information on leasing to convince you of the effectiveness of this approach.

Overview of the Office Market

In most areas throughout the United States, there is a surplus of office space. This situation is the result of overbuilding by optimistic developers who had available financing for their projects. Many investors were lured to real estate by the favorable tax environment. Prior to the 1986 tax reform, higher-income individuals were able to shelter paper losses on real estate. These people invested in real estate with the hope of hedging inflation and creating real wealth.

Anticipated demand for new office space was severely overestimated in many areas. As a result, many office markets now require three to five years—or even longer—to reach a more balanced supply-and-demand relationship.

Because of the oversupply condition, any professional with unwanted office space may find it difficult to locate occupants for that space. In most markets, there are more offices available than there are professionals to rent the available space. These conditions create an environment in which tenants are able to negotiate more favorable terms on their lease arrangements.

In some areas of major cities, however, a particular type of office is not in oversupply. A seven-story medical building in Southern California can remain fully occupied because of a scarcity of developable sites in the property's neighborhood. Such scarcity can prevent an oversupply condition, thus accounting for a building's success.

You should be leery of entering into a lease agreement that seems too good to be true. You may be buying into a problem lease in which the owner fails to uphold the terms of the lease and/or the underlying mortgage. The best office lease arrangement is one in which the landlord and tenant both receive equitable treatment, thus motivating both parties to comply with the terms of the agreement. After all, a lawsuit with either a landlord or tenant over the use of your office is often counterproductive. Your office facilities should add to your productivity, not detract from your practice of medicine or the running of your business.

Typical Lease Terms in Medical Buildings

An understanding of commonly offered lease terms is necessary when analyzing how to make use of excess space. Common lease (rental) rates vary across the United States based on local conditions, but many of the lease terms other than a monthly rate are similar and are consistently used by managers across the country. The rights and obligations of the parties to the contract will depend on whether the landlord provides all services, utilities, and maintenance (as in a *full-service lease)* or whether the landlord simply leases the land to a tenant who will build a building (known as a *ground lease).*

Many different variations of lease arrangements can be found, but most medical office leases negotiated are full-service leases in which the landlord provides the physician with a turnkey solution to his or her space needs. Part of the job of a property manager is to make certain that capable janitorial, maintenance, and security personnel are provided for the building's occupants.

Physicians are not the only professionals currently choosing full-service leases. Companies ranging from computer sales to governmental agencies may also find the advantages of full-service leases more attractive. Tenants can have leased space with either a full-service or no-service lease. Most office tenants, however, require full-service lease arrangements so that they can focus their efforts on their primary business and not on locating and maintaining qualified vendors to fulfill their janitorial, maintenance, and security needs.

Leases: A Legal Perspective

Moynihan, in his book, *Introduction to the Law of Real Property,* defines the modern lease as:

> both a conveyance and a contract. It is a conveyance because it creates in the tenant an estate for years, but it is also a contract because of the covenants or promises made by the respective parties. The landlord covenants either ex-

pressly or impliedly that the tenant will have quiet enjoyment of the demised premises. The landlord will frequently make additional express covenants, depending on the nature of the property, with respect to repairs, furnishing of heat and other services, noncompetition with the lessee, and many other matters. (P. 69)

In turn, Moynihan continues, the tenant normally agrees to pay the rent on time, to use the premises for a specified purpose, and not to sublet without the landlord's consent. The tenant also agrees to leave the premises in good condition at the end of the lease term. Leases for business properties often include such additional covenants as those relating to taxes, insurance, repairs, and improvements; provisions concerning accidental destruction of the premises, defaults in rents, and condemnation proceedings against the property may also be addressed in those instruments.

"Thus," Moynihan concludes, "the modern lease is a highly complex instrument in which the contract element is a substantial, if not the predominant, ingredient" (p. 69).

Courts of law have not normally looked at leases in the same way as they have other bilateral contracts, most of which operate under the mutual dependency of promises. However, in a lease contract situation, if one covenant of a lease is not fulfilled by the landlord (such as promised repairs), then this nonfulfillment does not relieve his or her tenant of the obligation to pay rent. Instead, it will give rise to a cause for breach of contract by the landlord.

Subleases and Assignments: A Legal Perspective

As Kratovil, in *Real Estate Law*, explains, "Unless the lease provides otherwise, a lessee may assign his lease or sublet the premises" (p. 435). If the lease forbids an assignment without the landlord's consent, it does not necessarily prohibit a sublease. As a general rule, a commercial lease prohibits both assignments and subleases without the landlord's consent.

Kratovil continues, "Whether a particular instrument is an assignment or sublease does not depend upon the name given the instrument by the parties. An *assignment* simply transfers the leasehold estate to a new owner, the assignee. A *sublease* creates a new and distinct leasehold estate in the sublease. If the lessee transfers the entire unexpired remainder of the term created by the lease, the instrument is an assignment. If the lessee retains part of the term, however small the part may be, or transfers only part of the leased premises the instrument is a sublease" (p. 435; italics added).

The difference between an assignment and a sublease is critical, because an assignee becomes liable to the *original* landlord for rent. A subtenant, on the other hand, is liable only to the sublandlord (who is also the tenant to the original landlord).

The following will illustrate this point: Landlord L leases certain premises to Physician T for a term beginning on May 1, 1986, and expiring on

April 30, 1991, at a rent of $1000 per month. On July 1, 1988, Physician T executes to Physician X a "sublease" for a term beginning on July 1, 1988, and expiring April 30, 1991, at a rent of $1500 per month. Although the document was called a sublease, it is legally an assignment.

Here is an example of the opposite situation: Landlord L leases to Physician T certain premises for a term beginning on May 1, 1986, and expiring on April 30, 1991. On July 1, 1988, Physician T executes to Physician X an "assignment" of said lease [except the term expires, one day before Physician's "T" lease expires]. Although the document is called an assignment, it is legally a sublease.

To protect themselves from tenants who sublease or assign a lease without permission, landlords often insert a restrictive clause into the lease agreement. One example of a restrictive clause used in a medical office building lease in Little Rock, Arkansas, is as follows: "*Sublease and Assignment:* Lessee shall not sublet any part of the premises or assign this lease without the prior written consent of lessor. Any sublease or assignment without such prior written consent shall be void and shall, at the option of the Lessor, terminate this Lease."

Of course, one's interest in restrictive clauses for subleases will depend upon one's position in the contract. If you are the owner and/or landord, you might consider the following as an excellent example of the protection of the landlord's rights:

> Assignment and subletting: Tenant shall not, either voluntarily, involuntarily, or by operation of law, sell, hypothecate, assign, transfer, or sublet this Lease, the Demised Premises, or any part thereof to be occupied by anyone other than Tenant or Tenant's employees without the prior written consent of Landlord, which consent may be withheld in Landlord's sole discretion. Any sale, assignment, mortgage, transfer, or subletting of this Lease which is not in compliance with provisions of this paragraph shall be void and Landlord shall have the option to terminate this Lease.

An assignment or sublease provision such as the above helps to protect the owner's control of the type of occupant that ultimately uses the premises. A property manager needs this control in order to assure the other occupants, as well as the owner, that the space will be leased for the type of use specified. The provision also helps prevent undesirable uses within the property. This provision does restrict the ability of the lessee to sublease or assign its lease.

A provision providing more flexibility for the tenant would be reworded as an affirmative statement with restrictive controls by the landlord: "Tenant shall have the right to sublease or assign this lease with owners' written approval; said approval shall not be unreasonably withheld."

Whether you, as a prospective lessee, can obtain sublease and assignment rights such as in the example above will depend upon your ability to negotiate this provision into the lease agreement. If the building is tightly controlled as to the type of occupants, you will probably not obtain an affirmative statement, but might be able to obtain the phrase, "Said approval shall not be unreasonably withheld." Inserting this language into your lease would allow for some flexibility when it comes to negotiating for renting to a sublessee.

The terms of the underlying lease will dictate the offer to a prospective subtenant; however, final terms will evolve through negotiations and can be more or less favorable than the terms of the underlying lease. The correct procedure when preparing to sublease or assign your space or to occupy another space under an assignment or sublease is to first consult your attorney about the terms of the underlying lease.

If your lease does not have a provision stating the lease will be terminated upon a proposed sublease or assignment, then approach the building owner before finalizing the sublease or assignment. Ideally, one should contact the landlord prior to advertising the space. It is important to give the manager of the building advance notice and an understanding of what you intend to do with the space as soon as possible. Do not surprise the manager with a completly signed sublease or assignment and then to expect him or her to immediately approve the document.

It may be wise to reevaluate the language of all leases to determine if they contain provisions that might be challenged as being a breach of the implied covenant of good faith and fair dealing. From a property manager's point of view, legal decisions such as the one to be illustrated will make landlords more vigilant in exercising their restrictive rights over a tenant attempting to sublease.

Tenants who have been most effective in dealing with a sublease or assignment have (1) understood the rights of landlord and tenant under their particular lease by reviewing their leases with their attorneys and (2) made known their intended action before finalizing any agreements. A property manager will normally react more favorably if a physician advises the manager in advance that an attorney will contact him or her with the details of the documentation. When leases do not contain cancellation provisions in the event of a proposed assignment or sublease, tenants may not be hesitant to discuss their desire to sublease or assign their leases.

The Courts and Recapture

As with all contract law, the terms of a lease contract itself can be contested in the courts when there is a dispute between the parties to the agreement. Some leases contain a recapture provision, which allows the landlord to terminate a tenant's lease upon receipt of notice from the tenant that he or she proposes to assign or sublet all or part of the lease premises.

Recent developments in the California courts have required commercial property owners and managers to reevaluate their sublease and assignment lease provisions. A California appellate court has decided that a landlord cannot enforce the so-called recapture provision, which is commonly included in assignment and subletting clauses of commercial leases.

Carma Developers, Inc., v. Marathon Development, Inc. ("Carma"), was just such a case. Attorneys have commented:

> "In Carma, the recapture provision allowed the landlord to terminate the entire lease upon either a proposed assignment or subletting. The tenant requested the landlord's consent to a proposed sublease of a portion of the tenant's premises. The tenant was in the fourth year of a 10-year lease and had expended $400,000 for tenant improvements. The landlord elected to terminate the lease based upon the recapture provision. The tenant vacated the premises and sued for breach of contract, negligent and intentional interference with prospective economic advantage and breach of the implied covenant of good faith and fair dealing. The trial court found breach of contract because the recapture provisions were commercially unreasonable and violated the implied covenant of good faith and fair dealing. (Steiner, Jeffer, Mangles, Butler and Marmaro Law Firm, personal communication, August 29, 1989)

A verdict was found in the tenant's favor and a settlement of $315,000 was awarded.

The appellate court, in upholding the trial court's decision, found that the recapture clause was void for two reasons. First, the clause was void as a matter of public policy because if enforced, the clause would constitute an unreasonable restraint on alienation. Second, the court held that the clause was commercially unreasonable and therefore breached the implied covenant of good faith and fair dealing. An appeal of the Carma decision is pending before the California Supreme Court.

As attorneys point out:

> The Carma decision leaves open several questions regarding the enforceability of recapture provisions and related limitations on the tenant's right to assign or sublet.
>
> The court in Carma does not address the enforceability of provisions through which the landlord shares in the profits derived by the tenant from a permitted assignment or sublease. However, the California Supreme Court in Kendall v. Ernest Pestana, Inc., one of the leading cases in this area, suggested that a reasonable profit-sharing clause would be enforceable. (Steiner et al., personal communication, August 29, 1989)

Whether or not you are conversant in real estate law, what this example points out is the absolute necessity of having a competent real estate attorney in your corner. This area of the law can be highly technical and contentious. Having an attorney point out pitfalls before you sign an agreement is the best strategy.

Practical Application

No professional wants to pay rent on space that cannot be used productively. Therefore, a physician should either negotiate a flexible front-end lease with cancellation rights, and operate his or her practice until the lease expires, or prepare to enter the sublease market and attempt to find a replacement tenant for any excess space.

You may want to handle finding a tenant yourself. Certainly any physician can run an advertisement in the local paper for his or her available space. If market conditions are favorable, a suitable prospect may be found quickly. More typically, however, available space exceeds physicians ready and able to use the space. "On-campus" locations (so called because of being situated adjacent to a hospital "campus") are typically in high demand and in some cases may provide an opportunity for the physician to profit from the sublease. Incurring a profit or loss with the sublease is determined by the current market conditions as compared with the market conditions at the time your underlying lease was signed.

Whereas an attorney can protect your interest by reviewing your current lease and making certain the sublease or assignment is properly drafted and executed, a real estate agent specializing in commercial leasing is the best source for prospects and determining the market rent for your space. In many larger metropolitan markets, lease brokers specialize in office space leases and, sometimes, only medical office leasing. These professionals normally work on a contingency basis and charge a percentage of the rents to be collected under the lease they negotiate. The percentage fee will vary depending on the lease or assignment and may be on a decreasing scale with longer-term leases. A flat fee may be arranged if the term of the sublease is not sufficient to warrant a broker investing his or her time to recruit a new tenant. If the remaining term of your master lease is less than two years, then a flat fee to the lease broker would probably be most appropriate.

Medical Time-Share Arrangements

The shared office concept was developed by office building owners and managers when vacancy rates escalated. The concept has proved to be an incubator of sorts for smaller tenants starting businesses, allowing them to later become larger tenants in regular office environments.

The influx of time-sharing suites in the medical profession, as well as in other professional settings, is intended to utilize a pool of resources which each individual could not secure as economically as they could under the shared concept. The shared office can be as informal as two or three professionals sharing expenses in an office complex or as structured as multilevel executive suites in major metropolitan areas which provide a broad array of executive services. Cooperative office projects provide ready-to-rent offices available on short-term arrangements.

Managers recognize three advantages to having a time-share office suite in their building: it provides the ability to establish a relationship with growing professionals, the ability to lease smaller offices to shorter-term tenants, and the opportunity to offer support to other tenants in the building.

In the medical area, the time-share or shared-office concept has proved to be an effective marketing tool to help a hospital accommodate a physician in transition. The time-share office allows the hospital to find a home for a physician and bond that physician to the hospital campus. For that reason, hospital administrators normally view the time-share concept as an extension of their recruiting and marketing division rather than as a free-standing economic entity. Some time-share enterprises are independently owned and so must quickly reach a certain occupancy level in order to be profitable. Some independent operators focus on favorable lease or mortgage terms to help them bridge the start-up period of reaching a break-even level of occupancy in the building.

Medical time-share office suite projects have not been well documented. However, traditional office projects have been offering a version of the time-share in a form many managers call executive suites or shared-service suites. Although these facilities do not sell an actual time period in the premises, as do recreational time-shares, a fixed level of service and space use is leased in return for a monthly rent.

One traditional shared-service program was well documented recently in the magazine *Real Estate Today*. The program described three tiers of service to fit a wide variety of needs in the market. The first tier was aimed at businesspeople—operators of new businesses, sales representatives, and people who work out of their homes—who needed an address and a corporate identity but not an office. For a monthly fee, tenants received such services as personalized telephone answering, reception, mail and package receipt, use of an address and telephone number on their business stationery, and a directory listing in the building lobby. Five hours of conference room time each month were included in the monthly charges.

The second tier of service was designed for new one-person businesses and short-term tenants, whereas the third tier serviced other current tenants in the building. The users of the second tier of service ranged from a psychiatrist who needed a private office away from the clinic to a local representative for a regional computer consulting firm. Most of the tenants who signed up for the third tier of service were smaller tenants and physicians who had two offices.

Medical buildings on hospital campuses are increasingly using the medical time-share concept. Physicians' suites are operated by the hospital and combine individual practices and/or small group practices. The suites have the capability to provide several doctors at a time with examination rooms, patient access, office services, and procedure rooms. The hospital typically equips the facility to handle the basic needs of the general practitioner. If equipment is needed for a specialty, then the physician must purchase this equipment or work out an acceptable agreement with the hospital.

A time-share unit may additionally include access to radiology, a stat laboratory facility, chemical analyzer, hematology analyzer, and EKG. The mission of the time-share suite is to allow a doctor to put on his or her coat and start seeing patients as quickly as possible. Minimizing the administrative headaches of locating space and securing equipment is the goal of most physicians, especially those in transition.

The advantages of time-share suites for the occupants are threefold: they eliminate the need for front-end capital, they eliminate the need to manage personnel, and they provide proximity to the hospital campus for maximum efficiency.

Hospitals rarely utilize the medical suites for the sole purpose of direct profit. Instead, the suites produce an environment for recruiting and keeping physicians and for temporarily placing physicians who are in transition.

The group of doctors in transition may include the following: a physician who has just completed residency; a physician whose practice has been sold and who is considering retirement but wants to continue seeing some patients; a physician with outdated and worn-out equipment, but who is close enough to retirement that replacing the equipment is not feasible; a physician from a smaller area who wants to expand his or her practice skills in a more metropolitan area; a physician whose practice group has disintegrated and needs to use a suite; and any physician between practices.

Overview of a Medical Time-Share Suite

An example of one medical time-share arrangement is illustrated in Table 19.1. The arrangement is nothing more than a menu concept, in which the tenant has access to certain standard items on the menu with optional access to other items, depending upon need and the nature of the specialty involved. These programs are normally sold in blocks of four hours (half days) with a minimum of a six-month lease.

The leases available in half-day units include all utilities, janitorial services, and basic telephone services (including direct hospital lines) as well as the additional services listed in Table 19.1.

Hospital administrators have come to believe that investing in a medical time-share facility is productive because it allows physicians to (1) expand practice accessibility while allowing patients easy access to the hospital; (2) increase the number of patients seen by offering services in the area near the facility; (3) provide flexible hours to meet the practice schedule in an affordable fashion by leasing just the time increment needed; and (4) broaden the referral base to include physicians practicing on the hospital campus.

Other examples of medical time-sharing projects have appeared throughout the United States with varying success. A Chicago project mentioned in an October 1987 *American Medical News* article is operated by a company that sublets one floor of prime office space in a medical building in the heart of the city's business district. Each physician or dentist who rents space there comes a few days each week. The approximately 50 physicians have main offices in other parts of the city, but to patients who visit the time-share suites it appears that a large group practice is in residence. The company runs the waiting room, supplies a recep-

Table 19.1 Example of Time-Share Facilities

Patient Care Areas

1. Exclusive use of two of the six functionally equipped examination rooms, including:
   A. Examination table with drawer warmer and airlift examination stool
   B. Diagnostic wall transformer with otoscope and ophthalmoscope
   C. Flexible, multipurpose task lamp
   D. Blood pressure cuff, stethoscope, oral thermometer
   E. Basic consumable soft goods (swabs, sponges, Band-Aids, etc.)
2. Use of single-channel electrocardiograph
3. Use of procedure room, including:
   Multiposition electronic power examination table
   Private patient bathroom
   Storage for personal instruments

Other Areas

1. Use of conference room
2. Use of physicians' private lounge and work area, complete with desk space and separate phones
3. Use of kitchen and break room

Laboratory

1. Access to in-house laboratory facilities, including basic laboratory equipment: centrifuge, microscope, hematology analyzer, and blood drawing station (*does not include services of laboratory technician*)
2. In-house tests billable to the physician at a cost-per-test rate comparable to outside reference test fees
3. Use of additional equipment and facilities, including:
   A. Four conveniently located x-ray viewers
   B. Storage for consumable pharmaceuticals
   C. Storage for patient charts and medical records
   D. (Future item: data link to hospital data base)

Reception Area and Business Office

1. Pleasant, attractive patient waiting room
2. Receptionist/front business office area, including:
   A. Built-in desk and work area to accommodate three people
   B. Reception/cashier functions (including telephone support five days per week)
   C. Copier, typewriter, and general office supplies
3. Business manager, providing the following:
   A. Transition planning and support
   B. Practice promotion (planning, writing, and design of copy)
   C. Assistance in patient-related business management services—that is, establishing policies and promotion of patient relations
   D. Service as a purchasing agent for the physician, locating goods and services at the best pass-through pricing
   E. General supervisory and ancillary support to facility

Optional Services Available (billable monthly)

1. Patient billing
2. Insurance billing
3. Transcription services
4. Registered ancillary personnel
5. Items not included in the lease-per-hour fee:
   A. Direct cost of practice promotion (media services, printing, etc.)
   B. Patient record-keeping forms and charting system
   C. Preprinted paper goods (letterhead stationery, prescription pads, etc.)
   D. Outside laundry
   E. Long-distance telephone services
   F. Surgical instrumentation
   G. Pharmaceuticals
   H. Dispensable soft goods

tionist, and, for an extra charge, takes care of the billing. The physicians pay half the standard rent for the area and can create new referral relationships with their fellow time-sharers. A wide range of specialties is located in the same time-share facility, and executives and office workers on their lunch breaks can take advantage of physicians who are close to their places of work.

Two additional time-share arrangements are managed by Lifespan Healthcare Services. Edina Medical Clinic, located in a Minneapolis suburb, was started in 1985 by a group of internists. They began with several internists, a group of gastroenterologists, a nephrologist, a cardiologist, a urologist, and an endocrinologist. The mix of physicians has changed over time, but the facility has consistently included a variety of subspecialists while providing space at a reasonable charge.

A board of directors composed of physicians with ownership interest in the clinic sets the time-share rates and makes decisions about other major policy issues. Daily management functions are handled by a manager hired by the board. The clinic has its own laboratory and sells these services to the physicians on a wholesale basis. The physicians bill their patients for these laboratory procedures at their own fee schedule rates.

Physicians sign a one-year contract and pay for a set amount of appointment times throughout the year, whether they use the time or not. The typical time slot is four hours, from 8 a.m. to 12 p.m. or from 1 p.m. to 5 p.m.

The clinic is currently relocating to a medical office building in order to improve the space's efficiency and location.

Started in 1985 as a women's clinic, the Isles Medical Group, also in Minneapolis, currently has four obstetrician-gynecologists and six internists. The Isles Clinic has evolved from a total time-share clinic to a hybrid variety, with a mix of time-share users and a regular practice that bills third-party carriers. Unlike the Edina Clinic, the Isles Clinic has not utilized a physician board of directors, though its physician board does help create a network of contacts necessary to bring in enough time-share users.

What Drives Medical Time-Shares

The success and motivation for the medical time-share arrangement is illustrated by the story of a 35-year-old general surgeon in a rural area who needed a way to grow professionally. He was ready to move and wanted a place to house his practice and some of his existing staff. A local community hospital was able to quickly establish the surgeon in practice and minimize the administrative side of his practice through the help of the physician's suite manager. Most physicians who follow the proven marketing practice developed by the office manager will see their practices grow substantially in a short time. Marketing a physician's practice is one of the jobs of the medical time-share manager.

According to one medical time-share manager, the practice of time-share for medical practitioners is driven more by its recruiting value than its direct profitability. Because some institutions are using these facilities as a recruiting tool, a physician should recognize them as an excellent resource to build patient bases, either in multiple areas or as a market-testing tool; if the market is a profitable one, then the physician can secure a more permanent location. The hospital referrals should easily be worth the typical minimum commitment of six months.

Conclusion

When considering your options for office locations, keep in mind two areas that are often overlooked. Medical time-share programs present options in larger markets that allow you to open new areas of practice without obligating yourself to long-term lease arrangements or considerable outlay for new equipment. Many times these programs are sponsored by major hospitals as a way to attract doctors in transition. These programs pool equipment and office staff in a package that allows the group to utilize resources more efficiently than they could as individuals in private practice.

Physicians may also find space currently leased to another physician or related professional who is underutilizing the space. Usually someone with underutilized space is glad to sublease excess space to minimize the amount of rent they are responsible for in the lease agreement. There are differences between subleases and assignments, so physicians are well advised to consult a real estate attorney when negotiating with the original lease holder.

Suggested Reading

Kratovil, Robert, *Real Estate Law.* Englewood Cliffs, NJ: Prentice-Hall, 1974.

Moynihan, Cornelius J., *Introduction to the Law of Real Property.* St. Paul, MN: West Publishing, 1962.

Page, Leigh, "New Twist on Time-Sharing System Lets Sole Practitioners Share Space, Staff, Equipment." *American Medical News* (October 1987):17.

Toler, Pamela, "Lease More Than Just Space." *Real Estate Today* (January/February 1990):66.

20 | Office Design: How to Optimize Patient Flow, Staff Convenience, and Ambience

JOANNE MOSER, RNMN

This chapter will cover the basic body of knowledge needed to develop your office environment. Several excellent books are available and your designer can guide you as well. Basic information about space planning, some specific information about specialty areas, and the design process itself will be covered. Interior design will be covered in detail in the next chapter.

Where to begin

All successful businesses begin with a good business plan. You and your business advisor should develop a business plan that includes short- and long-range goals. Focus on where you want your practice to be in five years: space planners like to assume that they can plan all contingencies 10 years or more in advance, but the reality of modern medicine, with its inherent technological and social changes, prohibits planning much beyond five years. One assumption it is safe to make is that your practice will be dynamic, which means change. Planning intelligently for change is the crux of a successful office space.

The time to hire a space planner is when you begin to look at space. The designer can help you decide which space will be the easiest to build out and the most conducive to meeting your needs. How do you choose a designer? There are several types of professionals from which to choose. An architect is a licensed, well-educated professional. It is essential to use an architect if you will be constructing a building. A space planner is typically an interior designer, also well educated, and may be used when tenant improvement work is all that is required. An interior designer will additionally perform all interior design work, such as choosing your color scheme and furnishing your office. No matter which category of professional you choose, one element is imperative: *choose a person with expertise in medical design.* No other type of design experience is comparable. Interview several candidates. Review their portfolios. Check their references. Choose someone with whom you can work well, and make sure he or she has the time to commit to your project. Naturally you will want to review the candidates' fees. Designers charge in several ways: hourly rate, square foot rate, a project fee, or an hourly rate with a not-to-exceed figure. The most desirable fee system for you will be one where the design cost is set. If you are very clear on the scope of the project, the designer may agree to structure the fee that way. When you request proposals, specify how you want the fee structured so that you can compare the proposals. Additionally, if the designer will be purchasing furniture or furnishings, the proposals should specify the discount allowance. Compare these, as well as the fees and you will have a complete idea of the cost to you. When you have all the information, you can make an intelligent decision.

Space Plan

The space plan begins with the building itself. Here is a checklist to use when evaluating a building.

1. Is the building easily accessible by car, bus, or taxi?
2. Are signs displayed effectively?
3. Is there adequate parking?
4. Are there enough elevators to serve the building?
5. Are there core facilities (e.g., restrooms, drinking fountains, public telephones) for your use?
6. Is there adequate square footage? Can it easily be configured to meet your needs?
7. Does the building have adequate power, plumbing, and air conditioning/heating to meet your needs?
8. Is the building constructed to accommodate the weight of your equipment?
9. Are there construction restrictions?
10. Is there additional adjacent space available for future expansion?

Some of these requirements are self-evident, and some will require the input of your space planner. Inadequate parking is the most frequent problem with office buildings. For example, in Los Angeles a 5 to 1 ratio of office to parking square footage is needed for medical office buildings—that is, if your suite has 2000 square feet, you will need 10 parking spaces. Not only do you need to meet this criterion, so do the other tenants. In mixed-use buildings the total number of parking spaces may be reduced. You need to ascertain that at least the required number of spaces are available to you at all times. Patients will not drive around for 10 minutes looking for a place to park; they will go elsewhere.

Core facilities usually consist of restrooms, a central telephone and power room, janitorial service area, hot water heater, public telephones, and a drinking fountain. If a building does not have these facilities, you will have to incorporate them into your space and pay fully for their use. It is to your advantage to have a building with core facilities and share their expense with other tenants. It will also decrease the amount of space you will need within your own suite.

The building structure must be able to meet your power, plumbing, and equipment needs. This is another good reason to have your designer look at the space with you. If the building cannot structurally accommodate your 2000-lb x-ray table, it would be good to know this before you sign the lease. The designer can also assess the overall dimensions of the space you are considering, location of windows, ceiling height, and other structural elements in deciding on design possibilities and constraints.

Ascertain if there are construction restrictions defined by the building owner. If the owner will allow construction only after hours to prevent noise and use of the elevators by workers, your cost to build out your space will be considerably higher.

You might choose a building with many of these problems anyway, just because the location is so desirable. At least by asking the proper questions, you will know what to expect and how much it will cost you.

The Design Process: The Programming Phase

The first step your designer will take in developing your space is to collect data regarding your needs.

1. Define your business goals, both short and long range.
2. Identify the staff you will need initially and in five years. Define their job functions. If you already have staff, involve them as much as possible in the planning phase. If you have job descriptions, share them with the designer.
3. Define the various departments in your office and how they will interrelate.
4. Identify the equipment you anticipate using and the salesperson who can supply specific information regarding size, power, water, and other requirements.
5. List any special requirements you have, such as oversized doors, soundproofing, special lighting, ventilation, shielding, or decorative items.
6. Describe the desired ambience of your office. Do you want it to be comfortable, elegant, casual, slick, or homey?
7. If you can, list the type of rooms you want and their approximate size.
8. Identify your budget so the designer knows right away how to gear the project.

The designer will take all the information you have offered and initially develop a simple bubble diagram (Figure 20.1) and a program (Table 20.1).

The bubble diagram simply illustrates the flow and functional relationships. Once this is reviewed and approved by you, an initial space plan will be developed. It should include room names, sizes, furniture, and major equipment layouts. Have the designer explain in detail everything about the plan. This is the time to critique and make changes; it costs virtually nothing to change walls now. Ask as many questions as necessary, and

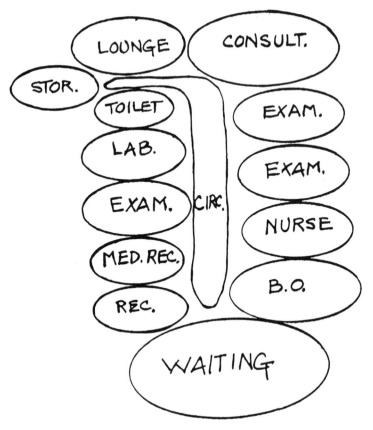

Figure 20.1. Bubble diagram.

Table 20.1 Designer's Program

Program	Quantity	Size (ft)	Total (ft)
Area			
Waiting room	1	10 × 15	150
Reception	1	10 × 10	100
Business office	1	10 × 15	150
Medical records	1	7 × 10	70
Consultation	1	10 × 12	120
Lounge	1	8 × 10	80
Examination rooms	3	8 × 10	240
Nurses' station	1	8 × 10	80
Laboratory	1	8 × 10	80
Toilet	1	6½ × 7	46
Storage	1	6 × 8	48
			1164
Circulation space		+ 20%	233
			1397

remember that blueprints are as difficult for you to read as x-rays are for the designer. If you have staff, have them review the plan too.

The basic medical office will have a waiting room, reception area, business office, examination rooms, consultation office, nurses' station, storage room, and medical records area. It may also include a toilet room, procedure room, x-ray room, darkroom, laboratory, employee lounge, janitorial closet, electrical and telephone room, and specialty areas such as a physical therapy room, cast room, chemotherapy infusion room, lens-fitting room, visual field room, dermatology light room, and so on. This chapter will address only basic practice areas and highlight some common specialty needs.

The waiting room should be spacious without being oversized. It must accommodate all possible patients and visitors. If you will be seeing 30 patients in a six-hour day, or five patients per hour, you will need seating for 10. Table 20.1 allows seating for one hour's appointments, plus family who accompany patients, and includes a factor for late appointments. Each person will require 15 square feet, so a waiting room of approximately 150 square feet should be designed. Some practices will require additional space for a children's play area.

The reception area needs to accommodate all the staff who will ultimately work there, plus room for a copier, fax machine, computer terminal, typewriter, and, perhaps, medical records. Each employee will need a minimum of 40 square feet plus space for equipment. If you have two receptionists, you will need at least 80 square feet.

A typical consultation office is 10 x 14 ft, which will accommodate an executive desk (36 x 72 in.), credenza, bookcase, executive chair, and two side chairs. A 10 x 12 office will basically accommodate the same furniture if the desk is smaller (30 x 60 in.). See Figures 20.2 and 20.3.

Some physicians dislike the barrier of a desk between themselves and patients. A lounge type of seating arrangement (Figure 20.4) with a sofa and chairs can be substituted. The desk area can be built in along one wall with overhead storage above the desk. Examination rooms are as variable as stars in the sky. A minimum size for an examination room is 8 x 10 feet, with a maximum of 10 x 12. An 8 x 10 room is becoming the standard as the cost of square footage increases. Examination rooms are typically designed as in Figure 20.5.

Allowing the door to swing into the room increases patient privacy. A small changing area can be created with a cubicle curtain on a track. A mirror, shelf, and hooks provide a place to hang clothes and comb hair. A minimum of three electrical outlets are needed in an examination room (see Figure 20.6). One outlet is to power the table, one is for a lamp, otoscope, or other equipment, and one over the counter for additional equipment, such as a desk-top otoscope.

In California the handicap code requires 18 in. clearance on the swing side of a door plus 5 ft. clear around a door for a person in a wheelchair to approach the door and open it independently. In an 8 x 10 examination room the door must then swing against the wall. Privacy is provided with a

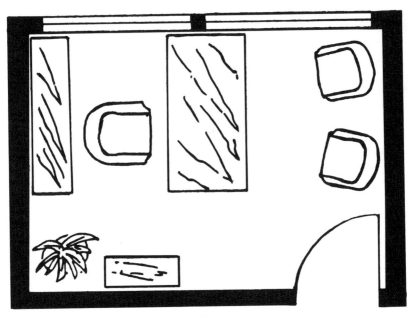

Figure 20.2. A 10′ × 14′ consultation office.

Figure 20.3. A 10′ × 12′ consultation office.

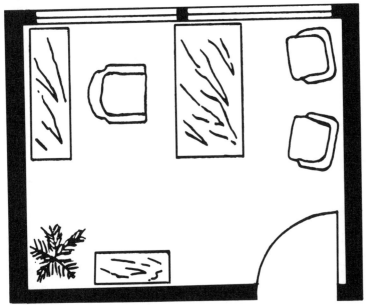

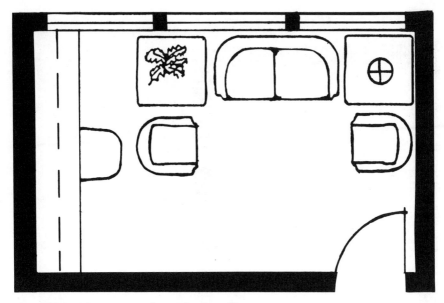

Figure 20.4. A lounge type of consultation office.

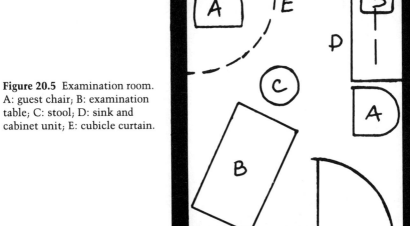

Figure 20.5 Examination room.
A: guest chair; B: examination
table; C: stool; D: sink and
cabinet unit; E: cubicle curtain.

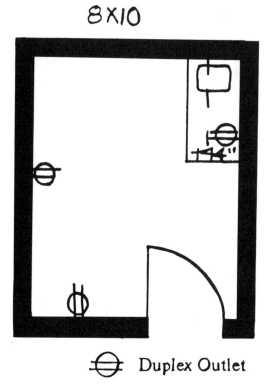

Figure 20.6. Electrical Outlets.

cubicle curtain as shown in Figure 20.7. In this instance, the room is private enough for dressing.

A writing desk or area in an examination room is essential in some practices. It is difficult to fit in a writing desk, but a pull-down writing surface can be used. Extensive charting should be done in another room so that the examination rooms are not held up and to keep the patient flow going. If a writing desk is necessary, increase the room size to 9 x 10 ft.

A larger examination room may be needed if you want family members in the room, if your patients are in wheelchairs, or if you need to circumvent the table for examination (e.g., if you are an orthopedist). A 10 x 12 room is used for eye examinations in conjuction with mirrors. A 10 x 24 wedge-shaped room is still used by some ophthalmologists for examining children.

Examination rooms usually have a four-foot cabinet unit with a small stainless steel sink with a gooseneck faucet and wrist-blade handles for handwashing. The lower cabinet usually has drawers, whereas the upper cabinet has adjustable shelves behind doors.

Most doctors prefer every examination room to be set up exactly the same way such that the patient is always examined from the right. Many

8 X 10

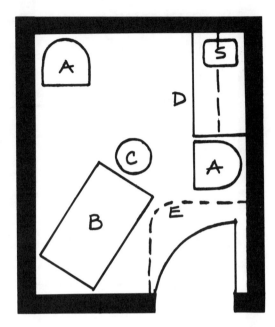

Figure 20.7. Examination room conforming to California code.

space planners will design mirror-image rooms so that plumbing is back to back. It is less expensive to build this way and you must decide if you are willing to pay for the convenience of identical rooms.

The nurses' station (Figure 20.8) provides an area for the staff to handle charts and make phone calls. In addition, an area is needed for cleaning and sterilizing equipment and preparing medications. The paperwork and the equipment/medication functions can be split into different areas (top) or combined in one area (bottom). Storage is sometimes combined with the sterilizing function.

In the paperwork area a counter either at desk height (30 in.) or counter height (36 in.) should be provided for each nurse. Additionally, space for a telephone, computer terminal, and filing space should be allowed. Overhead cabinets are often used for storage of paper supplies. The area needs to be close to the examination rooms and accessible to the physician. Sometimes space is allowed for the physician to chart and dictate notes.

The cleaning/medication function requires counters 36 in. high with storage below and above. A sink is needed for cleaning supplies. If medications will be mixed in this area a separate space with locking cabinets should be allowed. An under-counter refrigerator is usually adequate for storage of medications. The medication refrigerator must be used only for medications—food and lab samples must be refrigerated in their own refrig-

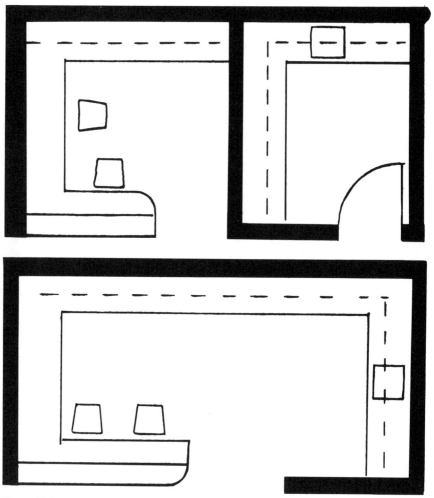

Figure 20.8. Two nurses' station plans.

erators. If toxic medications are being mixed, a venting hood must be installed.

The storage area should be commensurate with storage needs. In most offices a small 5 x 6 room is adequate. In orthopedic practices where casts, splints, and crutches are stored, a much larger area is needed. Storage areas need to be lockable to prevent theft. It may be a sad commentary on society, but some patients will feel entitled to supplies for which they have not been charged.

In small practices medical record storage is often incorporated into the reception area. If this is the case, use an area out of the patient's view. The best way to store charts is in an open filing system, which is the most easily accessed, but the charts are unsightly. Too many offices have huge chart files right behind the receptionist, in plain view of all the patients. If you plan to expand your practice within the next five years, have a separate medical records storage area. Not only will the receptionist be pulling charts, but so will the billing clerk, nurse, and transcriptionist. If the charts are in the reception area, you will have a traffic jam. Medical records do need to be adjacent and accessible to reception and also accessible to other staff members.

The business office will be used by staff performing billing functions, transcription, and other secretarial duties. It often also houses the computer, postage machine, copier, computer printer, and patients' financial files. Each staff member will require a 30 x 60 in. desk with a 48 in. return, a secretarial chair, one or two side chairs, and a file cabinet. This translates into a minimum of 70 square feet per person plus space for the other equipment. If the office has a full-time transcriptionist, a separate room is desirable so he or she can concentrate without interruption. In offices with two or more physicians, a separate office at least 8 x 10 ft will also be required by the manager.

Circulation space or a hallway is as important as other areas. A hallway has to be at least 44 in. wide to meet the fire code; handicap code requires a width of 60 in. Practically speaking, 60 in. is desirable for heavily trafficked halls, whereas a 48 in. width is reasonable for a short, less frequently used hall, codes permitting. Alcoved areas in halls are useful as weighing areas, subwaiting area, x-ray reading areas and around high-patient-volume areas, such as cashiering. Some practices require a quiet 20 ft hall for visual screening.

Other Areas Found in a Medical Office

X-Ray

X-ray is one of the most cost intensive spaces in an office. It will require leaded walls and maybe a leaded floor area, a floor sink, and additional electrical service usually requiring its own panel. The equipment is heavy and the weight of the equipment should be checked against the structural integrity of the floor. The ceiling height in most x-ray rooms is 9½ ft. A room at least 10 × 12 is necessary. A shielded area for the x-ray technician can be provided either with a leaded wall with a leaded window or this wall can be purchased with the equipment. A darkroom of about 5 × 7 needs to be provided. Processing equipment may be on countertops or freestanding. Both a water source and drainage needs to be provided. Pass boxes are usually built into the walls. Space for storage of x-ray films should be allowed either in medical records or adjacent to x-ray storage; it would be unsightly within the x-ray room itself. If an x-ray technician is utilized, then a desk area should be included.

The company that is providing the equipment will lay out the room for you and provide a detailed power plan. You will need to have a physicist's report prepared specifying the location and weight of the lead to be used. The x-ray licensing agency will have the equipment and room tested prior to its being used. Application must be made to the agency well in advance of the room's construction. The door leading into the x-ray room should be at least 3½ ft wide, with 4 ft being preferable. Not only does it provide wheelchair access, but it also allows the equipment to be installed easily.

The laboratory may range from a small counter with a microscope and centrifuge to an elaborate, separate area. Typically an office laboratory is for the purpose of performing stat laboratory work. All laboratories need counters at 36 in. with a power strip, storage for supplies, a dedicated refrigerator for reagents and specimens, a sink, and dedicated electrical circuits for certain equipment. An area for collecting specimens, such as a blood drawing area, and an adjacent toilet will be needed. An area for completing paperwork should be provided. All of this can be accomplished in a relatively small room (8 × 10 ft). The space needed is totally dependent on the volume and type of tests being performed.

One or two toilet rooms are often found within a suite. They are essential to some practices, such as urology, obstetrics, and pediatrics, and are desirable for most practices. If core bathroom facilities are adequate, individual toilet rooms may not be necessary. Toilet rooms in general are expensive to build because of the sewage lines. For example, to comply with the handicap code in California, restrooms must be a minimum of 6½ × 7 ft. If this code does not apply, a 4 × 5 ft room is adequate. A toilet room generally contains a lavatory, toilet, and some storage for supplies. If the toilet room will service a laboratory, a pass box can be built into the wall.

A procedure room is a larger space designed for special procedures, usually minor surgery. This room should be at least 10 × 12 ft. A counter with upper and lower cabinets should be placed along the 10 ft wall. A larger sink with foot controls is desirable. An electrical outlet in the floor centered in the room allows a power table to be plugged in without the cord laying across the floor. Outlets on each wall will power equipment and view boxes. Electrical outlets above the counter can be used for additional equipment. If this room will be used for treadmills, EKGs, or other procedures, dedicated circuits must be provided. Specialized equipment may have specific power requirements that differ from customary wall outlets. A ceiling-mounted surgery light centered in the room will require power and additional bracing because of its weight.

If you will have more than three employees, a lounge will be necessary. It can be a 7 × 10 ft room with a sink, counter, cabinets, microwave, and under-counter refrigerator. Outlets over the counter for a coffee pot and the microwave are necessary. A small table and chairs for eating will be needed. Some larger offices also have a coat closet and lockers for personal storage. Naturally the more employees you have, the larger the room needs to be.

If your building does not offer core facilities, you will need a janitorial area, space for a water heater, and an electrical and telephone room. The janitorial closet usually has a slop sink and storage area for supplies. The water heater can be placed in this room. Unless you have whirlpools or showers, a small 5 to 10 gallon water heater is sufficient. The telephone area generally requires a 4 to 6 ft wall space for the telephone board. The electrical panels require a 3 ft wall. A 4 ft space for servicing these panels must be provided in front of the panels. The telephone and electrical area can be combined but should be separate from the janitorial closet and water heater. They can often be incorporated into a hallway as a shallow storage area behind doors.

Orthopedics

Orthopedic practices will require all of the basic areas plus additional storage, x-ray, and cast rooms, larger examination rooms, and frequently a physical therapy department. Orthopedic examination rooms are usually 10 × 10 ft, with the examination table placed in the center of the room so that the physician can extend limbs out for examination. Electrical outlets are placed at 48 in. for x-ray view boxes. Additional storage may be required. A cast room can be 10 × 12 ft with either built-in storage for cast materials or an adjacent storage closet. A larger sink with a high gooseneck faucet allows room for a bucket to be filled. Plaster traps are essential in any sink that will have cast material put in it. Outlets for view boxes should be provided. The x-ray room should be directly accessible to the cast area. Some orthopedists prefer a larger x-ray room so that an x-ray can be taken with the patient in a wheelchair.

A physical therapy department usually has an open room for gym equipment and a mat area. Curtained areas or small private cubicles for treatments are needed. A whirlpool area with a water source and floor sink for drainage must be provided. The floors and walls in this room must be impervious to moisture and the floor must be slip resistant. A large-capacity water heater or instant water heater must be installed. Space, power, water, and drainage need to be allowed for hot-pack machines and ice machines. Some office space will be needed for the staff. A separate storage area for linens and supplies can be combined with laundry facilities if necessary. Walls need to be reinforced for any wall-mounted equipment, such as wall pulleys. Mirrored walls in the gym area help patients improve their exercise performance. Shower and locker areas are sometimes provided for patients.

Pediatrics

A basic office design can be used for pediatrics with the addition of a play area in the waiting room, some type of screening area for measuring vision, hearing, and weight, and a toilet room. Some pediatricians prefer a single reception area serving separate well- and sick-child waiting rooms. A "rash room" may be incorporated for children with contagious diseases. Examination rooms can easily be 8 × 10 ft because the examination table is along one wall. Baby scales are sometimes placed in examination rooms. An adult scale can be in a central area for older children. At least one room should accommodate a pelvic table unless the practice will be restricted to very young children. Some physicians will also want a separate room for long-term patients, such as those receiving I.V.s. A procedure room is necessary for suturing but can be somewhat smaller than 10 × 12 ft. A toilet room is a must in pediatrics. Laboratory and x-ray rooms may also be needed by the pediatrician. The medication area may be larger in this practice and need a mid-sized refrigerator. All electrical outlets should be childproof.

Obstetrics and Gynecology

Ob-gyn office space is usually set up as a typical practice but will also include toilet facilities, a small laboratory, ultrasound room, fetal monitoring area, and procedure room. Because all patients are weighed and most have urine testing, a central area for this function is desirable. The ultrasound room needs to be adjacent to the toilet but does not need to be larger than 8 × 10 ft. Some doctors do fetal monitoring in the examination rooms, but some prefer a separate area with a recliner so that examination rooms are not tied up. An 8 × 10 room is adequate.

Ophthalmology

Ophthalmology is set up somewhat differently from other practices. The basics are the same but because of the equipment, the planning is more involved. The eye examination rooms will either be 10 × 12 ft rectangular or 10 × 24 ft wedge-shaped rooms. Equipment, sinks, and outlets must be placed in exact accordance with the equipment. A close relationship must exist between the designer and the equipment supplier. The rooms must have dimmable lights controlled by the physician at the examination desk. This is one instance where it is essential that all rooms be designed the same. A visual fields room can be an 8 × 10 ft room, again with dimmable lighting. A darkened area may be incorporated for patients who are waiting with dilated eyes. The surgery area should accommodate additional equipment with special power for laser equipment if it will be used. A lens-fitting room can be 8 × 10 ft with adjacent storage for lenses.

Surgery

Surgery offices contain the basic office areas but usually have fewer examination rooms and a larger surgery area. Additionally, space for surgery scheduling is provided as well as an enlarged sterilization area. Depending on the volume and type of surgery, the surgery room may just be larger— say, 12 × 14 ft—or an outpatient surgery department may be designed.

In-office surgery is becoming more common as hospital expenses rise. An in-office surgery area needs to be well designed and in many states is licensed and regulated. In general, the following areas need to be included: a preoperative area, a surgery room with a sterile supply room, a recovery room, a nurses' station, a janitorial closet, a cleanup room, a sterilizing room, a toilet room, and a supply area. Most facilities include a doctor's changing room with a shower. If it is a true outpatient surgery department, a nurses' changing area, shower, and lounge will be required.

Let us assume that this is a small surgery area in a plastic surgeon's suite. In this case, the preoperative area would have recliners, curtained areas for clothes changing, and some type of lockers. The surgery room could be 12 × 14 ft with a wall of cabinets for storage and a sink with foot controls. A scrub sink outside the room is desirable. Swinging doors that can be held open for a patient in a wheelchair are needed. Opening off the surgery room should be a 6 × 10 room for sterile supplies. Adjacent to the surgery room should be a recovery area with lounge chairs. A nurses' station with a full view of the recovery area is necessary. Emergency equipment should be readily accessible in the recovery area. The other areas mentioned should all be in close proximity. The surgery area should be separated from the rest of the office by doors. Appropriate power and construction should be provided. For example, for infection-control purposes a hard-surface ceiling painted with washable enamel paint is required. Seamless flooring is also required.

Proper Office Flow

Now you should have an idea as to the number, type, and dimensions of the rooms in your office. How do these rooms fit together? What is the best way to arrange them? There are three parties involved in the flow pattern; the patient, the staff, and you. The patient wants to enter the office, notify reception of his or her presence, take a seat, enter the clinical part of the office, have any necessary screening, be examined by you, schedule any tests or surgery, make arrangements for payment of the bill, make another appointment if necessary and leave. The patient wants to accomplish this as efficiently as possible without feeling rushed. Those on your staff want to perform their jobs as easily and effectively as possible, and you want to see patients as efficiently as you can. In general, the waiting room and reception are contiguous. The screening areas come before the examination rooms, and the examination rooms are close together and close to the consultation area. The business office and/or cashier is not to be missed on the way out. In many practices the laboratory and x-ray room are at the end of a suite, unless they are an integral part of the screening process, in which case they are close to reception. The lounge, janitor's closet, and so on can be the farthest from the central activities. The nurses' station is in most cases contiguous or adjacent to reception as there is constant interaction between them. Most doctors want a private entrance, which must be accommodated.

Building Process

Now you should have some idea of what your office would contain in terms of the general layout. You will initially receive a space plan from your designer which, at this point, you have reviewed many times. You may have made changes and now have approved a final plan. The next plans you receive will be detailed construction drawings. In addition, a budget should be developed. Once the plans are complete, the project can be bid upon and a final budget approved. The following are the plans you should receive and review.

Electrical outlet, phone, and computer plan. This plan will identify all locations and types of outlets. Standard outlets are 12 in. above the floor unless otherwise specified. Review these plans carefully. Outlets are relatively cheap to install during construction, but are expensive to add later. Check phone and outlet locations in conjunction with the furniture and equipment plan. Plan for the future by having outlets for future equipment and staff.

Reflected ceiling plan. This shows all light fixtures and switching. If you require lights on dimmers, make sure they are included. Check the switching for your convenience.

Construction plan. This plan shows the exact location and height of all walls. Dimensions are usually to the center of the wall, so a room shown as 10½ × 10½ ft will actually have 10 × 10 ft inside dimensions. Partial-height walls will be shown. The ceiling height should be detailed. Plumbing fixtures will also be shown, as will cabinet locations.

Heating/ventilation/air conditioning (HVAC) plan. This will show the location of air vents and returns. Check the zoning so your examination rooms are warmer than other areas.

Cabinet elevations. All cabinets will be drawn as you would view them when standing in front of them. Check for adequacy of drawer space, height of counters, open space for desks, and space for equipment.

Construction details. This will show how walls, door jambs, window details, and any other construction details are to be built. In general, you need only your designer to review these with you. If you have requested soundproofing, these details will show how that will be accomplished.

Finish plan. The finish plan shows all paint, carpet, flooring, laminate, wallcovering, window covering, and cubicle curtains. It should be presented to you with a color-coded board with the actual samples on it. Your designer will have discussed this with you and obtained approval from you prior to doing the plan.

There will be plans in addition to these, but these are the basic plans for the contractor to use. Any subsequent changes to the plans initiated by you will be very costly. Make sure you review them carefully.

The next step is to provide sets of these plans to three contractors for comparative bidding. This usually takes two to three weeks. Either prior to this or concurrent with this, the plans should be submitted to the building department for approval. The building department checks the plans for conformance to codes and for fire safety features. During construction, they will monitor all the trades and make sure construction is to code. It is to your advantage to use this service.

After a contractor has been chosen, construction can begin. Depending on the complexity and size of the project, construction takes 45 to 90 days for tenant improvement work. It is cheaper to build out space in a shell building than to remodel existing space where you need to pay for demolition.

Once your space is complete you can obtain your certificate of occupancy and business license, and then you are ready to practice. One final point: make sure you receive a complete set of as-built drawings. You will need them for any future work you have done.

Summary

Space planning is a cooperative effort between you and your designer. It requires special expertise from a medical space planner. You will gain an education far beyond what you learned in school and this will be the first step you take in entering the world of business. You will have helped to create the environment that will enhance all the skills you have in delivering health care. In many ways your office is the embodiment of your philosophy of medical care. It should reflect your business goals and should last for at least five years or until you are ready to expand and change again.

Suggested Reading

Malkin, Jain, *Medical and Dental Space Planning for the 1990s.* New York: Van Nostrand Reinhold, 1989.

21 | Equipping and Furnishing Your Office

JOANNE MOSER, RNMN

Furnishing and equipping your office is every bit as important as designing it. Your furniture and equipment allow you to do your job in an efficient way. The right equipment and furniture enhance your image with your patients and allow your staff to function optimally. The wrong choices can result in decreased productivity, patient discomfort, and a poor image. This chapter will be divided into two sections: one dealing with equipment and the second dealing with furniture and decor.

Equipment

The equipment for your office falls into three categories: equipment essential for the practice of medicine or surgery; equipment essential to the functioning of your office, such as your telephone system; and equipment you would like, but which is nonessential.

Essential Medical Equipment

You probably have some idea of the type of equipment you want and may be familiar with specific manufacturers. Any large city will have several medical supply houses. They generally have showrooms where you can evaluate equipment. Practicing physicians in the community may also be able to give you some input on equipment they have found valuable. The medical supply house should be able to give you a checklist of all common equipment and supplies, including everything from surgical instruments, bandages, scales, and examination tables to surgery tables and lights. This is a good way to identify all the essentials you will need. A visit to the showroom can help you compare brands of major equipment. Check the styling, features, quality, warranties, availability, and access to servicing.

Once you have developed a solid list of the essential equipment and supplies you want, have two supply houses bid on it, if possible. You will also want to consider the service history of the supply house. Are they reliable? Will they have your equipment on time? Check with other physicians for references. You will need to continue to use them for medical supplies.

If you have no access to a medical supply showroom, you may be able to get help from the purchasing agent at the local hospital. An equipment consultant can also be used and is very helpful, especially if you have a lot of complicated, expensive equipment to purchase, such as ophthalmology equipment. They will present various types of equipment, evaluate it with you, and get competitive prices. This can save you money in the long-run.

Involve your designer in the color selections for major equipment such as examination tables. Insist on limiting the choices to neutral colors, because trendy colors date equipment. I was recently asked to redecorate an office with 12 dental operatories outfitted with pumpkin orange equipment. The cost to repaint and recover each chair and light was $800.00. That was a lot of money for a poor color choice made 12 years ago. Major equipment should last 10 to 20 years.

Standard Medical Equipment

Table 21.1 is a small checklist of general equipment needed in an office. This is a very basic checklist; most equipment supply houses will have an exhaustive checklist. Utilize an equipment consultant if your equipment is complex.

Essential Office Equipment

The essential office equipment includes a telephone system, medical records system, and a call-light system. Many physicians use a telecommunications consultant. The telephone company can supply one, and many independent consultants exist. You will want a system that will correspond with your five-year business plan, which meets your immediate needs, and allows for growth. The consultant should demonstrate the system to you. As with any other equipment, check availability, warranty, servicing, and references. Call at least two other offices where the system has been in place for a year or longer. No other single system can cause as much frustration as can a poor phone system.

Your designer should help in selecting the color of the medical records shelving so it will coordinate with the rest of the office.

The call-light system can be either a true light system or a manual flag system. A light system is installed during construction and has a panel with several colored lights indicating the status of the examination procedure. One color indicates that the patient is ready for examination, another that the patient is being examined, and another that the room is empty. The panels are placed above each exam room, in the consultation office, and in the nurses' station. This allows the physician and staff to keep the patient flow moving efficiently. The systems are expensive but very useful.

A manual flag system uses various colored flags indicating the room status. This flag system is placed next to the exam room door and must be visible by the staff and physician. Many physicians and large medical groups successfully use this system. You will have to decide which system will best suit your needs and your budget.

Table 21.1 Medical Equipment Checklist

Typical Adult Examination Room
_____ 1. Pelvic examination table
_____ 2. Wall-mounted examination light
_____ 3. Wall-mounted or desktop otoscope and ophthalmoscope
_____ 4. Blood pressure equipment
_____ 5. Surgeon's stool
_____ 6. Mayo stand

Other Medical Equipment
_____ 1. Adult scales
_____ 2. EKG machine
_____ 3. Autoclave
_____ 4. Wheelchair
_____ 5. Portable oxygen
_____ 6. Emergency cart
_____ 7. Portable I.V. pole
_____ 8. X-ray view boxes
_____ 9. Centrifuge
_____ 10. Microscope
_____ 11. Audiometer
_____ 12. Eye chart
_____ 13. Digital thermometer
_____ 14. Sundries

Typical Surgery Room/Procedure Room
_____ 1. Power surgery table
_____ 2. Ceiling-mounted surgery light
_____ 3. Hyfrecator
_____ 4. Mayo stand
_____ 5. Cryosurgery unit
_____ 6. Suction machine
_____ 7. Surgical instruments
_____ 8. Surgical supplies

Other Equipment
_____ 1. Treatment table (used in pediatrics, orthopedics, neurology, and physical therapy)
_____ 2. Stepstool
_____ 3. Baby scales
_____ 4. Children's eye charts
_____ 5. Adult scale with hand pole (for children)
_____ 6. Colposcope
_____ 7. Ultrasound equipment
_____ 8. Fetal monitor
_____ 9. Cast cutter
_____ 10. Casting equipment
_____ 11. X-ray equipment
_____ 12. Crutches
_____ 13. Sigmoidoscope

Nonessential Equipment

Nonessential equipment should be purchased after you have practiced for a while. Many doctors open practices with every gizmo and gadget available only to have them collect dust in the storage room. A computer system is a prime example. A manual billing system can work well for your first year or so in a solo or small practice office. This gives you time to evaluate what you really want and need. In addition, you will have staff who can give you invaluable input regarding the best system for your office. When evaluating your computer system, follow the same guidelines that you used in purchasing your telephone system.

All outlets and space for future equipment should have been planned into your office during the office design phase. That is why your five-year plan is so important.

New Versus Used Equipment

You may have a choice of buying new or used equipment. Some equipment, such as Mayo stands, practically never wear out. Examination tables generally last 15 years and longer. Used equipment can offer substantial savings but must be purchased carefully. First you must know the cost of new equipment so you have a point of reference. Let us take an examination table as an example. If an examination table is in good condition but is bright yellow, it will cost half the price of a new table to repaint and recover it. If the price of the used table is half that of a new table, you might as well buy a new table. New tables may also have features you want, such as a warming drawer for a vaginal speculum.

Some medical equipment suppliers buy and refurbish equipment for resale. They offer warranties for it and are available for future service. The important aspects of used equipment are age, condition, availability of parts and service, and warranty. If these conditions are acceptable and the equipment is priced right, used equipment can be a bargain.

If you are considering buying x-ray or other involved equipment, have an installer evaluate it for you. A physician recently wanted to purchase a used x-ray unit. The cost to move and install it in his office was $5000, but inspection showed that it was not U.L.-approved: the unit was essentially worthless.

Financing

Your accountant should advise you regarding the financing of both your equipment and furniture. You may simply borrow the money from the bank, lease the equipment, or choose other options of financing. Your accountant is best qualified to structure your financing and advise you on future depreciation strategies.

Ordering Equipment

Some equipment can take up to six months to receive so be sure to order your equipment in a timely manner. If your supplier advises you of the lead time necessary to obtain equipment, you can avoid such a situation as having your office ready for business except that your otoscopes haven't arrived. In this case, however, many suppliers will lend you equipment to use until yours is ready.

Arrange the installation with the supplier so that it coordinates with the progress of construction. Someone must be in attendance to receive, inspect, and direct equipment installation; most suppliers will assist with this. If a piece of equipment is to be installed by a contractor, the contractor should receive the equipment and work with the supplier. An example would be a ceiling-mounted surgery light, which must be braced into the ceiling and wired directly into the electrical system. All equipment should be checked for damage before it is accepted.

If you have used an equipment consultant, he or she should receive and place equipment for you. Make sure you know how long an installation will take; one x-ray room takes approximately one week to install.

Summary

Equipment purchases are based on your five-year business plan. It is best to begin with essential equipment first and add new equipment as needed. Used equipment can be a bargain if you know exactly what you are getting. Make sure the ordering and installation is handled in an organized and timely fashion.

Furnishing Your Office

Many of the concepts discussed in the equipment section will apply to this section as well, but additional considerations apply here.

It is very important to use a design professional for your interior design. Materials specified for commercial interiors need to meet strict fire codes and be commercially tested for office use. Residential carpet, drapes, and fabrics cannot usually be used in an office. They will not meet fire codes, and also, they won't wear well in an office. Think of the money you pay the designer as liability insurance.

You and your designer will need to establish a design concept. This may take place prior to construction if it is a newly constructed office. You need to convey to your designer how you want your office to look and feel. You may not be able to describe the exact style you want, but if you have seen another office you liked or a picture of one that appealed to you, your designer will be able to guide you in defining the design you want. Once you have decided on style, discuss your budget with your designer. The designer can then take that dollar amount and translate that into a working budget with exact quotations for your approval.

Ambience

The ambience of your office is specified by you and created by you and your designer. Your waiting room creates the first—and often, the most lasting —impression of your practice. This is the area you want to emphasize.

There is much written about healing environments and the ability of soothing color schemes to calm patients. In general this is true, but there are many exceptions. Your office doesn't have to be bland and it doesn't have to be trendy. It should reflect your philosophy of care, the type of practice you have, and your patient population. It should be durable, and easy to maintain, and comfortable for patients and their families. There are no restrictions on design other than the practical ones we have discussed.

The color scheme creates a dominant note to the design, so it is appropriate to focus briefly on color choices. We know very little about color perception and how it affects human beings. For instance, we aren't sure at what age infants perceive color. It is thought that children like more saturated colors, such as the primaries. Also, we know that the aged eye perceives yellows more intensely. Some research has shown the warm colors such as red excite people, whereas cool colors such as blue and green have a calming effect. What we don't know is how individual experiences and tastes affect our likes and dislikes of color. I happened to have trained in several Veterans Administration hospitals, which universally paint all walls green. There is nothing inherently wrong with this color, but to this day I shy away from it. You can use any color scheme you like, keeping in mind your type of practice and your patient population. Avoid using trendy colors in the basic elements of your office, such as cabinets, counters, and carpet. It is better to use them as accent colors, so that you are not stuck with them when they are no longer in vogue.

The lighting of your office is crucial to your color scheme, considering that color is perceived only when light is applied to it. Be sure your designer specifies the correct light source for you. Daylight offers the truest color rendition and is naturally therapeutic. Daylight can also cause glare, heat gain, and fading. It has to be used with thought given to your climate and sun orientation. Incandescent light (regular light bulbs) also give good color rendition, but energy conservation codes limit their use. Fluorescent fixtures have become a building standard, and a "daylight" bulb is available which not only will provide good light and color, but also it is the most flattering and truest for skin tones as well. You don't want your patients to look sicker than they are.

The overall ambience of your office is chosen by you -- it can be calming, soothing, fun, whimsical, elegant, exciting, colorful, or whatever you want. In any case, it should reflect your philosophy of medical practice.

Finish Materials

Finish materials include paint, wallcovering, wood stains, plastic laminates, carpet, flooring, base, and window coverings. They can vary in price from $5 to $150 per square foot. They need to be chosen wisely and be consistent with your budget. There is a material to meet your budget—the question is, will the material correspond with the ambience you want?

Your designer will help you decide how to spend your decorating dollar, keeping in mind your five-year plan. If you plan on staying in this office for only a few years and moving to a larger space, it doesn't make sense to buy expensive carpet that will last 10 years; instead, spend your money on furniture you will take with you. Be sure to ask for options in your budget—for instance, using a less expensive wall covering to give you more money for artwork. There are many ways to adjust your budget and still maintain your design concept. As with all plans, request a complete copy of the finished plan for future reference. Also get a maintenance guide for maintaining carpet, window coverings, wall coverings, fabrics, and so on.

Furniture

You will need waiting room furniture, which includes seating, tables, lamps, plants, artwork, and a magazine rack. Clerical areas will require secretarial desks, files, secretarial chairs, and guest chairs. Laboratory areas and nurses' stations will require secretarial chairs or drafting stools. Examination rooms will require guest chairs and chart holders. Your consultation office will need a desk, bookcase, credenza, guest seating, and an executive chair. This should cover all your essential furniture needs. Furniture comes in a variety of styles, qualities, and price ranges. Your designer will direct you in selecting the best furniture for your needs. In general, furniture will last from five to 15 years; desks, tables, and other wooden items will last 10 to 20 years or longer. It is best to get at least a medium quality of furniture. Cheap furniture looks cheap, will last only a few years, and is usually not a good investment. Many doctors buy inexpensive furniture with the intention of upgrading in a few years, but they never get around to it and their office never looks attractive.

Waiting Room Furniture

Seating can be provided by the use of individual chairs, sofas, or other lounge seating. A majority of the seating should be individual chairs. Most people don't want physical contact with a stranger and won't sit next to one on a sofa. Sofas, however, do soften the appearance of a waiting room and avoid the "bus station" look. In some offices—such as those that specialize in plastic surgery or psychiatry—lounge seating can easily be used exclusively as the patients are more physically capable. As a general rule in all other waiting rooms, seating should be firm with a seat height of 18 in., which is easy to get in and out of, and should provide good lumbar support. Wooden arms are easier to maintain than are fabric-covered arms. Fabric should be attractive and durable. Patterned fabrics hide spots and soil better than do solid-color fabrics.

Tables are needed to anchor seating arrangements and provide surfaces for magazines and lamps. Wooden tables should have laminate tops or be covered with glass to avoid scratching. Artwork and live or silk plants finish off a room. Poster art, if framed and matted properly, is an inexpensive way to provide artwork. If you have the budget for quality artwork and feel comfortable having it displayed in your office, it can contribute tremendously to the overall appearance. Custom artwork such as weavings, oils, and monoprints are also available. You can add to the artwork gradually, but at least start with it in the waiting room.

Specialty Waiting Rooms

Most waiting rooms are decorated to appeal to a broad range of tastes. Walls should have softly patterned wallcovering or simply a textural wallcovering. Strong patterns need to be avoided, especially in ophthalmology, otolaryngology, and other areas where patients may have visual or balance problems. One exception to this generalization is the pediatric office. Pediatric waiting areas should be fun, whimsical, nonthreatening, practically indestructible, and above all, safe. Wallcovering in this room should have pattern and movement. A tremendous number of children's wallcoverings are available. Most pediatricians request a pattern that appeals to a range of ages, not just babies and very small children. Brighter colors can also be used. In addition to adult seating, children's seating should be provided. Some play area should be incorporated. At the very least, this may consist of children's chairs and a table. Some safe toys (washable) and activities should be provided. Many pediatricians request a play pit—that is, a carpeted play area. Also, commerical playhouses are available which are designed expressly for waiting rooms. This type of design welcomes children and denotes that the practice is geared toward them. To ensure safety, all edges should be soft and rounded; nothing sharp should be used. Plants should be nontoxic if they are present, which is inadvisable. Seating should have no button tufting or other removable parts. All electrical outlets should have covers. Doors opening into the waiting room should have a glass panel placed so that small children can be seen. Artwork should be securely mounted. Oversized objects, such as large plastic crayons and mobiles, can add an extra dimension to the art. Seating is usually covered in a washable vinyl.

The pediatric waiting room should be fun, safe, and comfortable. It is one of the designer's favorite rooms to work on and can result in some very creative designs.

Obstetrics

Ob-gyn is another practice that offers unique design opportunities. The patient population is fairly well defined, which allows the design to be more specific in its appeal. The color palette can be softer and more feminine, as can the style of furniture. Floral patterns can be incorporated into the design scheme, though one should not overdo the floral influence; women do like patterns other than flowers.

The furniture needs to be predominantly armchairs that are wide and easy to get into and out of. Because many patients will bring children with them, a small play area is desirable. Although vinyl is probably the most practical upholstery fabric to use, it is not the most attractive. One should order additional fabric for future reupholstery needs. Many OB waiting rooms will have one or two rocking chairs for nursing mothers.

The OB office should be comfortable, soft, and appealing to women.

Wheelchair-Accessible Waiting Rooms

Many practices include a large patient population in wheelchairs. Of course, the physical plant must accommodate wheelchairs. Wheelchair-accessible telephones, water fountains, elevators, doors, and toilet facilities should be available. The waiting room should also accommodate the patient in a wheelchair. The carpet should be a low pile and glued directly to the floor. Plush carpet with thick padding is very difficult to wheel over. If the practice has many patients in wheelchairs, the reception counter may be dropped to a 30 in. height. The waiting room should have additional aisle space for easy maneuvering and an area without seating to accommodate a wheelchair. Benches with a 20 in. seat height are very convenient for patients with leg casts, who can sit on the bench and elevate their leg. The higher seat helps them to get up easily.

A waiting room designed with thought and care will be appreciated by all of your patients. Designing the waiting area for your specific patient population shows your concern for the comfort of your patients.

New versus Used

If you are purchasing a practice complete with furniture, you need to determine the value of the furniture you are purchasing. The same principles of buying used equipment apply here. Office furniture can be refurbished just as equipment can. The refurbishing companies should evaluate the furniture and give you a quotation; you can then decide what to do. For example, if a good waiting room chair costs approximately $350 new and the used chair is in good condition, needs no refurbishing, and the price is $200, then you've saved money. If that $200 chair needs $150 worth of work, however, you might as well buy a new one. Like medical equipment, used furniture can save money, but you must know what you are getting for your dollar.

Ordering Furniture

Furniture has a typical lead time of 10 to 12 weeks. It needs to be ordered in a timely fashion to avoid late delivery. Your designer should be responsible for receipt and inspection of the furniture as well as placement according to the furniture plan. This should be coordinated with any construction and with your office opening. Furniture installation usually takes only one or two days. Do not install furniture when there are still tradespeople present —too many accidents can happen.

Consultation Office Furniture

Your consultation office should blend with the rest of the office but reflect your own taste and style. The basic furniture you need is a desk, executive chair, guest seating, and bookcase. A credenza is not essential, but most physicians need the additional storage. Choose a style and quality you like very much. Good office furniture, though expensive, can last 15 years, with good desks lasting longer than 30 years. Your chair should be very comfortable and fit you well; sit in a sample chair before ordering one. Your guest seating should also be comfortable. Patients like to see their physicians' diplomas, and your office is the best place to display them. You can arrange your office in any of the ways shown in the previous chapter. Make your office as much a reflection of you as possible—it will become your home away from home for a long time.

Summary

The ambience of your office reflects your philosophy of care. It takes much thought and work from both you and your designer. A successfully designed office will have a good flow and a good feel to it. It should be supportive of your practice, your staff, and your patients. Furnishing and equipping your office represents a tremendous financial investment. Like any investment, it needs to be well planned in accordance with your business plan, and you need to know the dividends you can expect from it. It should enhance your practice of medicine and be an environment that you are happy to work in every day.

Suggested Reading

Malkin, Jain, *Medical and Dental Space Planning for the 1990's.* New York: Van Nosfrand Reinhold, 1989.

22 | Hiring and Firing Staff: Developing Job Descriptions that Support Your Practice Objectives and Recruitment Techniques

PETER KANE

Hiring the wrong person can cost an organization over $100,000, not counting the wasted time and effort. Unfortunately, this error happens all too often. Selecting the right candidate for a position is a process that must be *managed* to minimize the hiring risk and ensure a winning decision. This chapter addresses the technique of thinking ahead by developing job descriptions.

"I need a receptionist" is a simple statement, right? Wrong! The physician office practice, whether large or small, invariably needs much more than a receptionist. After all, a receptionist, as defined by Webster's, is "one employed to greet callers." Once the greeting is done, what happens? The office practice receptionist will undoubtedly do much more than greeting. He or she may schedule appointments, open the mail, accept payments, record them, make payment arrangements with patients, compose letters, respond to patient correspondence, maintain logs of patient activity, complete patient charge slips, order office supplies, escort patients to examination rooms, hand out instructional materials, and myriad other duties depending on the size and complexity of the practice.

The point is that if you seek a receptionist for your practice, the title alone will not get you the personnel with "the right stuff" to get your job done. Your first step should *not* be to pick up the phone and call your local newspaper to place an advertisement. Considerable homework needs to be done first, including development of a detailed job description. This job description will help you to write the newspaper advertisement that brings applicants that are truly qualified. Being explicit in your job description and, subsequently, in your advertisement about the nature of the job will dramatically minimize your time spent screening letters and résumés prior to the interview process.

The key to a successful hire is how well the job is defined. A common mistake, to be discussed in more detail later, occurs when the boss intuitively knows what the job is—that is, the boss knows what he or she wants—but fails, often miserably, to communicate his or her expectations to the person hired for the job. Many organizations today are going beyond the traditional job description format of job summary, job description, and job qualifications in order to ensure a complete communication link between employer and employee. Such things as candidate profiles are being developed which include the degree and type of experience preferred for the position, the education mandatory to perform the role, and the specific skills needed to accomplish the goals established for the position.

Job offers to prospective candidates are customarily based primarily on the applicability of education and experience to the job in question, along with other, more subjective, criteria, such as personality traits, and communication skills. The *acceptance* of the job offer, however, is more often than not a function of the prospective employee's understanding of what duties the job actually comprises. This includes all the so-called minor details of the job. If you haven't done your homework—a detailed, written job description, which becomes your recruiting discussion document—you run a serious risk of omitting from your employment discussions key ingredients of the job, any one of which could destroy an otherwise good fit between employee and employer.

For example, let us presume that you run an advertisement, receive 35 responses, interview seven people, and select Ms. Jones for your receptionist job based on her outgoing personality, her professional demeanor, and her three years of well-recommended experience as a receptionist at her previous job. After her first week, in the course of teaching her the details of her job, you show her the list of delinquent patients whom she is supposed to phone and request payment. She balks. She had no idea that this would be part of her job and tells you she simply cannot make those kinds of calls. The cost to the practice is significant when one considers the cost of the ad, the time to review each résumé and application, the time-consuming process of setting up and conducting interviews, responding appropriately to those not selected for the job, and most importantly, the physician's time away from seeing patients. Clearly this is an extreme example; nonetheless, without a job description that details each and every major responsibility and many of the minor ones, such a scenario is all too common.

Job descriptions are also excellent tools for use in the new-employee orientation process. Newly hired employees, given a copy of their position's description, can better understand the position's responsibilities and their place within the organization.

The third reason for taking the time to define the job in the form of a written job description is for employee performance appraisal purposes. Writing a job description prior to hiring, and reviewing it in depth with a prospective employee, ensures that there is no question about what the job responsibilities are. It is also highly recommended that you allocate a percentage of effort, time, consequence of error, or complexity to each task area (totaling 100%) on the job description and place the items in order of importance. This weighted scale will contribute to the employee's understanding of not only the job content, but also each task's importance to you, the employer. Once this is done, you and your staff are "in synch"—all doubt about whose job consists of what and its import to the practice is gone.

In the employee evaluation process, job descriptions are invaluable. Employees have a right to know, in advance, the criteria, goals, and expectations that will be evaluated in the course of their job. Certainly, the job description contributes to this understanding of what will be evaluated and what will not. I can testify to the countless times employees have said, "I was never, ever told *that* was a part of my job." Candidly, that kind of statement is usually the precursor to a grievance or external legal action. During the evaluation, the performance of directly job-related duties, (according to the job description) should always be discussed and evaluated before other common evaluation areas such as attendance (absenteeism), ability to follow instructions, initiative, innovation, appearance, and so on.

Furthermore, a number of legal issues could come into play, leaving your practice vulnerable. First, however, it is important to point out that no law requires that an employee be provided a written job description; however, discharging an employee for failure to perform some aspect of his or her job, and not having a written job description on file that has been previously discussed with the employee, can have disastrous legal consequences. A court finding of wrongful termination or a regulatory agency—such as the Equal Employment Opportunity Commission or the Fair Employment and Housing Commission—finding of discrimination could force you to reinstate the employee to his or her same job and pay all back wages; in the extreme, such a judgment could assess punitive penalties on the employer, as an organization, and on those *individuals* found directly responsible (usually owners, officers, and directors).

Consider again the recent hire of Ms. Jones for receptionist. The best scenario shows Ms. Jones voluntarily resigning because she does not want to make those "awful collection calls." The worst scenario has Ms. Jones declaring to her attorney that there was never any discussion about calling delinquent patients, either in the advertisement or the interview process, and that she, by accepting your job, lost out on several other equally promising positions in well-respected physician practices. Naturally, her attorney sees substantial dollar signs after listening to this rendition. A jury will probably have a very sympathetic response to Ms. Jones.

The development of job descriptions and regular, periodic reviews are therefore essential to well-managed, productive medical practices. They prevent misunderstandings between employee and supervisor in terms of not only what the job is, but whose job it is to perform specific tasks. They let the employee know how their job fits in with others' in the practice, they help specify the importance of each job duty, they act as productivity tools to ensure the employee's entire job is being completed, and finally, they help prevent the ultimate "misunderstanding" that results in a discharge and potential litigation and/or negotiations with federal, state, or local regulatory agencies that administer discrimination and fair employment laws.

In even the most mundane unemployment compensation hearing, the supervisor/employer or employer representative will be asked by the administrative law judge (who will probably have little or no knowledge of your business) to "Describe for this hearing the job duties of the employee." When you pull out a written job description and read from it for the record, the judge will know you have done your homework. If the dispute concerns a job duty, the judge will ask your former employee if he or she knew of the written job description and had ever seen it or received a copy. This means that employees should acknowledge receipt of their job description, by signature, and this should be a part of the employee personnel record.

There are a number of other extremely important reasons to have job descriptions. For management development, they will help identify training and development needs of employees in their current positions and provide requirements needed for promotion and career planning. In an organizational analysis they will allow comparison of relationships of various positions within and across organizational functions. Also, in compensation administration, job descriptions are essential to establish internal and external pay equity. The many compensation surveys are conducted by phone with pay data being provided based on the title of the job. Remembering Ms. Jones, if a survey were conducted on her job (receptionist), and it was not made clear to the caller that Ms. Jones also makes collection calls (a higher-value skill), the pay rates and data shared between you and a colleague would not fairly represent her position. Again, having that comprehensive job description in front of you during those sensitive salary surveys can help prevent mismatches in job comparisons (common in telephonic salary surveys).

The mere possession of a job description is only half the battle: the employee must acknowledge receipt of his or her job description in order for you to win your court battles. The environment today finds employers constantly in a position of having to prove, through a signed document, that the employee was indeed informed of the policy, rule, job description, or whatever. If you should find yourself in a legal conflict without dated, written support for your position, whatever that may be, you will most assuredly become familiar with the "my word against your word" phenomena. The fact that you are the employer and a well-respected physician in the community will not influence the outcome.

Any written document, including a job description, must be kept current. Job descriptions entered into evidence in a court setting do not mean much if they are five years out of date and there is no record of revisions being routinely made. Consequently, as jobs change, as your practice grows and duties are assigned and reassigned, ensure that job descriptions are updated routinely, discussed with the employee, and made a permanent part of the employee's file. Use the annual employee performance appraisal process as an opportunity to mutually update job descriptions. It is often remarkable for both parties to see the volume and magnitude of changes that have taken place in the span of one year. Consider asking the employee to participate in the updating process by coming to the evaluation/ appraisal meeting with an updated job description for discussion. General guidelines for developing job descriptions are listed below.

1. Each primary duty should be described in three ways: What is the duty performed? How is the duty performed? Why is the duty performed?
2. The statement of each function should be brief and to the point. Articles such as *a, an, the,*and so on, may be omitted.
3. Each responsibility statement should begin with an action verb and should be written in the present tense (e.g., Order back-office supplies).
4. Specific titles, departments, and terms used in performing functions should be used. Short definitions of job-specific terms may be necessary.
5. Ambiguous words should be avoided. *Sometimes, on occasion,* and *frequently* do not accurately describe the amount of time spent on responsibilities. If possible, quantify the time required to perform specific functions.

Developing and maintaining accurate job descriptions for each position in the physician office practice can pay dividends for years to come through loyalty, esprit de corps, low turnover, low unemployment insurance claims, nonexistent wrongful termination suits, no calls for labor unions, low worker's compensation claims, low medical insurance claims, and high productivity with long-term employees.

Suggested Reading

Executive Compensation Services, Inc., *Position Description Manual.* Fort Lee, NJ: ECS, Inc., 1988.

Executive Compensation Services, Inc., *Salary Management Handbook.* Fort Lee, NJ: ECS, Inc.

The Human Resources Yearbook. Englewood Cliffs, NJ: Prentice-Hall, 1989.

Comptan, Jo Ann L. "Strategy for effective hiring minimizes risk." *HR News* (February 1990) : B13.

23 | Implementing Effective Personnel and Office Management Procedures

PAULA P. DEAN

The nurses, secretaries, and bookkeepers who work for you are the backbone of your practice. Your patients will judge the quality of care they receive based on their interactions with you and your staff. Managing these employees effectively will not only build your practice, but will also give you a sense of satisfaction as an employer.

Effective personnel policies and office management procedures should be established from the outset. It is easier to develop these policies and procedures as you begin your practice than to attempt to implement them after your office staff has established behavior patterns. Setting realistic parameters and expectations for your staff is critical to the ultimate success of your medical practice.

Several key areas should be addressed: interviewing and hiring the best-qualified people; determining pay rates and pay increase guidelines; offering benefits that will attract and retain your good workers; establishing office rules and policies that meet your practice goals; and setting job expectations and appraising performance. Each of these areas will be addressed in this chapter.

Employing the Best People

The job market in health care is booming, but the number of people who can fill these jobs is diminishing. Qualified applicants are at a premium, and the labor shortage is expected to worsen. By the year 2000 the number of new workers between the ages of 16 and 24 will drop by 8%, whereas the demand for health-care workers will increase by 53%.

Finding the right employee takes more than placing an advertisement in the local newspaper: you must first define what you want in a coworker. You must have a clear idea about not only the tasks the individual will perform but also the personality characteristics that will mesh with your particular practice philosophy. This should be done, in writing, before you begin the process of advertising or interviewing.

First, define the technical skills you will require. Educational level, prior work experience, applicable work experience, and specific technical skills should be clearly defined. Determine whether the qualification is mandatory or if you are willing to train an applicant in a specific skill.

Second, define the personal characteristics. In many ways, personal attributes, the "intangibles," are more important than the technical skills. Technical skills can be taught, but it is far more difficult to change a person's innate behavior. Some traits that might be considered are pleasant demeanor, good organizational skills, good oral communication skills, good grooming, eagerness to learn, and initiative.

The most common method of finding a good employee is to place an advertisement in the classified section of the local newspaper. This method can work well, but there are many other productive methods to attract applicants, including contacting local professional societies and employment agencies, word of mouth, networking, contacting other medical offices, and participating in career fairs.

After you have developed a pool of applicants, review the résumés and compare them with your written qualifications for the job. When you have found a promising candidate, telephone that person and conduct a brief interview over the phone. Try to match their answers to your qualification list. Listen to the person's tone of voice, and be attuned to the impressions you develop during the telephone interview; remember that your patients may also get the same impression. Try to be both sensitive and critical. Use this opportunity to further screen your candidate. Ask any questions that may have surfaced as you reviewed the résumé. It is helpful to develop a list of questions ahead of time that can be asked of each candidate. State and federal laws require that you ask nondiscriminatory questions, so phrase each question in a nondiscriminatory way. For example, if you are concerned about an applicant's ability to get to work on time each day because of potential child-care problems, you could ask, "Are there any personal circumstances or plans in your future that might interfere with your ability to come to work on time?" A list of legally appropriate interviewing questions is given in Table 23.1.

After you have made the decision to conduct a formal, person-to-person interview, schedule it during office hours. Ask other staff members to interview the person, too: more than one assessment can be valuable in hiring the best applicant. You should perfect four essential interviewing skills: listening, asking questions, taking complete notes, and being aware of verbal and nonverbal traits.

Ask each candidate about his or her education, work experience, and desire to work for you. Ask prepared questions (see Table 23.2), listen, take good notes, and record your observations and feelings. It is important to let the applicant do most of the talking, while you listen objectively. After you decide to hire a candidate, check the person's references thoroughly *before* you make a job offer.

Determining Pay Rates and Other Salary Issues

Probably one of the most difficult tasks is determining how much to pay your staff. Each practice group should clearly identify how much they are willing to pay. A key question that must be answered is, Do I want to pay

Table 23.1 Sensitive Questions and Their Alternatives

Too direct or sensitive	Less direct or sensitive
Why were you fired from your last job? *or* Why are you looking for another job?	What are some of your reasons for considering other employment at this time?
Did you have trouble with your boss?	How would you describe your boss?
Why did you leave school before you got your degree?	Was there any particular reason you decided to leave school when you did?
To what do you attribute your poor employment record?	I see you have changed jobs several times. What were your reasons for seeking new opportunities? *or* Everyone has problems with some aspects of their job. Could you describe some of the things that posed problems for you on previous jobs?
Did you get along with your coworkers?	Could you describe your relationship with a coworker or colleague to whom you were particularly close?
What didn't you like about your last job?	Most situations have some aspects that are not as pleasant as others. Were there any less pleasant aspects of your last job?
Are you free to move?	How would you feel about moving to another city at the present time? *or* If you were relocated to another area, what problems would this present for you?
You mean to say you're unemployed?	At present you're not employed, then, is that correct?
Why would you think you are qualified to go into research and development, with your background?	Would you comment on how you feel you could use your background in our research and development area?

Source: Thomas L. Moffatt, *Selection Interviewing for Managers* (Madison, WI: Science Tech Publishers, 1987).

my office staff less than, the same as, or more than the average medical practice in town? Each approach has its own benefits and drawbacks.

Some physicians choose to pay a lower base salary but enhance the pay package with semiannual or annual bonuses based on the employee's productivity and the practice's profits. Others elect to pay a low base wage but include a rich benefits package; still others elect to pay higher wages and offer enough benefits to entice staff members to make a career in that practice. The most common methodology in determining pay levels is to participate in a local salary survey of key medical office positions and then

Table 23.2 Sample Interview Questions

Honest and candor

What would your present or previous supervisor say is your weakest area?
A variety of positions often become available in this company. What would you really
   like to do?
What particular professional advantages do you feel you will gain by working for this
   company?
What prompted your decision to leave your most recent employer?
What would your previous supervisors say are your best assets?

Motivation

How close are you to reaching your potential?
What position in this company would you like to work toward in the next year?
How would you describe your own standards of performance?
How do you feel about your career progress to date?
What do you think you will be doing five years from now?
Specifically, how do you plan to achieve your career goals?
To what kind of supervision do you respond best, and why?

Organization

How do you plan your day at work?
How do you determine the priorities for your day's activities?
How do you stay current with the new techniques in your field?

Resourcefulness

What can you tell me about the company and position for which you are applying?
To whom did you go for help and counsel when you encountered a tough job problem?
What changes did you make in your recent job during the time you held it?
Describe a time you were given an unfamiliar job responsibility: what did you do?

Stability and dependability

Please describe your personal record of punctuality and dependability.
What average length of time do you feel an individual should stay with an
   organization?
What elements do you consider when contemplating a job change?

Value system

Give me your idea of the perfect supervisor.
What qualifications would you look for if you had to hire someone to fill the position
   for which you are interviewing?
What do you think is going to make the difference between success and failure on the
   job?
What are two things that are very important to you in a job?
If you were given the choice between two employers offering the same pay and
   position, what would determine your choice?
Describe the best manager you ever had.

Table 23.2 (*continued*)

Describe the worst manager you ever had.
Tell me about the kind of rewards that make you feel adequately recognized for your contributions.

Ability, stability

How do you handle repetitive tasks?
What are the personal qualities this job demands?
Tell me about a time when the boss was absent and you had to make a decision.
Tell me about an occasion when you chose, for whatever reasons, not to finish a particular task.
If you could have any job in this company, what would it be?

Willingness

Do you ever find it necessary to go beyond the call of duty to get a job done?
What role do you play in ensuring a smooth working environment when your boss is away?

Flexibility

What type of people do you get along with best?
Describe the toughest situation you ever faced at work.
When have you rescheduled your time to accommodate an unexpected workload?
Have you ever dealt with the general public?
When was the last time someone or something made you very upset at work?

Written communication

Tell me about the kinds of documents you type at work.
Do you ever compose letters for others?
What was the most complex document you ever produced?
What forms or documents have you developed for your department?

Teamwork

How do you establish a working relationship with new people?
With what kind of people do you like to work?
With what kind of people do you dislike to work?
How do you feel about people who do not like their jobs?
How do you define a conducive work atmosphere?

Source: Corporate Interviewing Network, San Diego, CA.

determine salaries based on the pay philosophy of the medical group. In many states, the local chapter of the Medical Group Management Association (MGMA) conducts annual salary surveys for its members. This is a good starting point, but it should not be the final decision-making tool. Position titles can be very deceiving; consequently, a physician should make an effort to match the job responsibilities—not the job titles—to the salary data. Reviewing the brief job description supplied with the survey document is essential in matching your job to the survey data.

After determining the minimum salary for a given job, you should also determine the maximum salary your practice can support for that position. Too often the maximum levels are never defined, and over time, a medical office may find itself paying many more thousands of dollars for an employee than is reasonable. This practice can severely affect other employees in your office who earn less but who have greater educational or technical skills. Therefore, general guidelines or salary ranges should be established for each job.

Next, rank the jobs by levels of difficulty. The key medical office jobs might be ranked as follows: Level 1: medical records filing clerk; Level 2: receptionist/scheduler; Level 3: biller/insurance processor; Level 4: nurse; Level 5: office manager. The salary ranges associated with these positions should reflect your understanding of the job skills necessary to perform the jobs. For example, a filing clerk deals primarily with the medical records and must have an aptitude for numbers, alphabetizing, and organizing details. Generally, there is little or no work experience necessary for this type of position. Your filing clerk may have some patient contact, but it will be limited. The billing clerk or insurance processor, however, must be able to deal effectively with patients, insurance carriers, and claims personnel, in addition to having good number skills, mathematical computation ability, an understanding of billing processes, and good organizational skills. Communication skills and good patient relation skills are important attributes for a billing clerk. Obviously the pay levels or ranges for these jobs should reflect the differing job responsibilities. Table 23.3 is an example of a pay scale chart that reflects both the community standard of pay as well as the differing job duties.

For the purposes of fairness and consistency, each pay range has approximately the same amount of pay growth in the pay range. In this case, each job has about a 30% pay growth potential from the minimum to the maximum pay levels. Of course, the process does not end with the formulation of pay scales. Each year, the pay levels should be reviewed and, if

Table 23.3 Pay Scale Chart

| | Hourly pay rate | |
Position	Minimum	Maximum
Medical records file clerk	$ 5.00	$ 6.50
Receptionist/scheduler	6.00	7.80
Biller/insurance processor	8.50	11.00
Nurse (LVN or LPN)	10.00	13.00
Office manager	12.00	16.00

necessary, adjusted (usually upward) to meet the pay philosophy established for your practice and the general cost-of-living increases in your geographic area.

Bonuses

Bonuses can create positive incentives for the staff, contributing to the motivation and productivity of your employees. To be used effectively, however, bonuses should be awarded based on fair evaluations of each employee's value to your practice. This can be difficult to accomplish, particularly in a small office. However, the benefits can far outweigh the time and effort that must accompany a performance evaluation. Factors that should be considered in an evaluation are the quantity and quality of the work performed, quality of patient relations, innovation or creativity, cooperation, attendance record, and organization. You may choose to annually evaluate the performance of each staff member and grant bonuses based on these evaluations. You should clearly explain to your staff how the bonus system will work, what will determine the amount of bonus, and the maximum bonus amount given. A short policy might read as follows:

1. The XYZ Medical Group believes in rewarding those employees who have contributed to the success of the group. The bonus program was implemented to provide additional income to staff members who perform their jobs in the most effective and productive ways possible.
2. The XYZ Medical Group will consider each employee for an annual bonus, which will be given in December of each year.
3. The bonus will be determined by physicians in the XYZ Medical Group. Such elements as quantity and quality of work, quality of patient relations, cooperation, attendance, and organizational skills will be evaluated to determine the staff member's bonus award.
4. The minimum and maximum amount of bonus will be stated each year, based on the profitability of the XYZ Medical Group.

Overtime Compensation

Under federal laws, employees who are not exempted from overtime regulations, as defined by the Fair Labor Standards Act (FLSA), must generally be paid 1½ times their salary for hours worked in excess of 40 hours in one work week. Some employers choose to give employees time off in lieu of paying overtime salaries. Compensatory time-off plans are a very troublesome area for employers, and employers are surprised when compensation claims for overtime pay are filed by disgruntled employees. Further, when a physician has an informal time-off arrangement with nonexempt staff members he or she is often surprised to find that these "agreements" generally do not satisfy the FLSA or state laws. Consult legal counsel if you plan to implement a compensatory time-off program for your nonexempt staff.

Employee Benefits

There was a time when employee benefits played a secondary role in attracting and retaining qualified employees. Today, however, with spiraling medical costs, applicants seriously consider benefits in their decision to accept or reject a job offer.

The first step in setting up a benefits program is to select a competent insurance broker who can guide you through this legislatively complex arena. A good broker will assist you in designing your benefit package and be able to find programs that meet your goals and your pocketbook.

Many groups offer a basic benefits package of medical insurance, vacation, sick pay, and holiday pay. Medical insurance is the most common benefit offered; it can also be the most expensive for the employer. A broker can outline the various medical plans available for your group, with the associated cost for each. Some groups pay for the employee portion of the premium but have the employee pay for any dependent costs. Others also pay for the employee's family; some groups choose to offer group medical insurance but have the employee pay the full cost. Again, your group of physicians must decide on its pay and benefit philosophy and develop a plan accordingly.

Vacation programs generally allow an employee one or two weeks of paid vacation each year. If the office is small, it may be best to require the employee to take his or her vacation at the same time as the physician's. In any event, it is important to schedule the time off well in advance of the date.

Under California law, any accrued but unused vacation is considered a vested benefit and must be paid to the employee when the employee terminates. It is illegal to remove unused vacation at the end of the calendar year. If you do not want to accrue a potentially sizable liability, you should encourage staff to use all earned vacation each year. It is advisable to consult with an attorney about applicable laws in your state.

One method is to not allow employees to accrue more than the annual allowance. For example, if an employee earns two weeks of vacation each calendar year and uses only one week of vacation, he or she may accrue only one additional week. Thus at any given time, an employee can have accrued a maximum of two weeks of vacation pay. This accrual method must be put in writing and consistently adhered to in order to satisfy the requirements of state law.

Sick Leave Pay

National statistics show that an employee will miss an average of five workdays per year because of illness or injury. Some medical groups pay their employees for the occasional absence due to sickness. It is important to clearly state your established policy and then abide by it. If you decide to allow an employee to accrue a specific number of sick days, record the accrual as well as the usage. It is best to work on a calendar year and set a limit on the amount of sick time an employee can accrue. The following is an example of a sick leave policy:

1. Each full-time employee is eligible to receive pay when absent because of illness or injury.
2. The employee can accrue one sick day each month until 10 days are accrued.
3. An employee who is absent because of illness or injury may apply for sick pay if he or she has any amount of accrued but unused sick leave.
4. It is expected that this benefit will be used only for its intended purpose. Any employee who abuses the policy may become ineligible for sick-leave pay.

Holidays

Each medical group should establish which holidays it will observe and publish the list of holidays for current and new employees. The medical group physicians should determine whether holidays will be a paid day for all staff, for full-time employees only, or for none of the employees. The most common holidays are New Year's Day, Memorial Day, Independence Day, Labor Day, Thanksgiving Day, and Christmas Day. Some organizations grant a "floating holiday" or the employee's birthday as a paid holiday.

Establishing Office Rules and Guidelines

Myriad issues must be considered when setting up a group practice. How well your office functions is a direct result of the office rules, guidelines, and expectations you set. This section will attempt to address the major areas of concern.

Work Hours/Lunch and Break Times

Establish office hours that are convenient for the patients and reasonable for you and your staff. Employees should understand the office hours and the work schedule you have arranged for them. The employees should be told that you expect them to be on time every day; tardiness can cause problems with other staff members and patients. Lunch schedules should be determined, and they should be consistent for everyone.

Ten-minute breaks in the morning or afternoon will allow your staff to rest and rejuvenate themselves for the next work period. Federal laws require that an employee be given a minimum one-half hour lunch break, prior to completing five hours of work, and a 10-minute rest period for every four-hour shift.

Uniforms/Dress Code

Your expectations regarding an employee's appearance, grooming, and dress should be clearly communicated. You should openly discuss and enforce your rules on appropriate dress, shoes, hairstyle, jewelry, and use of perfume.

The medical group should determine whether they want the staff to wear uniforms. Lab coats or jackets can create a professional image for the office that is expected by patients. When uniforms are required as a condition of employment, the medical group should discuss who will incur the costs of buying and maintaining those uniforms. A number of state laws as well as the Fair Labor Standards Act address these issues. Consequently, if your group requires the employees to wear uniforms, the group should be certain that its uniform policy complies with state and federal laws.

Smoking

Smoking, besides being a health risk, is quickly becoming a social taboo in the United States. As a health-care provider, you have additional incentive to promote a healthy work environment that encourages patients and staff to adopt a healthy life-style. "No smoking" signs in the waiting area, along with the absence of ashtrays, will discourage patients from smoking. Staff who smoke should be told where and when they can smoke, if the practice does permit smoking on the premises.

Legislated Leaves

State and federal laws mandate that an employer must allow an employee time away from the job for several purposes. These include military and jury duty, appearing as a court witness, and in some states, pregnancy leaves of absence.

Military Leave

Federal law mandates that employers must allow qualified employees who enter military service to take leaves of absence from their jobs. These employees must be reinstated upon discharge from military duty if they comply with the reinstatement rights outlined by the law. The reinstatement provisions require that the employee apply for his or her former position within 90 days of discharge. Reservists and National Guards also have reinstatement rights. A legal opinion should be sought if your medical group is uncertain about its responsibilities in this regard.

Jury Duty

Many states require that an employer allow an employee time off from work to serve on a jury. The employer, however, is not required to continue the employee's wages while he or she serves as a jury member. Many employers find it useful to specify a number of paid days for jury duty. Employees can then notify the courts of limitations in their jury duty benefit, thus averting the possibility of long periods of jury service.

Witness Duty Leave

An employee who is required to testify as a witness in a court case must be granted time off from work to fulfill his or her civic obligation. The employee does not have to be paid for this time.

Pregnancy Leave

Some states require an employer to grant an employee a leave of absence during late pregnancy and/or after childbirth. Generally, the length of leave is determined by medical necessity as stipulated by the employee's physician. The period of physical disability is normally the time granted for pregnancy leave. Many state laws stipulate a period of time an employee must be granted pregnancy leave.

Some employers choose to grant additional personal leave beyond the woman's actual physical disability to allow her to bond with her child prior to returning to work. This time is generally unpaid but allows the mother to return to work with a minimum of emotional conflict. Many women today must work to support their families. The most productive employee is one who has resolved personal commitments and can balance family and work obligations. Many companies set a limit for physical disability and personal leave at three to six months. In these cases, the employer must hold the job for the employee's return, utilizing temporary personnel or other arrangements during the leave period.

Setting Job Expectations and Appraising Performance

Communicating fair, realistic, and clearly defined job responsibilities and expectations is critical to the successful functioning of a medical office. Some expectations should apply to all members of the office, whereas others are specific to a job. Examples of office-wide expectations involve how to answer the phone, how to handle an angry patient, and general office behavior and attitudes.

Employees want to know how they are performing and if they are meeting your expectations. Appraising performance is often difficult and time consuming, but generally the office and the employee both benefit from the appraisal. A brief checklist of items to evaluate might be the following:

1. *Professional or technical competence.* Does the employee understand and perform the fundamentals and procedures of the job?
2. *Productivity.* Does the employee produce work on a timely basis and effectively use his or her own time and the time of others?

3. *Quality of work.* Does the employee demonstrate accuracy, thoroughness, neatness, and clarity?
4. *Dependability.* Does the employee follow through on assignments? Is his or her attendance within established guidelines?
5. *Patient relations.* Does the employee demonstrate respect, a caring attitude, and helpfulness toward patients, coworkers, and the general public; observe patient confidentiality; and show cooperation and courtesy?
6. *Judgment/decision making.* Does the employee consider relevant facts and make logical decisions?
7. *Communication.* Does the employee exchange ideas, information, and messages readily and effectively?

It is best to write an appraisal of an employee when you have uninterrupted time to objectively review his or her past performance and write an accurate and meaningful evaluation. Documenting both the assets and weaknesses of employees throughout the year is also helpful. Ideally, the annual appraisal should summarize those expectations that you have communicated to your employee on prior occasions. The appraisal should contain no surprises. Confrontational discussions of the performance appraisal probably indicate communication problems or lack of understanding of job expectations.

The evaluation should also include a brief discussion of areas for improvement or learning that you would like the employee to achieve in the future. Describe specific means to accomplish these goals and set a deadline for achieving each goal. Most employees are anxious to do a good job. It is up to the employer to state the expectations and help the employee achieve the goals.

Disciplinary Actions

If an employee is not performing the job to your stated expectations, steps should be taken to correct the problem. The goal should always be to identify the area of concern and correct the problem. Most employees, when told about a concern, are very willing to modify their behavior or to perform a task more effectively. However, they cannot improve if you fail to tell them about the problem.

The first step is to discuss the issue. Many times an informal discussion is enough to correct the problem. The employee should be told specifically what the problem is, what you expect, how he or she can meet your expectation, and the consequences of failing to comply. If the problem persists, the employer or supervisor should document the issue in writing and give a copy to the employee. The consequences of failing to comply (e.g., termination) should again be clearly stated. If the problem continues, the physician should seriously consider terminating the employee.

Documentation is an important element of any involuntary termination. It helps to protect the employer from litigation while informing the employee of the seriousness of the offense.

Firing people certainly is not an easy or enjoyable task. There are six things you should do once you decide to fire an employee:

1. Do it soon—postponing this decision does not make it easier.
2. Document the reasons for the decision. Use good judgment, and be sure you are firing the person for good reasons.
3. Conduct the termination in a humane, caring way. Do not demean the person, and always do it in a private office.
4. Stick to the facts and keep the meeting short and simple. Long justifications or convincing arguments are not helpful to you or the employee.
5. Attempt to have the person leave your office with dignity and goodwill.
6. Explain your decision to the other staff members while being as supportive of the terminated employee as possible.

Summary

Office policies and procedures are essential to a successful practice. The philosophy of the group and the clarity of the policies, however, require clear, consistent, and regular communication between the staff and the physicians. Weekly staff meetings should be scheduled, with an agenda outlining the main topics of the meeting. Both physicians and staff should attend these meetings, and concerns, new or changing policies, schedules, and so on, should be openly discussed.

Services such as health and medical care must be sensitive to and focused on patient relations. Office policies and procedures should be geared toward attracting new patients and retaining existing patients. Staff members can contribute to the success of the office by increasing their awareness of the patient and suggesting new or improved policies or office practices that enhance the patient's experience.

24 | Developing Hospital Affiliations

VICTOR G. ETTINGER, MD

Once you have decided on the community in which you wish to perpetrate the knowledge you gained in training, the need to obtain hospital privileges becomes apparent. Joining a hospital medical staff is a simple but time-consuming task, and if you are applying to several hospitals for appointment, then the task is more than just incremental. Once on staff, you will need to participate in certain hospital activities that ensure the quality of patient care, the future development of the medical center (all hospitals are medical centers now, even if they only have 10 beds), and so on. You will also want to cultivate relationships with other physicians, both as referral and referring sources.

If you are going into practice on your own, you will certainly benefit from the support services that many hospitals provide to entice unsuspecting doctors into their sphere of influence. Their help can be quite useful as long as you remember that you get nothing for nothing. Many of the onerous tasks associated with joining a hospital staff and participating in medical staff activities can be mitigated if you are prepared. If you are joining an organization such as an HMO or a large group practice, they often will be able to smooth the way.

The credentialing process is tedious but inescapable. It usually takes about three to six months, so it behooves you to start the application process three months prior to finishing your training program. This will enable you to open your office, or join your group, as soon as you return from the last vacation you will be able to afford for the next six to 10 years.

Time can be saved if you gather all the materials together *prior* to starting the application process. Most hospitals will supply a checklist of needed items (Table 24.1) with their 1200-page application form. You will need at least one picture for each hospital. I strongly recommend that it be current and that you are properly groomed. I know this sounds "uptight," but this picture is the first image that your future colleagues will have of you. You have only one opportunity to make a first impression, and negative attitudes can take years to reverse. Thus the picture taken at your graduation soiree may not convey the image you would wish to someone who does not already know what a swell person you really are.

The most difficult task may be obtaining letters of recommendation from physicians (most often the magic number is three) already on the hospital staff. Many times you will have to get letters from doctors who are not in the practice group you will be joining. Therefore it is worthwhile to

Table 24.1 Sample Application Checklist

Picture
Signature
Privilege card
Current DEA
Current
Proof of place of practice (i.e., lease agreement, business license)
Medicare Attestation
Statement of confidentiality
$250 application processing fee
Certificate of insurance (a billing statement does *not* meet our requirements)
Radiology certificate, if applicable
ACLS certificate, if applicable
Base station certificate, if applicable
Full mailing addresses of all references, physicians, and institutions
Time gaps
Medical references (not associates)

meet as many people from the hospital staff as possible prior to making application.

You will also need letters from the directors of all of the programs in which you have trained. This is often the bottleneck in the process. This epistle should clearly document the number and types of procedures you have successfully completed as well as stating the usual gibberish about what an outstanding resident, fellow, or postdoc you are. Substantiation of your procedures has become a very important part of the process because of the large number of under-employed lawyers who like to sue hospitals and doctors.

You will need copies of all state licenses, narcotics license (ie, Drug Enforcement Agency—DEA), board certification, Advanced Cardiac Life Support (ACLS) certificate, etc. A list of other hospitals applied to will be requested, as will a copy of your malpractice insurance certificate. Depending on the state in which you will be practicing, the cost of insurance will range from several thousand dollars to over $100,000 per year for about $1 million to $3 million of coverage.

It may be necessary to fill out a privilege card listing those procedures you will wish to perform on patients in the hospital. In order to prove that you are within a hospital's boundary, you may need proof of your office address, such as a signed lease or business license; this is necessary even if you are joining an established group. Finally, at some point you will have to sign the Medicare Attestation form stating that you will not try to cheat the government, and that the patients' diagnoses are accurate. This form is mandated by the federal government because Big Brother (and Big Sister) is convinced that all doctors are out to rip off the system. Of course, we do not know anyone in government who is dishonest, do we?

The cost of applying to a hospital may range from nothing to several hundred dollars. This covers the clerical expenditures, helps increase the medical staff coffers, ensures the seriousness of the applicant, and pays for the chief of staff's trip to Tahiti. It may also discourage some from applying to many hospitals.

In the past, many hospitals required personal interviews. This is not the rule anymore, but some holdouts remain. The purpose of this perfunctory process (here is a little quiz to keep you in shape) allows the credentialing committee to:

a. see if you have two heads
b. see if you have green skin
c. waste their time
d. waste your time
e. see how you react under extremely stressful circumstances
f. decide if they like your tailor
g. all of the above
h. none of the above
i. some of the above

In addition, it allows you to:

a. meet some of your future colleagues
b. see if they have three eyes
c. note if they have plaid skin
d. see how they waste their time
e. see how they waste your time
f. see how they react under extremely boring circumstances
g. decide if you want to switch tailors
h. all of the above
i. none of the above
j. some of the above

After you have joined the medical staff, you will want to meet other physicians in your community. The best place to do this is in the physicians' lounge or dining room. It will be beneficial to arrange with the director of medical education for you to give a talk on a topic that will enhance your image, preferably something that makes you unique to your community. Make the time to go to the offices of *all* of those doctors who might be sources of referrals. It will be helpful to go to as many hospital department meetings as possible and have one of your colleagues—one who knows you for the superb physician you are—introduce you as new to the community and imply what a phenomenal coup it is that you have decided to join this particular staff. The doctors in the emergency department are also important for you to get to know, because they can help you rapidly build your practice by sending you all the deadbeats no one else will take. This is part of the dues we all pay, and the ER doctors will remember you and send you the paying patients, too, after a while.

As a medical staff member, you will acquire certain formal responsibilities. Some are required by certifying organizations, and some are specific to a particular hospital and to which level of staff membership you wish to sustain—active, associate, or courtesy. All hospitals require a minimum attendance at departmental meetings—usually 50% to 75%—as well as at full staff meetings. You may be required to cover the emergency room in your specialty for a specified number of months or years. This helps you acquire patients for your practice. In addition, you will probably need a minimum number of admissions and/or consultations to maintain your desired level of membership.

Many hospital administrations realize that starting in practice is a fear-filled, expensive proposition. In recent years, many institutions have become major sources of support services to new physicians. It is critical, however, to remember that no matter what you are told, there are *always* strings attached—overt as well as implied. Hospital administrators do *nothing* out of the goodness of their hearts (as a point of fact, one of the great questions debated at medical meetings is whether or not hospital administrators even have hearts).

Hospitals will be most agreeable to help primary care physicians and those specialists who will most likely utilize it to perform procedures. If you are going into infectious disease, dermatology, allergy, or endocrinology, forget it; go to the bank or your parents. The hospital may help you with low-cost loans (in exchange for your firstborn), finding and renting office space, finding another physician to join or with whom to share space, and even practice development (previously known as advertising—a very dirty word in medicine). In addition, if the director of staff development got out on the right side of the bed, you may be able to receive help with home or car financing.

Much of what I say in this chapter may have little to do with the world of medicine as you will come to know it. The credentialing process is likely to continue as it is now, though I expect it to become more and more cumbersome as the government and the lawyers progressively interfere. I also foresee a time when the hospital committee requirements will be so time consuming that outside medical or paramedical groups will be hired to do the work in a timely fashion. Hospital support services may go the way of physician autonomy, if (when!) doctors become employees of these institutions of health. It is safest to recognize that medicine is very big business and that the people with the money control the process. Thus the most satisfying part of medicine may be the relationships one develops with colleagues and patients.

25 | Practice Fees and Financial Policies

RON ROSENBERG, PAC, MPH

This chapter will provide an overview of the process of setting fees and financial policies. I will discuss the resources available to the practice for determining the market value of the services it provides.

In addition, I will examine the issues present in the business relationship between a practice and its patients—issues that are often not discussed directly with the patients. Also, I will suggest areas to be covered by the practice's financial policies.

Historical Context

Most physicians never analyze the true nature of fee-for-service medical practice. In such practices, a service is provided in exchange for a fee. Over the years, customs have developed that have shaped the way services are priced and fees collected. Several key events and trends have shaped the reimbursement environment in general and the issues of fee levels and financial policies in particular.

Relative value studies (RVSs). First developed in the 1950s, these systems of identifying and valuing physicians' services allowed for a universally understood and standardized method for physicians to set their fees. In 1974, the Federal Trade Commission succeeded in obtaining a ruling that the use of an RVS was "price fixing." Physicians were required to turn in their RVS books, and the California Medical Association stopped the development of the system. These events removed the one standardized method of comparing and quantifying the value of services. Even though relative value studies were again allowed and developed in the 1980s, other changes in the reimbursement environment diminished their importance.

Medicare. This federal government program, which funds health-care for the elderly, has had a great impact on the pricing of physicians' services—often more of an impact than is healthy for the practice.

Many physicians have allowed Medicare's reimbursement policies to influence the fee-setting and financial policies for the non-Medicare portion of their practice. For example, Medicare does not pay for all services, and many physicians have stopped charging private insurers for those services not covered by Medicare. As another example, Medicare has capped the allowable payments for services, but not uniformly; physicians who set their fees based on Medicare's maximum allowables will overprice some services billed to commercial insurers, thereby punishing patients, and underprice others, thereby punishing themselves.

As a publicly funded program, however, Medicare is a goldmine of data. By making informed requests for Medicare data, a physician can develop a data base that though not sufficient for setting all prices, is a great help.

Competition. During the 1980s medicine has felt the impact of competition. Rapidly escalating costs forced employers, as well as government, to search for ways to constrain costs. Also, the perceived physician shortage of the 1970s gave way to the perception of a coming surplus, at least in urban areas, in the 1980s. This perceived surplus is specially acute in some specialty areas.

One effect of cost containment and increasing competition has been the appearance of new ways to deliver care and systems to tighten expenditures. Managed care systems, second opinions for surgery, and pre-authorization requirements are but a few of these.

The net effect has been the introduction of price sensitivity into the medical marketplace. Its effect on practices has often been manifested as a shrinking bottom line, making assertive, accurate management more important. An often overlooked aspect of practice management are the areas of financial policies and fee-setting.

The following information is not meant as an exhaustive text on these topics; rather, it is a perspective from which to assess your own practice and initiate the kind of changes that will improve your practice's income. At the same time, you will allow your patients to get full value from their health insurance and reduce their out-of-pocket costs for your services. If the policies are applied carefully and effectively, another effect will be an improvement in your patients' satisfaction with their care.

Financial Policies

Most practices have reimbursement policies that they have "slid into" almost by default. For example, if one asks practice personnel about their policy on cash collections, the responses usually vary among personnel, and even when the responses are similar, the extent to which the policy is enforced will vary. The following sections address several policies to consider.

Cash Collections at Time of Service

Most physicians say they want to collect as much of their fees as possible at the time the service is provided. Although this is a sound policy, the question is, What *actions* are taken to collect the money? Is there a stop at the end of the patient's flow through the office where the fee is requested?

Before their appointments, are patients aware that payment is expected at the time of service?

Acceptance of Credit Cards

Money is expensive. The longer you wait for payment, the less the money is worth. In today's society, people are used to paying for essential goods and services or luxuries when they do not have the cash—they simply use credit cards. Physicians have traditionally carried patients' unpaid balances, but there is no reason to continue to do so. Credit cards (Master Card, Visa, American Express, Discover) are an easy way for patients to handle their medical bills, at least for office services and minor surgical procedures. Finally, patients' unpaid balances can interfere with the therapeutic relationship. The debt is seldom mentioned but the patient knows it is there, and it affects follow-up care and compliance with therapy. Thus for the financial health of the practice and the therapeutic health of the patient, it pays to make it as easy as possible for patients to pay their bills quickly. Credit cards assist in that goal.

Assistance in Filing Insurance Claims

Does the practice file insurance forms for patients? If so, for what types of services? These questions are best answered by analyzing the services provided. Hospital or procedural services are best filed by the practice. These services are more complex in terms of third-party payments and may require closer monitoring of receipts, including appeal of inadequate or denied payments. Medical services such as office visits are less critical, and those revenues may not be lost by having the patients file their own claims.

Your general rule may be that the only patients you assist by completing their insurance forms are those who because of age, language, or other problems cannot complete them and those whose services were surgical in nature and total more than some threshold amount ($400 may be a reasonable level).

Participation in Medicare

Many factors must be considered when deciding to be a participating physician in Medicare or any other insurance program. These include the following:

A. The percentage (or prospective percentage) of your patients covered by Medicare or the insurer in question.
B. The maturity of your practice (or the portion of your practice covered by the insurer in question). Is your practice full, or are you searching for new sources of patients?

C. The quality of the insurer (or the local fiscal intermediary in the case of Medicare). Does the insurer process claims quickly and efficiently and is it available to the physician to answer questions and provide information?

D. The benefits of participation. Are there higher payments? More patients? Faster payments? Less paperwork?

E. The long-range effects of participation in the plan (or participation in insurance plans in general) in your community. The power of the insurers to set financial policies in a community depends on a critical mass of practices participating in their programs. For example, some communities have a much higher proportion of managed care patients covered under capitation agreements, whereas in others their managed care patients are covered in fee schedule relationships. Still other communities have very few managed care systems. These variations are the result of many factors, but an important one is the ability of the managed care plans to enroll physician providers under the terms of a participating provider agreement.

F. Your philosophical position. What is your position on the government in medicine? On the socialization of medicine? On the power of the insurers to dictate how care is delivered? After all of the financial and marketing considerations, these philosophical positions generally have a great influence on a practice's decision to participate.

In the case of Medicare, a financial analysis is a critical step in the process. Factors that determine the benefits of participation to a practice include the following:

A. The level of the practice's maximum allowable actual charges (MAACs). Nonparticipating physicians are limited to these levels for Medicare patients. The MAACs are determined by the charges submitted to Medicare during the base period April to June 1984. If a provider was not in practice or did not provide a particular service during that base period, his or her MAAC for that service is based on the median charge submitted from the community during that time. The MAAC is allowed to rise slightly each year, and the MAACs set by median charges in a community are generally well below the market level.

B. The collection rate of the practice for its Medicare patients. For participating physicians, Medicare pays 80% of the allowable payment. The practice collects the 20% copayment from the patient. Therefore the practice's collection rate applies only to the 20% copayment. For nonparticipants, Medicare pays the patient 80% of the allowable payment, and the practice collects 100% of its fee (up to the level of the MAAC for that service) from the patient. Therefore, the practice's collection rate applies to 100% of the bill.

In calculating the financial impact of participation, a spreadsheet program on a personal computer is helpful. Set up the spreadsheet as in the example below:

A	B	C	D	E	F	G
CPT code	Freq.	MAAC	Medicare par prev.	Medicare nonpar prev.	Customary	Collec. rate
90050	28	$73	$55	$53	$65	78%

Then perform the following calculations for each current procedural terminology (CPT) code:

PAR	NONPAR
Frequency (28) × par. prevailing ($55) = $1540	Frequency (28) × MAAC ($73) = $2044
MC pays you 80% = $1232	$2044 × 78% (coll. rate) = $1594
You collect 20% from patient (at 78%) =$240	
Total collection = $1232 + $240 = $1472	

The result is that for CPT code 90050, at a 78% collection rate, you are better off financially as a nonparticipating physician, as you collect $1594, compared with $1472 for a participating physician. You must perform that calculation for each CPT code for which you bill, and perhaps at varying collection rates. The sum of all of the calculations will give you the total financial impact of your decision to participate.

It should be noted that there are significant changes occurring in the Medicare system. A National Fee Schedule, in the form of a Resource Based Relative Value Study (RBRVS) is being implemented over a five year period. Changes affecting reimbursement in general, and Medicare reimbursement specifically, include:

1. Calculated relative values for services that will increase the value for "cognitive" services such as patient visits and consultations, and decrease the value for surgical services. These changes will definitely affect Medicare reimbursement, and, to a lesser extent, payments from other third-party payors.
2. Adjustments that will "blunt" the geographic variations in Medicare reimbursement between areas with the lowest and the highest Prevailing Charges.
3. Decreasing limits in the amount a Nonparticipating Provider can bill to a Medicare patient above the RBRVS allowable. The current version of the regulations places that balance billing limit at an effective rate of 9.25%.
4. As part of the National Fee Schedule, certain changes in the definitions and guidelines in the CPT coding system.
5. A standardized interpretation of reimbursement policies by all Medicare carriers, ending the variations in reimbursement for the same services from locale to locale.

The final Relative Values for services, the geographic adjustments, and the changes in coding and reimbursement policy are all subject to the political process, and will invariably change many times. These guidelines for financial policies should be assessed in light of those changes, as they occur.

Participation in Blue Shield

The decision to participate in Blue Shield has considerations similar to those for Medicare. The patients covered by Medicare include all those over a certain age, whereas the Blue Shield population is more variable. What is the market share of the "Blues"? How many of your patients are covered? How many would you lose if you do not participate? (This is a function not only of the rule by which the patients must abide—that is, they must see only participating physicians—but also of the availability and participation policies of other providers of your specialty in your community.)

How does Blue Shield's participating physicians' fee schedule compare with your fees? A financial analysis similar to the one described for Medicare will assist you in determining the financial impact of your decision, especially when you factor in the marketing implications of participation.

Professional Courtesy

Providing services at reduced or no charges to physicians, other health-care providers, and their families is an old tradition in medicine; however, there is no reason to provide such courtesy to their third-party insurers. Always obtain information on any insurance these patients have, bill the insurer as you would for any other patient (accepting assignment of financial benefits so the check will come to you), and then write off any balance after the insurer pays. You will have provided the courtesy to the patient so that he or she has no out-of-pocket expense, and you have recovered the revenues due from the insurer.

Fee Reductions for Other Reasons: "Insurance Only"

As with professional courtesy, reducing the amount a patient pays is best done with accounting procedures. Bill at the full fee, make a good-faith effort to collect from the patient (send at least three bills), and then write off the uncollectible amount. You may tell the patient with a financial hardship that you are required to bill them but that you do not expect them to pay more than their insurance pays. You *should not* apply this policy to all patients, or even to many patients.

The third-party payors write contracts with employers so that the co-payment—the portion of the bill for which the patient is responsible—not only reduces the insurers' costs, but also holds down utilization of services by the policyholders. Some insurers consider providers who accept insurance only as guilty of fraud. When Medicare finds a provider with a *policy* of accepting what Medicare pays as payment in full, they will consider that the provider has a lower fee than actually charged. For example, for a $120 charge, Medicare allows $100, pays the provider $80, and the provider does not collect the $20 copayment from the patient. Medicare then assumes that because the provider accepts $80 as payment in full for the service, the amount for which Medicare is responsible is only 80% of that, or $64, and may request the provider to refund $16. This changes the provider's allowable payment for that service to the $80 total.

Financial Counseling

If your practice has financial policies and you expect your patients to follow those policies, *all* of your patients should be counseled. The counseling should start with information on your financial policies summarized in a patient information brochure. Your policies on collection at time of service, insurance billing, plan participation, payment plans, and other matters such as office hours, after-hours coverage, and anything else you want your patients to know about your practice should be included.

At the patient's first visit, the policies should be reviewed with the patient, and at that time any questions or requests for fee or payment schedule exceptions may be resolved. By being clear with the patients about your financial expectations, you will have fewer problems and fewer deviations from policies.

Payment Plans

Acceptance of credit cards can avert many extended payment plans. However, when a patient has an unpaid balance and cannot discharge it with a credit card, a payment plan may be required. For small balances (under $100) you may simply want to set up payments appropriate to the financial situation of the patient.

For larger balances, you may want to add interest payments to the amount owed. There is no reason not to make this routine for payment plans, as money is not free. The longer a balance owed to you remains unpaid, the less the money is worth. For payment plans with interest, you should have a signed agreement that fully discloses the balance owed, interest rates, payment amounts, and total of the payments plus interest. Samples of these forms are available at office supplies stores and may be available from medical supply companies. It is wise to have your attorney and/or accountant review the form you use in light of federal and local truth-in-lending and consumer laws.

Does the Practice See Medicaid Patients?

Medicaid is partially funded by the federal government, administered by each state, and pays for medical care for low-income people. Each state's program has a fee schedule by CPT code and pays anywhere from 20 to 35 cents on the dollar compared with most practices' fees. Payment of Medicaid claims is generally very slow. Although the payment level is low, most physicians feel an obligation to see some Medicaid patients. The questions that must be answered are, what is a reasonable number to see, and how can you attain and maintain that level?

Factors that will enter into the determination of the amount of Medicaid patients to see include the maturity of the practice (ie, how full is it, and if you see a Medicaid patient, will it keep a full-paying patient from getting an appointment?) and the availability in your community of alternative sources for the type of medical services you provide.

Many practices limit the number of new Medicaid patients they see to keep their Medicaid patients below a certain percentage of their payor mix (eg, 15%–20%). This is often accomplished by assigning a limited number of new patient visits per week for Medicaid.

Information Collection

Demographic, insurance, and financial responsibility data must be collected when a patient is brought into the practice. The information collected should include the following:

A. Full name of the patient and of each family member, with the name of the insured person noted
B. Address and phone number, with a photocopy of the patient's driver's license or other identification with the address
C. Complete insurance information, including a photocopy of the insurance ID card
D. Credit card information, including card name, number, and expiration date, and a signed preauthorization for charging unpaid balances to the card
E. Financial responsibility statement signed by the patient or patient's parent or guardian promising to be responsible for the fees. This is especially important in the case of underage patients brought into the office by divorced or separated parents.

This information should be updated annually.

Information on Hospitalized Patients

Patient demographic and financial information collected at hospital admission is notoriously inaccurate.

If the hospitalized patient is new to the practice, a staff member from the practice should obtain the same information described in the foregoing section. This should be done while the patient is in the hospital. If the patient is already established in the practice, the information should simply be verified.

Summary

You and your staff make decisions relating to these areas every day, usually without the benefit of a clearly, deliberately stated policy. Even when there is a clear policy, it may not have been adequately communicated to each patient in the practice. Has the patient received a written copy of the policies in the form of a patient information brochure, preferably prior to his or her first visit? Are patients counseled at their first visit to ensure that they understand the practice's financial policies? Are the appropriate policies reviewed with the patient at the time they are telephoned to confirm their appointment? These steps will help to increase compliance with your financial policies.

The practice that has clear policies and explicitly communicates those policies to its patients will have the fewest problems with patient accounts becoming exceptions to those policies.

Fees

"Physicians charge too much!" But how much is too much? How does anyone—including the physician—know if a fee is appropriate? What are the bases of physicians' fees?

An important distinction here is the difference between *charge* (or *fee*) and *reimbursement*. In most cases a provider can charge for any service at any fee level, but this is separate and distinct from what a third-party payor will pay—or what is fair and equitable to ask a patient to pay—for that service.

Most providers determine what services are billable and how much to charge for those services based on what they hear in the hospital doctors' lounge. Other providers base those decisions on what they have always charged. Still others charge based on which services Medicare pays for and at what level. There is seldom an investigation into what specific services are separately billable according to the CPT system or a review of available data on community fee levels.

You can take several steps to determine fee levels that are appropriate for you.

1. Know your practice. A provider with a full practice can be more cavalier about fees and other financial policies than can a young practice that is in real competition for survival.
2. Learn how the CPT system describes the services you provide. You cannot set fees rationally unless you know what is included under the CPT codes for your services. Read the definitions of *levels of services* and *consultations*, as well as the remainder of the introduction to the

current year's CPT book. In addition, read the guidelines for the medicine and surgery sections and the notes in front of each subsection of procedures you provide.
3. Obtain all available data on the community fee levels for the services you provide (see below).
4. Review your fees at least annually.
5. Use Medicare data, but use it as data, not as gospel or as a model on which to base your practice.
6. Use other payor data!
7. If possible, have only one fee schedule. Trying to adjust your fees for each payor will be confusing, lead to errors in billing, and may even be seen as fraud. The only exception to this dictum is if you are not a participating physician in the Medicare program. In this case, you are limited to your MAACs for Medicare beneficiaries. Most practices in this circumstance have two fee schedules.

A Methodology for Fee Analysis

Collecting Data

For any practice that goes to the trouble of collecting it, information is available from the sources listed below.

Medicare. Obtain from Medicare the data for your specialty. Be sure to request the complete set of codes, not only the ones for which you have customary profiles. Request the following:

Your customary profiles (the median charge you submitted to Medicare for that CPT code during the preceding year)

Your MAACs and the gap-fill MAACs for those codes for which you do not have your own MAAC (even if you are a participating physician)

The true 50th percentile charge

The true 75th percentile charge

The capped 75th percentile charge (the Medicare prevailing charge) for both participating and nonparticipating providers (also called the *allowable charge*)

Remember, the true 75th and true 50th percentiles are actual percentile analyses of Medicare charges in your region, including those submitted by nonparticipating providers limited by those providers' MAACs. The true 50th and 75th percentiles are therefore somewhat lower than a "true" analysis of all charges in the community.

Obtain these data each year; Medicare re-analyzes and recalculates the profiles and allowables annually.

Commercial insurance. These data are the most difficult to obtain. If Blue Shield or any of the other commercial insurers in your area release their schedule of allowables, this is an extremely valuable piece of information. Generally, the only way to obtain these data is to analyze your own collections from these payors.

Managed care. HMOs and PPOs will often provide their payment schedules to prospective providers. Recognize that these will be reduced by some percentage and will not include all CPT codes, but you can increase these fees by 15% to 25% and approximate insurance company allowables.

Workers compensation. The Workers Compensation fee schedules are relatively complete and generally follow a relative value study. Although the allowable payments are low, this fee schedule is valuable as a component of your data base, as are the managed care data. You can increase the fees by some percentage to determine true market value.

Relative value study. Use a relative value study as the basis for your data base. Both the Florida and McGraw-Hill studies use the entire CPT system. The McGraw-Hill study is available on floppy disk, making it an ideal basis for your analysis.

Analysis

Using a computer spreadsheet, set up a matrix of fees for each CPT code used in your practice. For example:

CPT	My fee	RVS unit value	RVS fee @ $10/ unit	50th	75th	Custom.	Blues	HMO	Workers Comp.
90080	$85	11	$110	$82	$97	$75	$105	$90	$80

The CPT code 90080 is for "comprehensive service, established patient." Reading across the row of fees, you can see that this provider's fee, $85, is barely above the Medicare 50th percentile, well below the Medicare 75th percentile, even further below the Blue Shield fee, and barely above Workers Compensation. Even worse, the customary profile at $75 shows that the provider charges less than his or her already low $85 fee at least half the time.

Using this analysis to establish a new fee at the market level of the community, one could assume that the appropriate level would be slightly above the Blue Shield level, or $110. Dividing $110 by the RVS unit value, 11, gives you a conversion factor of 10. This will be helpful in establishing other fees.

Let us look at another example:

CPT	My fee	RVS unit value	RVS fee @ $208.33/ unit	50th	75th	Custom.	Blues	HMO	Workers Comp.
49000	$1200	6	$1250	$1125	$1190	$1170	$1125	$1210	$950

Analyzing this array for an exploratory laparotomy, the fees do not fit quite as nicely as in the first example. The Blue Shield fee is lower than the Medicare true 75th. The HMO fee is higher than both the 75th and the Blue Shield fee. The point here is that none of the data elements in this data base can be taken alone as a fee schedule. Because of idiosyncracies in each data set, there will be aberrantly low and high fees, which will show up in unpredictable ways.

Because various market forces affect fee levels in different ways, the fees for some services will vary geographically in proportion to relative value studies. Others will not, and other data must be used.

You must analyze each code you use, apply logic to the data available to determine the market value for that service, and set your fees according to where you want to be in your marketplace.

Summary

The quality of a practice's financial management can be evaluated by its handling of each of the issues discussed in this chapter. How the issues are handled is secondary to the inclusion of each of them in the practice's management system.

The physicians who are at least aware of the factors involved in valuing their services, and who have made conscious decisions on their financial policies, will receive the maximum income within the constraints of their financial and ethical guidelines.

Suggested Reading

American Medical Association, *Physician's Current Procedural Terminology*. Chicago, IL: AMA, 1990.

California Workers' Compensation Institute, *Official Medical Fee Schedule (California Relative Value Study 1974)* (rev. ed). San Francisco, CA: CWCI, 1989.

Florida Medical Association, Inc., *Florida Relative Value Studies*. Jacksonville, FL: FMA, Inc., 1989.

Relative Value Studies, Inc., *Relative Value for Physicians* (3rd ed.). Denver, CO: Systemetrics/McGraw-Hill, 1989.

26 | Strategies for a Successful Business Office: Understanding the Insurance Claims Process, Maximizing Your Reimbursement, and Controlling Your Accounts Receivable

MARK BABST, MBA, FACMGA
AND NEAL GREEN, MBA

Essentially, the practice of medicine consists of one individual providing a personal service to another. No two physicians are identical; consequently, no two practices are the same. Business techniques that work well for one practice may be an abysmal failure for another. However, in spite of their many differences, all medical practices must function within the same macroeconomic environment, and all are subject to the same external—and often similar internal—influences.

Although a handful of "keys" may be used in making a medical business office successful, there is no "magic door" that any one of them can open that guarantees financial success. Establishing a successful practice requires having a good understanding of the economic environment, on both the macro and micro levels, and then doing a number of different things very well.

Successful Collections

Some practices have been more successful than others in dealing with reimbursement for services. Although simple in concept, time and time again it has proven difficult to execute. Implementation is actually harder in smaller practices because they cannot afford to hire separate experts to perform all the various and necessary tasks. Most solo practices and small group practices rely on an individual office manager. It is extremely difficult to find a single person with all of the necessary knowledge, background, and skills to fill all of the many responsibilities of the job, which can include hiring, supervising, filing insurance claims, and collecting payments, among others. Therefore, smaller practices often have to settle for the best they can find at the price they are willing to pay.

Turnover of office managers is generally high and severely complicates the problem of consistency and continuity in shepherding the small practices' business growth and development. The external macro-environment, however, continues to evolve and become more complex. That no formal or widely accepted credentialing process exists for medical business office management further adds to hit-or-miss results in recruitment, hiring, and ultimately the practice's collections and financial performance.

Leaders and Teachers

Making sure that *all* of a practice's employees have at least a basic understanding of the various external economic and environmental factors is an important first step for collections success. This means that the physician or administrator must be a teacher. There must be a formal, ongoing program established to update the staff regarding dynamic environmental changes and to increase their practical knowledge. This process is too important to be left to chance. The doctor or administrator must first understand the basics of the macroeconomic environment in which the practice strives to prosper. This type of knowledge cannot be obtained merely by hiring an office manager from a competitive practice whose doctors drive more expensive cars—it starts with the practice's leadership.

Is there a formal leadership structure? For the physicians, is the title of "Managing Partner" or "Medical Director" (or its various equivalents) considered a burden and not to be taken seriously? Are all of the position's responsibilities delegated to staff lower down the organizational ladder? Does the managing partner have the temperament to lead and manage the practice as an iterative process, in which one learns by doing, or does he or she view this role as a hassle and headache and therefore demand often unattainable standards of perfection? People are the pivotal resource in managing any business. To effectively employ this resource requires leadership, of which many aspects cannot be learned from books or courses. However, there are many techniques that can be learned by reading, attending conferences and meetings, taking classes, and visiting other practices. For those physicians willing to meet the challenge, there is a plethora of resources available to help: national and local medical management associations, journals, books, seminars, consultants, provider manuals, and provider relations representatives.

The absence of physicians and executive-level administrators filling this learning and teaching role typically creates an obvious knowledge gap within a practice. The absence of internal communications serves to widen the gap. As the differences in knowledge at the practice's various staff levels become greater, the difference between the practice's realized collections and its true collection potential also increases. Without conscious leadership and strong business policies, money can be irretrievably lost.

When a practice suffers a loss of organization and revenues, the physician might decide to consult an office management professional. Many consultants approach this situation in a very didactic way: they present information in a classroom setting, and the physicians attend seminar sessions along with the nursing and business staff. The fundamental teaching of these consultants is often that leadership relies on open communication, which can often be clouded by poor listening skills and/or interpersonal issues. Frequently seen symptoms of poor communication by leaders of medical groups are high staff turnover, suboptimal performance by otherwise capable employees, and complaints of lack of training or understanding of job duties. Underperforming practices can blossom after just a few hour-long sessions or a retreat with a clinical social worker, psychologist, or practice management consultant. In these sessions the practice is considered a living organism that is dependent on the work and effective communication of many individuals. In effect, the practice becomes the "patient."

Components of Reimbursement Process

Successful collections come from an understanding of how the health-care industry works. A simplistic model of the health-care industry has four essential components: the patients, the providers, the payors, and the third-party administrators. This paradigm creates an easily understood conceptual foundation for all of the practice's staff. It is flexible enough to deal with a dynamically changing environment, and it offers even entry-level employees the intellectual structure to integrate the reasons behind a new task into a bigger framework.

A single educational model also facilitates ongoing training of new employees and retraining for existing employees, maintains the pool of knowledge, and continues to reinforce and disseminate information within the practice.

The patient component is, of course, self-explanatory. The provider category includes the physicians, hospitals, pharmacies, and nursing homes as well as home-care nurses and agencies, ambulatory surgery centers, drug companies, free-standing scanners, and so on. Some are organized into chains or belong to big conglomerates, whereas others are small, independently run businesses.

The payors are the various parties who earn the money used to pay the providers. There are three general categories of payors: business/industry, government, and the individual patient or his or her family. The payors are the source of pressure for cost containment. Every dollar a company spends on medical insurance is an expense that must be passed along, via higher prices, to its customers. Thus an increase in health-care costs affects either the company's profitability or its ability to compete in the marketplace. Similarly, every dollar that government spends on Medicare or Medicaid must be raised by taxation, in one form or another. All of the various cost-containment efforts and access restrictions—via managed care entities, prior authorizations, and so on—have been instituted in response to payors' demands to curb the upward spiral of health-care prices.

Third-party administrators are the various business entities that reimburse the providers with the payors' money. Insurance carriers, fiscal intermediaries, and union benefits administrators fall into this category.

Until recently, most health insurance companies assumed the actual financial risk for the medical care of their beneficiaries. They did this by spreading the risk of paying for any one person's illness among many people. Using sophisticated statistical techniques to tabulate the incidence of various diseases as well as the risk factors and costs of treatment, insurers were able to calculate how much to charge each beneficiary in premiums. This process is called underwriting and is performed by a special category of statistical experts known as actuaries.

With the cost of health care rising nearly 20% per year, the insurance companies suffered tremendous underwriting losses during the 1980s. They passed these losses onto their payors in the form of increased premiums. The payors found themselves economically squeezed between massive premium increases on one hand (to both make up for prior underwriting losses and compensate for the current year's price inflation) and their contractual obligations to their employees, both current and retired, on the other hand.

One response to the high costs of traditional indemnity insurance has been the development of administrative services only (ASO) contracts. This is most attractive for large employers or union benefits trusts. In this method, payors do not transfer the risk of illness to their insurance carriers. Rather, they have enough members on their own to take the risk themselves, and they purchase only claims processing, provider networks, and utilization review services from the insurance company. They may pass off the risk of certain catastrophic losses or illnesses, such as AIDS, by buying excessive loss coverage called *re-insurance*. ASO variations also fit well with the simplified model of the reimbursement environment.

The Computer as Tool

Another key resource in the practice management process, besides good leadership and a shared knowledge of how reimbursement works, is the practice's computer. The computer is merely a tool—albeit an important one—to effectively manage the practice. All too often, particularly in large clinics or academic faculty practices, the response to low collections or high overhead is to buy a newer, more powerful, and invariably more expensive data-processing system. Generally the new computer does exactly what the old model did—perhaps faster—with no appreciable effect on collections, but with a significant increase to the costs of doing business. As part of an organism that includes a shared and accurate understanding of the environment together with effective leaders and organization, the computer hardware and software can be critically valuable tools. Unfortunately, purchasing the very best computer system without these organizational prerequisites in place can leave the practice with a very expensive and, most likely, underutilized asset.

Should You Submit Claims?

For some practices, it is essential to submit claims to the patients' insurance carriers. Other practices choose to do this as a courtesy for some of their patients. Still others avoid it entirely by providing their patients with all of the necessary information to submit their own claims. Some, particularly multispecialty groups, find themselves in all three situations at once.

As in most areas of business administration, there are no steadfast rules to follow. Specialty practices, particularly surgeons generating high per-episode charges, must send assigned claims to the carriers. Most patients cannot give a surgeon an out-of-pocket payment of thousands of dollars and then wait for their insurance companies to repay them. However, family practitioners, pediatricians, and internists generally request payment at the time of service. In return, they give their patients itemized receipts, often called *superbills*, which patients can attach to their insurance forms and submit directly to the responsible party. Obstetricians often require the patient to pay the total obstetrical care package by the seventh month of pregnancy. Following the delivery, an unassigned claim is submitted to the patients' carriers as a courtesy.

Whichever way a practice decides to handle this issue, it should be implemented with the prior knowledge of the patient. This means that the receptionist, when scheduling a new patient, should be trained to say (along with other essential information, such as the office's location), "The group prefers that you make payment at the time of service; is that okay with you?" This, or some alternative script that fits your particular practice, will avoid embarrassing the patient and can help increase collections and minimize the group's receivables.

Payment at the Time of Service

A policy of payment at the time of service can be very important, especially in the case of a patient's first visit to a specialty consultant. Because there will probably be no ongoing patient-physician relationship (and frequently the specialist is confirming bad news), many of the charges for these one-time-only visits may be carried in the practice's accounts receivable for a long time.

The ability to accept credit cards can be a great convenience for the patient and can accelerate the practice's cash flow. This form of payment will also encourage payment at the time of service. Almost every bank now offers what are commonly called *merchant accounts*, which allow credit card vouchers to be deposited, just like cash, directly into a practice's bank account. The bank's charge for these accounts is usually a small percentage (about 2%–3%) of the total value of the transactions, with a minimum monthly fee of $10 to $20. Experience of many practices has shown this to be well worth the investment. If this method of payment becomes well received by your patients, then by all means consider buying a point-of-service (POS) terminal, which will allow your staff to slide the patient's credit card through an automatic magnetic-strip reader for approval. It will save staff time and shorten your patients' waiting times.

Insurance Claims Process

Making the insurance claims process work from an operational perspective starts with the initial encounter and continues with ongoing maintenance of accurate and thorough information. This is often called the *front-end process*. The best way to accomplish this is with a well-designed patient registration form. All of the information collected is important for the creation of an accurate and clean claim form, or for good skip-tracing and follow-through in the event that the patient's account must be assigned to a collection agency. In the case of primary-care practices where both spouses are often insured, it is necessary to obtain both their birth dates to assist with the coordination of both plans' benefits under the industry standard first-birthday-is-primary rule.

Make certain that your receptionist has quick access to a photocopier, and request that all insurance, Medicare, or other identification cards be copied for the charts. This saves time if there is a problem with reading the patients' handwriting; there is no need to hold up the claim (and the practice's cash flow with it) while contacting the patient for clarification.

Maintain Current Patient Information

The receptionist should always scan the patients' completed registration forms to make sure that all of the questions are answered legibly. Frequently, patients simply skip entire blocks or sections of a form. The receptionists must be taught to understand the value of accurate registration information. Their review can catch obvious omissions as well as more subtle ones, such as inadvertently writing the current year after the day and month of birth, or Social Security numbers that appear to be missing a digit. They should learn to notice whether the Medicare patient has a spouse and if the registration form lists the spouse's work phone number without listing a second medical insurance policy. This one issue could significantly delay payment from Medicare on an assigned claim, now that Medicare is legally always considered the secondary carrier. By having participated in the fundamental and ongoing training processes, the receptionist will have a better understanding of why these are not just silly and bothersome forms, but essential source documents for the entire reimbursement function.

In terms of data-base management, it is also essential that the practice record changes in the patients' situations via updates of registration information. This function is often ignored, with a high cost in reduced collections and higher receivables. Bills and claims are often mailed out with obsolete information. If it is a surgical practice, a bill for many thousands of dollars might never be forwarded to the right address.

Another example of poor data-base management may result in a claim being sent to a former employer, thereby breaching the patient's confidentiality and exposing the practice to lawsuits. In the meantime, when the patient arrives for follow-up care he or she may complain and ask, "Why haven't you billed my insurance company yet?"

There is currently no sure-fire way to update every change in the patient's information, but at least 80% of the changes could be discovered by the receptionist casually asking returning patients, "By the way, have you moved or changed jobs or insurance companies since your last visit?" It is a friendly question, and if the answer is yes, the receptionist can simply have the patient complete a new registration form.

If your group provides ongoing chronic care that can result in significant account balances, it is wise to contact the patient's responsible payor during the initial visit to ascertain if there are any benefit limitations, restrictions, or prior authorization requirements. It is important for the caller to have a good understanding of the doctor's treatment plan for the individual patient. (This again comes from good communications and training by the physician!) It is useful to develop a practice-specific form that prompts the insurance verification staff person to ask questions such as: "What is the deductible, and has it been met this year?" "What are Mr. Jones's policy limits for inpatient (or outpatient, psychiatric, surgical, etc.) benefits?" and "Do we need to request a prior authorization number?" Your staff should always obtain the name of the insurance carrier's representative providing your practice with this information.

Once the staff has obtained this valuable information, it is the responsibility of the administrator and physicians to ensure that the communication structure exists within the business office to properly use it. The physicians should be notified of any financial impediments in the implementation of the treatment plan, particularly if an expensive hospitalization or operation is contemplated. The doctor can then make an informed decision for implementing or changing the treatment plan and counsel the patient about the various alternatives. Information such as prior authorization numbers must also be communicated to the billing unit so that they will be included on the appropriate claim forms.

During the last five years, the entire issue of prior authorization has become critically important for almost all third-party administrators and insurance carriers. It is an essential component of all managed care plans as well as Medicare, Medicaid, workers' compensation, personal injury, and almost every hospital admission.

Prior authorization is often required retrospectively within two days of an emergency admission or delivery of a baby. Inadequately addressing the need for prior authorizations will definitely result in decreased third-party payments to the practice and higher out-of-pocket residual balances for the patients. This can create disastrous public relations for the practice.

Not only does the practice's data base have to be updated regularly for accuracy, but its foundational pool of information must be adjusted to keep pace with the environmental changes that directly affect the billing and claims process. For example, the Medicare fiscal intermediaries in many areas are now capable of electronically *crossing over* or billing certain *Medi-gap* secondary carriers. To take advantage of this, doctors' offices need only to enter the Medi-gap carriers' ID numbers on the claim forms or on their electronic submissions.

Interestingly, even where this service is available and practices have all the necessary information, many of the Medi-gap carriers continue to receive expensively produced paper secondary claims. Unfortunately for these groups, lack of understanding of the correct procedure slows reimbursement, raises expenses, and increases the time required for accounts receivable follow-up.

Setting Practice Fees

The importance of a practice's fee schedule cannot be overemphasized. An improperly constructed fee schedule can cost a practice a sizable fortune over time. All too often a fee schedule is built around anecdotes or a chat in the doctors' lounge over coffee. This is far too important a fundamental to be treated casually.

Almost all insurance carriers and fiscal intermediaries understand only one language when it comes to fees: relative value scale (RVS). To use a fee schedule that is not based upon relativity is a fundamentally poor decision in today's environment. This is especially relevant for procedural specialists. Gone are the days when third parties paid 80% to 100% of whatever a doctor charged. Using something other than an RVS-based fee schedule will, in some cases, delegate by default the function of setting the doctor's fee to a clerk or computer in an insurance company's office. They will be happy to calculate, using an RVS, what they will pay, and then send the patient a note saying that "your doctor's charge for the service exceeds the community's usual and customary fees." On the other hand, in reviewing your claims, if they calculate that your fee is lower than what you could have charged using the RVS, they will never write you a note suggesting that your charges are too low.

There are a number of RVS systems available, but so far the "gold standard" has been the California Relative Value Scale (CRVS). The majority of third-party payors use this model in adjudicating your claims. Consequently, there is no good reason why physicians should not use it in constructing their fee schedules.

The CRVS may eventually be replaced by the Resource Based Relative Value Scale (RBRVS) being developed for the Social Security Administration to use for paying Medicare claims. It remains to be seen whether other third-party payors beside Medicare will use this new physician reimbursement system. Now, quite a few years after Medicare fully implemented the diagnostic related groups (DRGs) system of paying hospitals, there has not been an industry-wide movement toward that methodology.

It is important to implement an RVS-based fee schedule with a solid familiarity with billing patterns of your particular locality. It is not appropriate to apply New York or Los Angeles fees to Middle America. The rates used by local HMOs, PPOs, and other managed care entities can be helpful in determining appropriate local levels. An analysis of an area's Medicare profiles and MAACs can also be helpful. Remember to update fees at least annually.

Design and Proper Use of Superbills

Once the fees of the practice are set at appropriate levels, it is essential that the charge document be easy to use in recording those fees. The practice's charge document, or *superbill*, is very important for both intra-office communications and reimbursement. It must be kept up to date. Whenever an obsolete code is used, the third-party payor will typically insert the code of the next lower level of service. This process is also complicated by many third parties using their carrier-specific codes and by Medicare's intermediaries using regionalized, local codes.

In 1989, Medicare required linkage between the ICD-9-CM diagnostic codes and the CPT service codes. Eventually all of the third parties' claims adjudication systems will require this as a basis for automating their medical necessity verification programs. They will compare a patient's diagnosis and the doctor's services against a computerized set of clinical audit routines to identify patterns of overutilization. Medicare also recently began requiring consultants and specialists to list on their claims the names and license numbers of the referral source for each patient. The physicians' charge document, or encounter forms, must be modified to include these changes, and the data processing programs must be updated so these new data elements appear on the claim form.

Other key elements that might be appropriate to include on an encounter form are prior authorization numbers, workers' compensation case numbers, and an assignment of benefits. If the form is used as a superbill, then the doctor's name, license number, and taxpayer identification number are requisite, as is a section that shows the total charge amount, any payment received, and balance due.

These encounter forms should be organized graphically in a format that the doctors will find easy to read and use and that will be keypunch-ready when completed by the doctor.

Although the CPT codes are updated annually, several years can pass between the time when a test or procedure becomes a scientifically accepted component of the doctors' armamentarium and when it is assigned its own CPT code. This necessitates the occasional use of the unlisted (99) codes. When these are used without any accompanying explanation, the third parties have almost no idea which services the office actually performed. In almost all cases, these unexplained claims will be rejected unless accompanied by an operative report, test results, or a narrative describing the service. Using support documentation to prevent claims rejections or underpayments is also essential when billing for multiple procedures performed during the same operation, when modifiers are used on surgical claims, or when the total charged amount exceeds certain levels. It therefore pays to attach all of the documentation to the original claim. If your practice falls into this category, it will definitely require a well-organized billing group to match the documentation to the claim forms. The reduction in the outstanding accounts receivable, together with the elimination of the need to deal with all the requests for and generation of duplicate claims, will more than outweigh the inconvenience.

Unfortunately, these supportive documents cannot be submitted to the third parties electronically. The technology is not yet that advanced or affordable.

Many of the widely used medical practice billing computer programs that can submit claims electronically also contain various editing functions that, in effect, "kick out" such claims from the electronic submission routines, and automatically produce hard-copy versions. It is worthwhile investing in this feature; it can reduce the matching and other paper problems mentioned earlier and can assure you that hard-copy claims are generated whenever appropriate. It is extremely important to maintain the currency of this feature as the codes and the payors' policies evolve.

In the past, most third parties requested copies of consultation reports along with the claim, especially if the highest-level consultation code was used. This is no longer the case. However, virtually all confirmatory consultations (second opinions) must be accompanied by copies of the reports.

Critical care and intensive care services are specialties that should always provide as much documentation as possible. Usually the claims are extensive and expensive. Copies of progress notes as well as admission and discharge reports are often requested, so again, these should be attached to the original claim.

Today's reimbursement environment, with its battle cry, "cost containment," coupled with the ever-increasing practice overhead expenses, demands that the accounts receivable staff and procedures be stronger than ever. The third-party reimbursement for every episode of care must be maximized.

Medicare Reimbursement

State-of-the-art knowledge will result in increased collections from Medicare, as well. For example, the Health Care Financing Administration (HCFA) instructs Medicare fiscal intermediaries to pay claims within a specified period. Participating and nonparticipating practices have somewhat different payment time frames. Know the expected reimbursement timeliness for your practice, and start your delinquent claim follow-up procedures as soon as possible after a deadline for payment has passed. Big claim balances—for example, those in excess of $500—should trigger a phone call from your office. Use your office computer or photocopier to regenerate tracer claims after 45 to 60 days for the smaller-balance claims.

Review your Medicare MAACs and profiles annually. These profiles occasionally contain gross errors that can result in many thousands of dollars of lost collections. This must be reviewed each year because a mistake left uncorrected in one year will snowball and become the basis for erroneous reimbursement allowances in all subsequent years.

Compare your Medicare allowance with your charges, and calculate your average reimbursement rate. Use this as a gross screen, and whenever you are paid appreciably less, automatically generate an appeal. If your practice frequently provides speciality services such as cataract surgery and hip replacements to Medicare patients, use your profile as a reimbursement screen for triggering appeals. Some computer systems can store this data and identify underpayments. It is important to identify these underpayments whenever possible and file appeals with Medicare and third-party payors.

Different methods exist for tracking receivable balances in various stages of appeal. One methodology is to maintain an appeal list separate from the accounts receivable. Whenever a Medicare or Medicaid balance is appealed, it is deducted from the accounts receivable and entered on the rolling appeals list. Including these balances with the other receivables distorts the meaning of the total receivables balance, and this method of accounting recognizes that the balance is not readily collectable. Maintaining these balances on a special list allows the practice to continue to treat these balances as assets and to appropriately manage each appeal, and assures the doctor that these charges are not being ignored or lost to follow-up procedures. Whenever an additional payment is received as a result of the appeal, the list should be updated, the previous write off reversed, and the posted payment's special "payment on appeal" transaction code deleted.

If your practice accepts Medicaid, your billing and collection staff members must have an intimate working knowledge of all special forms, procedures, and policies that affect your practice. There is a definite cost for each claim and each follow-up call or tracer you send. Because the Medicaid payment levels are typically very low, it is important that your office submit the claim correctly the first time. It is too easy to pass the point of diminishing returns and spend, for example, $10 in office resources to collect a $9 balance.

Someone other than the primary biller should monitor all explanations of benefits (a.k.a. EOB forms) to spot patterns of rejections, denials, or underpayments. It may be possible, then, to set up a meeting with the intermediary's provider relations staff with the explicit agenda of analyzing these trends and patterns. Ask them to bring their own computer reports on your claims to the meeting. At the meeting try to avoid establishing an adversarial atmosphere; it is not their fault that your state pays only a pittance. The goal of the session is to make certain that your office's output (which becomes their system's input) is compatible in content and form with their processing needs. If electronic claims transmission is available and suitable for your practice, then use it. It will reduce your mailing and paper handling expenses, often edit out unacceptable claims, and speed up payment processing.

Follow-Up with Private Insurance

Private insurance follow-up is becoming increasingly important in managing a practice's receivables. Telephone follow-up is critical to effective management of private (or commercial) insurance carrier receivables. This broad category includes the Blue Cross and Blue Shield plans. The following paragraphs include some effective techniques that you and/or your staff can use. Instruct staff to call within 30 days of submission on all balances greater than $500. Make sure your claim has been entered in the company's processing system. If it cannot be located, immediately send a duplicate, via registered mail, directed to the attention of the person with whom you have communicated. Some carriers now accept fax transmissions. This sends the claim the same day and furnishes your office with verification of receipt of the claim. Your billing person should attempt to ascertain when your claim is scheduled for payment and should mark the date on the calendar to begin follow-up calls if the balance is not received by then. If you feel you are being given the runaround, ask to speak to a claims supervisor. In a cooperative manner, try to find out what is causing the delay in payment; it may be some critical information that your staff can readily provide. In most states, a written complaint to the insurance commissioner can serve as a tool of last resort. This is typically sent after allowing a reasonable period of time (90–120 days) for the claim to make its way through their medical review and adjudication processes. If you believe the insurance denials or underpayments to be unjust, then contact your local medical association to see if they have a claims mediation panel.

Make certain that correspondence concerning your patient's accounts receivable is answered promptly and thoroughly. The insurance companies often request additional information to complete their claims review; other times it seems that they send requests for data they already have as a tactic to delay payment. Regardless of their motivations, you will not get paid until your staff answers the mail.

Outstanding claims of smaller amounts (the dollar thresholds must be defined by each practice) can be effectively followed by sending duplicate claims as tracers. When doing so, use a large rubber stamp that prints "TRACER CLAIM" to distinguish it from an original.

Balances due from managed care systems—HMOs, PPOs, EPOs, and IPAs—should be handled in much the same way as are private and commercial insurance accounts. However, it is important to check the actual payments against the contract-promised payment levels. Furthermore, participating IPA gatekeeper groups often delay and underpay claims from outside consultants. The parent HMO can often bring additional pressure to bear on the IPA. Again, because these managed care systems pay less than the market rates, it is critical to make certain that each service is properly and maximally compensated. Depending upon the guidelines and structure in your particular state, you can report excessive delays or deliberate underpayments to either the insurance commissioner, the secretary of state, or the commissioner of corporations.

For outside specialty consultants, prior authorizations are of the utmost importance. Read them. An important distinction exists between a prior authorization for "evaluation" and one for "evaluation and treatment." The latter will allow for follow-up visits. If you see a patient for ongoing treatment who has an evaluation-only authorization, it is likely that all of your follow-up visits will be denied. In addition, you must find out if the authorization will allow you to order laboratory or radiographic studies. If so, inquire whether you are required to use one of their contract facilities.

Summary

The reimbursement environment changed dramatically during the 1980s, and the pace of change appears to be continuing—even accelerating. Maximizing reimbursements will require that a practice's leadership integrate these changes (i.e., new rules, regulations, billing requirements) into all levels of the organization. Practices must become adept at a number of new skills and be willing to accept new responsibilities. Orchestrating all of this will present new challenges to the practices' leadership. Those willing to invest the time, energy, and money to meet these challenges will be rewarded by maximizing their reimbursement for each unit of service in an environment increasingly oriented toward cost containment.

27 Computerization of Medical Office Systems: Defining Information Needs and Evaluating Available Hardware and Software

SUSAN M. OSTOYA

Defining the computing needs of the practice is essential prior to the start of any software or hardware search. Most large practices do this well in the form of a *request for information* (RFI), which is usually prepared by a committee formed for the purpose of evaluating software and hardware needs. The RFI is generally a well-thought-out product of weeks or months work by the committee, based on interviews and discussion with the end users. However, even small- to midsized practices can and should follow the same process in order to successfully evaluate computing systems. The important aspect to the process is to avoid being under- or oversold on a system based on budget or other factors. On the one hand, the practice may invest a great deal of time and money in a system lacking many basic requirements or on a system too soon outgrown. On the other hand, the practice must avoid buying a system too complex for its needs in terms of maintenance, the staff's ability to properly operate it, and extraneous features. This is not to say that a practice at some time in the future may not have to buy a new system. In fact, chances are that they will, because of the changing environment and growth of the practice itself. With each purchase, however, the practice should do enough soul searching to ensure that the new system will meet their needs closely for several years to come.

Factors to be considered follow several lines: billing requirements, reporting capabilities, third-party contractual arrangements, accounting needs, appointment scheduling, medical record keeping, current size of the patient population, and realistic projections in the growth of the practice. In considering requirements in each of these areas, prioritize each point of interest. Mark each item as being either essential or part of a wish list. When the actual review of available software begins, buy the package that most closely meets the essential items and use the pre-identified wish list to break the tie. Wish-list items are usually "whistles and bells." Avoid the all too common mistake of buying whistles and bells and no substance. That type of purchase is doomed to failure, results in frustration for physicians and staff, and fosters a feeling of scepticism toward vendors which could inhibit the successful installation of a new system.

Defining Information Needs

Before you compile any wish list, consider carefully the areas of the practice that are to be computerized. If the system to be purchased is the first one for the practice, this step can be especially important. Software is written and sold along application lines. The term *application* may be the vendor's term for the product he or she is selling, but it has its roots in way the software package is to be used. In the world of medical group practice the basic applications to be considered are those pertaining to billing, accounts receivable reporting, appointment scheduling, HMO administration and tracking, and medical records.

Examples of other applications that may apply to any business in addition to the medical industry are accounts payable, general ledger, payroll, electronic mail, and security. The organization's size and complexity will determine how many of these applications should be purchased. In order to determine what to buy, consider why the application should be purchased in terms of its benefits. There will be two criteria: the ease with which it can perform specific tasks and the type of data accumulation that allows for reporting.

In addition, consider what will be involved in getting each application up and running. A single application may take a few days' to several months' work before it is ready to use. The organization may need to prioritize software purchases and stagger their implementation. Some of the areas named may never need be computerized. Consider carefully whether the additional software will make certain business functions run more smoothly and take less time than if the same function was done manually or even contracted out. For instance, generally only an organization large enough to have a full-time staff accountant should consider purchasing a general ledger system, and many very large organizations may never choose to do their own payroll in-house, opting instead to use a contracted payroll service, whereas a one-physician office may do payroll manually. Never buy software now that you do not plan to use immediately; someone is always working on a better mousetrap. Waiting to buy nonessential software will accomplish two things. First, you will be able to choose from the very latest software, which may include features not previously available. Second, even if you ultimately decide to purchase the original package you chose, the price may be lower.

To allow you to understand the methodology in defining software requirements, I will use the billing system as an example. This is probably the most commonly purchased software in the industry. Billing software has been around the longest, and there are numerous vendors and packages from which to choose. The reason is that the sheer volume of data collected and used for billing makes the purchase of a billing system cost effective.

Data collected once can be used over and over for different functions. Consider all the obvious benefits that may sprout from storing basic data consisting of patient address and insurance information linked with all charges and services provided, compared with their manually performed counterparts:

Typing claim forms vs. computer-printed claims

Typing statements to patients vs. computer-printed statements

Automatic calculation of balance due from patients vs. manually maintaining running balances

Automatic totaling of charges daily, monthly, and yearly vs. manual day sheets and subsequent manual calculation of statistics

Automated reporting of procedure statistics and volumes (this is nearly impossible on a manual basis)

The list goes on, but these items demonstrate why the purchase of even the most basic billing system is so economically feasible. Think carefully about how your business office handles the basic billing functions of demographic information collection, logging of charges, billing, and collections. With respect to these aspects of data collection, what statistical information would be valuable to the practice? The statistical needs become the basis for evaluating the reporting capabilities of a new system.

Demographic Information

Demographic information, obtained at registration of the patient into the system, will contain everything you will want to know about the patient in general. Many software packages contain a standard set of items that may be collected, and the list of items cannot be changed. Standard items include name, address, phone number, insurance type, insurance company name, and policy information. Many systems also can store employer and spousal information. Will your practice require other information, such as ethnicity and primary language spoken by the patient population? Will it need to keep information about emergency contacts? Does the practice anticipate future contractual arrangements that may call for other types of information? If so, search for a system that has miscellaneous data fields that can be user defined, or a system that is capable of adding user-defined data elements.

What will you wish to do with the information collected, other than print statements and claim forms? Will you want

to print address labels?

to send form letters?

to generate statistics on use by zip code?

to generate statistics by ethnic group (often required for government reporting)?

to list patients with credit problems?

to list patients with incorrect addresses?

Anticipate the uses your practice will have for demographic information to add to your list of desired features in the billing system.

Encounter Data

Collection of encounter data—individual charges, pricing, and dates of service—should be reviewed both in terms of quality of billing data as well as reporting capabilities. A system should allow billing by different procedure-coding schemes, converting the code entered at the time of data entry to the corresponding coding required by the carriers to be billed. Also, encounter data should include any other elements required by third-party carriers, such as location of service and referring physician. Ideally, the system would store pricing in some kind of table or profile to prevent data-entry errors.

Individual practices will have other aspects that should be considered when defining needs:

What special contractual arrangements does the practice have that may need to be dealt with at the time of charge entry?

Are all services billable? Are there contracts such as employee physicals or capitated arrangements for which reporting is required but no charge is billed to the patient? Are there prospective payments?

What are the practice's policies on professional courtesy arrangements?

Are there other front-end contractual adjustments that must be made?

Are there any other front-end processing requirements in your practice?

From the reporting standpoint, the physician should consider the type of statistical data he or she would like to see related to charges. Generally, in order to obtain any report of dollars (revenue, income, or accounts receivable) as a function of elements that vary with different services, the system should allow those various elements to be entered at data entry time or have the capability to derive such statistics from internal tables or profiles. For example, a multispecialty practice may wish to have reporting by specialty. How would the system they purchase accommodate the need? A word of caution: concentrate on reporting requirements that actually relate to the application you are reviewing: in this case, receivables and productivity. Do not expect a billing system to provide reporting that would be more accurately or efficiently done by a different application, such as appointment scheduling or general ledger.

Different software systems maintain the detail of encounters for varying lengths of time. The most basic system may purge detail after the first claim is produced. Some print claims or statements, and have no reporting capabilities. Other systems maintain detail for a year or longer, until the balance is zero, or until the user decides to purge. Purging too, varies greatly, from automated purging to user-defined specifications for purge. How long the individual practice will need to keep detail depends on collection policies, how much patient accounting they will do for the individual patients, and reporting needs (for those systems that offer full reporting).

Billing/Collection Policy

The way different software packages handle billing and collection tasks varies as widely as do medical practices' patient accounting and collection policies. Ensure that the software you are considering has capabilities consistent with your own policies. Consider these items in regard to software requirements:

Is the group's policy to bill all types of insurance? To bill only certain types of insurance?

Is the patient always responsible for bills regardless of insurance coverage?

Will the patient receive a statement for services even though his or her insurance has been billed?

Will the business office do follow-up directly with the insurance company on the patient's behalf?

How will changes to claim forms be handled over the life of the contract in response to changing business needs or government requirements?

Will the business office need to produce tracers on insurance claims? Should the tracers be produced automatically or on demand?

Will bad debt accounts be transferred to a collection agency? What will the volume be? What capabilities will be needed? Will the patient's account's financial class be changed? Will the collection agency require ledgers?

How will patients be informed of collection policy?

Will a dunning message be needed? What will be the policy with regard to the minimum monthly payment or the length of time that may elapse between payment and transfer to a collection agency?

How will patients be informed of pending collection assignment?

How will your specific patient population affect your collection policy? If the population you serve is especially indigent, affluent, or non-English speaking, will you want special features available to accommodate these situations?

Staff Input

For practices already in business which are either buying the first system or considering a change from an old system, take advantage of the experience of the staff. Interview staff members individually. Find out from them exactly how they are performing each office function. Most important in this process is finding out why they are doing what they are doing. If a system is already in place, find out what the staff likes and dislikes about it. Compose a list of tasks that are being performed manually because the system cannot accommodate the need. Keep in mind that your existing system may be able to do certain things but that the staff may lack the training needed to do them; always check with the vendor if you are uncertain. Also, if the staff is doing certain things manually or finds the existing system's method for performing certain tasks cumbersome, ask how they would envision a system doing such tasks. Sometimes they will have good ideas to include in the RFI, or you may learn that the task simply requires too much subjective thinking to be computerized. You may be surprised at the ingenuity of some staff members and shocked by others. However, for this process to be effective, you must remain objective. The point is to elicit open and honest responses from the staff. Later you may determine that some procedures being followed translate into valid software requirements and other procedures translate into training issues. Do not assume that because someone has performed a task in a certain way for a long time that the method is either the only way or the best way to handle the situation. In other words, staff input is very helpful in getting ideas for software requirements, but do not necessarily take what they say as gospel. There is no point in perpetuating old, bad habits in a new software system.

At this point in your analysis of the business office, you should have some strong ideas about the information and computing needs for your billing system. Let us review the steps:

1. Break down the basic functions.
2. Analyze each function according to policy, output requirements, and reporting needs.
3. Interview staff for input and current procedures.
4. Compile the list of requirements and their respective priorities into a document called the request for information.

Even if you plan to meet with software vendors directly rather than mailing your request to them, you should still compose an RFI type of document to use in weighing the relative merits of each system. Record on the RFI whether each item is mandatory to your practice, would be helpful, or would be nice. You may want to go so far as to assign point values to each helpful or nice item. If you do not take the time to determine these needs at the outset, salespeople will tell you what you need and do not need based on their own system capabilities.

Use this same methodology in defining needs for other applications and to determine what other application needs exist.

Evaluating Software

The RFI will become the final tool in evaluating software. However, there are so many vendors and packages available on the market now that many can be eliminated from the beginning. Most important to keep in mind is that different packages are aimed at different marketplaces. Depending on the specific medical practice's target patient population, the software available will perform better, worse, or just adequately. The size of the group plays another important role, because the different packages also target different-sized medical groups. The major factors in this case are cost and complexity.

Prior to beginning the software search, gather some basic statistics. Provide software dealers and vendors with these numbers during your first conversations and you will narrow your search significantly. If the vendor does not explicitly tell you that your group size is inappropriate for a specific package, ask about the average group size of the system's other users and decide whether it is worth pursuing. Use the following numbers as guidelines:

how many physicians the group will have in total

how many full-time physician equivalents the group will have

how many nonphysician revenue-generating practitioners there will be

how many patient visits take place daily, monthly, or annually

the number of charges generated daily, monthly, or annually

how many active patients there are

the projected rate of growth in all these areas, if any, over the next year and the next five years

At this point, it is also important to keep in mind what the practice's target population will be, because this could also rule out certain vendors and systems. Many systems are geared toward specific types of practices, so define your type of practice by answering these questions:

Is the practice a community health clinic?

Will there be a high proportion of Medicaid or other government-sponsored patients?

Will there be a large number of HMO or PPO contracts to manage? If so, what degree of risk will the group agree to share? What will the reporting requirements be to the HMO, PPO, and the group to manage profitability? How will copayments and noncovered services be managed ideally?

Is the group a practice plan?

Is the group a free-standing clinic?

Is the group a partnership or corporation of specialists, or is it multispecialty?

Once the search has been narrowed, it is time to get more involved with the software vendor using your RFI as a guide. However, the RFI will not be the entire basis for a final decision. There will be other considerations such as system maintenance, staffing, user assistance with the installation, ongoing support for the application, and the available user documentation.

There are four basic concepts to understand about the types of software available. These types may be described as turnkey systems, tailored standard software systems, custom systems, and full-service systems. Vendors may offer any combination of these basic types as well as use a number of terms to describe their own version.

With a turnkey system the user is usually sold the software and the equipment needed to run it. It will have relatively few options, if any, and the implementation time is short. Implementation may take a week or less, and following hardware installation and user training there may be little or no further contact with the vendor. This type of purchase may be likened to buying off-the-shelf software. The advantages of a turnkey system are that it is the least expensive system to buy and is the easiest to operate and maintain over time. The software is usually stable and bug free because it has been well used and never modified. Its disadvantages are that it will be relatively inflexible and may not offer any potential for growth in terms of additional hardware. Also, chances are the software will never be updated, so as business needs change it may become necessary to buy another complete system. Turnkey systems are probably the best alternative for single-physician practices, specialty groups, or other small groups without complex contracts. Many turnkey systems are in fact targeted to a specific specialty. The cost of a turnkey system, including software and hardware, may be anywhere from $10,000 to $100,000 or more.

A tailored standard software system may be described as a system in which the software is standardized by the vendor but has built-in capabilities that provide flexibility, allowing the software to be tailored to the individual group's needs. These systems include options that can be turned on or off to suit the needs of the group. They may also depend on the user to build a number of data files that also will reflect the group's individual use of the system. A wide range of systems that vary in flexibility and limitations on use may be included in this category. The implementation of such a system may take weeks or months, and successful use of the system may require a substantial amount of staff time, in both implementation and ongoing maintenance. The amount of time spent in maintenance will depend on the complexity of the practice's needs as well as how well the system addresses those needs. The way tailored systems are sold and maintained by the vendor vary. Some will require a certain brand of hardware, which may or may not be sold through the vendor. Some systems will include updates to software as the system is enhanced over time, whereas others will require a new software purchase to gain enhancements. These systems may also be sold on a time-sharing or in-house basis. Time-sharing generally means that the group will not buy the hardware, but will rent space on a computer housed and maintained by the vendor. In-house purchases mean that the practice buys and owns the computer and its associated hardware and maintains the equipment either in its own computer room or under a facilities management contract. Time-sharing normally involves a lower initial cost to get the system running but higher maintenance fees over time, often dependent on the volume of space used by the practice. In-house systems incur a higher initial cash outlay in the purchase of the equipment and lower maintenance fees over time. However, these lower maintenance costs may be offset somewhat by costs incurred in expanding the equipment or upgrading it as needed for growth or additional software purchases.

Tailored systems offer software maintenance based on a monthly fee over the life of the contract which usually includes telephone support and visits by a vendor representative. Changes to the initial setup may be performed for a fee. These systems also may be targeted toward a particular type of medical practice. Tailored systems are more expensive than turnkey systems, both initially and over time, but provide a high degree of flexibility and growth potential and do not generally require that the group be particularly sophisticated in data processing or have a large data processing staff. However, be realistic, especially if you are considering an in-house system, because there will be operating expenses. Software costs alone for a tailored system may range from $50,000 to $500,000, depending on the number of applications and the sophistication of the software. The different tailored systems on the market are targeted for various practice sizes but have more flexibility as to the optimal group size. For tailored systems, your group statistics will be especially valuable in narrowing down the number of vendors for serious consideration.

Custom systems are only for the largest, most complex, and sophisticated medical practices. In a custom software package, the system will actually be designed and written completely to the purchaser's specifications. Such systems are somewhat rare these days because of the range of standard software available. Not only would such a system require a very long implementation—perhaps years—but it would be expensive. Also, this requires a data processing staff dedicated to the implementation because of the high volume of testing it would require. Over time, maintenance becomes difficult because the original programming staff will not always be available. Often this results in major rewrites of the software because another programmer may not be able to interpret what the originator was attempting to do in a particular area. Needless to say, this type of purchase is not recommended. Most custom systems seen in groups are "home grown," meaning that the group itself has hired the programming staff needed to undertake the project. Even after years of development such systems may end up as failures because of high overhead cost, lack of experience and foresight, and the difficulty in maintaining the system.

A full-service vendor generally has designed software and offers, in addition to the software, the staff to perform all the business office functions that make use of the application. Most common here are billing services in which physician groups send all charges and demographic information to the vendor, who has data processing staff to input the data and do the billing and receivables collection. This is similar to sending tax return information to an accountant and receiving the filled-out return without having to do anything but information collection. The cost for this type of service for billing is usually based on a percentage of collections, so the vendor has an incentive to collect as much as possible. The group must be able to send to the vendor complete and accurate billing information, and it should still have a staff business manager to work with the vendor as a liaison on an ongoing basis, because cooperation and coordination is crucial to the success of such an arrangement. Full-service vendors may be a suitable choice for almost any size of group, though the primary market is in hospital-based physician groups that may not otherwise find it effective in terms of cost or time to set up and manage a business office off site.

It is very likely that more than one of the above alternatives may be appropriate for a given medical practice. Using the RFI determines which systems within the cost and size ballpark will most closely fit your information needs. During the investigation of each system, attempt to determine the associated staffing required to operate it. Staffing may be an additional, hidden cost over the base price of the system. When checking the references of each vendor try to determine how these other groups are staffed to handle the system and how that fits in with your own staffing pattern or planned staffing requirements. These staff requirements may be composed of, but not limited to, data entry staff, billing staff, follow-up and collections, and phone contact with patients or insurance companies, in addition to direct computer operations. Remember that not all groups are alike; if the reference practice has a higher-than-expected number of staff, it may be that it has some unusually complicated data processing needs.

Among software systems are two underlying basic features. These are *real-time* versus *batch* systems. In a real-time system, transactions entered immediately update the data base, ensuring valid input of certain data elements. In a batch system, transactions are entered in a file that then updates the data base in a separate process, which is usually run each night. Data-entry errors are output to an edit list, which must then be worked on daily and corrections made to previous input. Real-time systems have the advantage of instant retrieval, whereas batch systems may allow faster data input.

Determine what training is required to efficiently operate the system. Do not create a training nightmare by buying a system far too complex for a small staff to manage. How will training be managed on an ongoing basis as needed as a result of growth or employee turnover? Will the vendor offer retraining or advanced training for a fee after the staff has adjusted to the new system? How much on-line help is available within the software itself? Does the vendor offer training materials that can be used in staff training? Also, be sure to review the vendor's own user manuals. The user manuals should be easy to read and, most importantly, they should accurately explain system prompting for the various functional aspects of the software. Remember, all the features in the world will not do any good if your staff cannot learn how to use them effectively. Overcomplication can lead to underuse of the system and unnecessary dissatisfaction with what would otherwise have been a good purchase in a different environment. Be honest with yourself when evaluating systems, and do not be led astray by high-tech features you do not need for a smooth operation.

In reviewing the results of your RFI with each vendor, try to find out how the system would handle specific, important processing points, especially if you have unusual requirements. Will the resolution be a straightforward feature, or will the processing be difficult? When speaking with the vendor's references find out if they are using the same feature and how it works for them. Although you cannot expect one system to meet 100% of your needs, it should meet about 95% of them. Usually some circumstances will be too complicated or specific to an individual group for a standard software system to accomplish efficiently. Do not be disappointed in a system that cannot manage those 20 special procedures you do that no one else does if it works like a charm on the other 1000 procedures you do.

Reference checking on vendors is important for several reasons. Of course, you want the vendor to have a reputation for a good product as well as good service. In addition, you will want to see the system in use at an actual practice site and be able to discuss the experiences and use of the system firsthand. Establishing a rapport with the vendor's other customers may be helpful during your use of the system, if you end up buying it.

Evaluation of Hardware

Chances are that the software you select will require a certain type of hardware as well as a particular brand. Turnkey systems usually run on PC hardware or on a minicomputer. Tailored systems may run on anything from a PC network to a large mainframe. The hardware purchase may be several times the cost of the software alone. Because most software runs on only certain types of hardware, the software selection and the type of hardware which must be purchased may be interdependent and be influenced by the difference in price of hardware by the various manufacturers. There are two schools of thought in system selection: the first recommends that you find the hardware you like, and then find software that is compatible. The second school says find the software you like, then find the hardware. In the first case, you may overlook excellent software because of the hardware bias. In the second, you may find excellent software running on hardware that is too expensive or made by a manufacturer who could go out of business any time. The hardware business is extremely competitive, as is the software business. However, if you cannot get parts, you could be out of business. Each group will have to make its own choice on the priority. It is probably best to find some middle ground. Be open minded about the software options, and then scrutinize the associated hardware manufacturer and choose from those who have a reputation for stability.

What does *hardware* mean? It is important to understand the basic components. The *central processing unit* (CPU) is the basic box, the actual computer itself. It contains the storage area (disk drives) for data and software programs and memory. The CPU is the brain of any system. The *terminals* are used to communicate with the CPU. Terminals are the eyes, ears, and fingers of the system, and include the screen (CRT, or cathode-ray tube) and keyboard. *Printers* are used to get hard-copy information from the CPU. A *telecommunications* system is a network of machines used to communicate over telephone lines with a CPU located any large distance from terminals. Everything must be linked to a CPU by cables, but cables are useful only if all terminals and printers are within about 50 feet of the CPU. For greater distances, data can travel over phone lines. Terminals and printers are plugged into multiplexors (muxes) and modems instead of the CPU, and matching muxes and modems at the CPU end are actually plugged into the CPU itself. The alternative to telecommunications equipment is fiberoptic cables, which communicate at light speed over great distances. However, at about $2 per foot, they are expensive.

Terminals, printers, and telecommunications equipment are known as *peripherals*. Although the vendor will always make recommendations on peripherals, sometimes the buyer may shop for alternatives for some of these items as long as the buyer can be sure they are of a compatible nature. A word of caution: although you may realize a great cost savings in doing so, the software vendor may not have any experience with other manufacturers and there may be substantial inconvenience when trying to get the peripherals working. Also, consider the reliability of alternative peripherals. Cheaper is not necessarily better.

If you plan to time-share, you will have less to worry about in terms of hardware configuration because the vendor will be managing the CPU for you. In this case, the type of hardware may be less important than it would be if you were actually buying the entire system, as with turnkey or in-house systems.

Based on your statistics gathered prior to beginning your software search as well as how many people you expect will need access to your system, the vendor will make an estimated configuration of the system. The configuration will include the size CPU you will need, the amount of storage space, the number of terminals and printers, and the type of telecommunications needs you may have. Most groups experience some growth in the data base over time, and your group may have specific needs that may cause additional growth. However, the vendor should make the configuration based on a projected time frame determined by you. What will it cost to add more hardware after that time? What are the expandable aspects of the hardware configured? If your reporting needs are greater than average, or if you plan such items as incoming interfaces, you may need additional storage capacity. Be sure to have these types of items calculated into your storage estimates. The same would apply if you will have multiple practice sites over time which will need to share one CPU. By informing the vendors of such plans, they will be able to configure the system more accurately and you will avoid huge unexpected expenditures down the line.

As with software, try to find out how complicated the hardware will be to operate. A system should be fully backed up each day—that is, a copy of all data and software is saved so that in case of a system failure, including power loss or disaster, data may be restored. How long will the daily operations take? Will you have the staff to operate a complicated system? What have the references' experiences been with regard to hardware operation, maintenance, and reliability? What level of service do they get from the vendor? Does the vendor's staff appear knowledgeable on hardware issues? Hardware problems can be extremely difficult to diagnose and they often appear to be software related. The vendor's knowledge and experience will count a great deal after a hardware purchase.

Conclusion

The value of the formal RFI will become apparent once the actual process of system selection has begun. There will be numerous pros and cons and give and takes as you review the various systems available. One system may do one item extremely well but do others poorly. Another system will do many things well but do poorly on one item that is very important in your particular practice. The RFI will be your objective resource to keep you from being swept off your feet in the showroom. The RFI will be your conscience, because it will represent your down-to-earth needs. Evaluating each system equally against the RFI is crucial in determining the finalists. Then let some subjectivity take over based on discussion with vendors and references, cost, and staff requirements.

Buying a computer system is a major decision. A good system will have an impact on income potential as well as patient satisfaction. Be realistic in your expectations of the system. You should expect efficiency, not necessarily staff reduction. Business office tasks should run more smoothly, timely, and completely with the new system. Be realistic about your practice's growth potential, and avoid buying a bigger system than you actually need.

IV | DEVELOPING AND MANAGING A PRACTICE

28 | Patient Appointment Scheduling

PATRICIA A. FOX

The appointment scheduling system performs a vital role in managing resources, maintaining patient relations, and improving the patient care process for both the patients and the providers. It is a powerful tool for building an information data base and serves as the gateway for the patient into the health-care process. Because the scheduling system serves all these functions, its design and implementation must be given careful consideration in the management of a health-care facility.

The basic concept underlying a scheduling system is simply to place the patient and the appropriate provider in the same place at the same time. However, as the requirements of all of the people affected by this process are examined, it becomes apparent that a truly useful and effective appointment scheduling system is necessarily much more complex. The scheduling system is frequently the first point of contact between a patient and the health-care environment. The efficiency and the ability of the scheduler to meet the patient's needs will set the tone for the initial relationship with that patient.

The scheduling system is also a tool for managing a provider's time. If the system facilitates bringing in appropriate patients for an appropriate amount of time with minimal idle time and minimal overbooking, it will help determine the provider's satisfaction with the care process.

These basic needs of arranging appointments for patients and effectively managing time for providers will be shared by all health-care facilities. However, the complex details of the scheduling process will vary with each implementation. It is therefore necessary to carefully evaluate a facility's needs and resources in establishing an appropriate system. The factors that must be taken into consideration when establishing a scheduling system along with possible approaches to the process will be discussed in this chapter. There is no one sure method for scheduling that will maximize practice efficiency. It is important to use creativity in the design of a process and to make it flexible enough to adapt to the growth and changing needs of the practice.

Evaluation of Needs

The first step in establishing an approach for a scheduling system is to evaluate the needs and identify the expectations of the users of that system. This will help to build a system that will enhance the patient entry process and assist in its efficient management. The more accurately all needs are identified at the outset, the more effective and useful the scheduling system will be.

The first component of the scheduling system to be considered in this evaluation is the provider. It is imperative to evaluate how providers spend their time and what information they need from the scheduling system to help them work effectively.

Concrete Elements

An analysis of provider time and how to manage it must include many factors, the first being what types of appointments they have and how long an appointment should take for each type of visit. An evaluation of types of visits has to be done for each individual provider. In compiling this information, it is helpful to create a table for each provider that lists the types of visits, their average duration, and a brief description of what the provider does at each type of visit. This information is one of the cornerstones of an effective appointment system. It not only supplies the information necessary to establish and manage a provider's schedule, but it also helps the support staff utilize those schedules effectively. It is one of the first building blocks in a powerful appointment information data base. As each factor involved in the process is analyzed, it is important to consider its effects or implications for all those who play a role in the system. For example, although information about visit types is generated by the providers, it quickly becomes a tool for the scheduler and a basis for statistical analysis by the administrator.

Once the types of appointments, the reasons for these visits, and the duration of each visit has been identified for each provider, it is necessary to determine the time needed for nonappointment tasks. How much time does each provider need for phone calls, rounds, or administrative duties? When is this time usually taken? To maximize the efficiency of a provider's day it is just as important to consider these needs as it is to consider appointment needs. These nonappointment tasks are important to the health-care process. They should be incorporated into the schedule so that they do not compromise appointment time. If allowed to cut into appointment time, these tasks could reduce productivity and the satisfaction of both providers and patients with the scheduling process.

Dynamic Aspects of the Practice

Once the concrete elements of a schedule have been compiled for each provider, it is necessary to identify and plan for the more dynamic aspects of the medical practice environment. Consider the rate of walk-in appointments and/or same-day appointments. In an urgent care setting, the bulk of each provider's time must be set aside for walk-in appointments, but the amount of time needed for walk-ins in other areas of the practice requires more careful evaluation. The history of walk-in appointments should be examined for an entire year's period. You may find that the walk-in rate for a department will vary from day to day as well as throughout the year. Based on this information, evaluate how much time should be allocated for these appointments and the staffing needed to handle this load.

The rate of no-show patients must be considered as well. As with walk-ins, the no-show rate will vary from day to day and throughout the year. It is also likely to vary by department and, therefore, so must the approach taken to accommodate these appointments. In a department where the no-show rate is minimal, it may not be necessary to make any accommodations in the schedules. However, in an area where the no-show rate is high and could mean significant idle time for the provider, then a creative solution must be found to minimize this result. One solution often used to address this problem is to overbook a provider's time. Although this will definitely reduce idle time, it is also likely to generate crowds in the waiting room and promote bad relations with the patients. A well-designed scheduling system should have the flexibility to allow for overlapping appointments. This will serve to reduce the impact of a no-show without angering all of the patients.

Changes in Scheduling

After evaluating how the providers spend their time for appointments and nonappointment tasks and tabulating the usual volume of walk-in and no-show patients, it is necessary to consider how often changes occur in a provider's schedule. Although the rules and guidelines for the schedules are established based on the above information, none of these rules can be made so rigid that they cannot bend. An effective system must have the flexibility to react quickly and appropriately to changes initiated by the provider.

If the provider will not be able to see patients on a day for which a schedule has already been established, then the system must have the ability to block out that day so no appointments will be scheduled. If appointments have already been made for that day then the system must also incorporate a mechanism or a procedure to cancel and reschedule those appointments and notify the patient. In addition, it is important that the impact of this procedure on patients be measurable to a certain extent, so that if it becomes significant, policies may be incorporated to reduce this occurrence. Each patient file should contain the number of times that patient's appointments have been cancelled by a provider. If this number becomes significant, then the rescheduling process should take steps to be sure that it will not happen again. Information such as this, when used by the scheduler, can be extremely helpful in maintaining good patient relations.

Another common change in a provider's schedule occurs when the provider decides to see patients on a previously unscheduled day. A mechanism must be established to add this schedule to the appointment process at any time.

By establishing the provider's basic needs, building a flexible schedule, and allowing for changes, the foundation has been laid to make appointments for the patients and to use the provider's time effectively. Next it is important to consider what information the provider should expect to receive from the system each day. The first expectation a provider will have is access to each day's schedule. This schedule should contain at least some basic patient information, the time of the appointment, and the reason for the visit to help the provider plan the day.

A less obvious—but just as important—expectation is that when the patient arrives his or her chart and all of the appropriate forms will be available. The scheduling system itself cannot account for these items. As the entry point for the patient appointment information, the scheduling system must initiate the requests for these items. Therefore, an appropriate and efficient means of communication must be established between the scheduling system and the medical records room.

In addition to evaluating the needs of the providers, the needs of the schedulers must be considered. Although the system needs to be complex to meet the providers' demands, for the schedulers it must be fast, efficient, easy to use, and contain all of the information necessary to make an appointment. The system must also assist the scheduler with the constant flow of information. How will the provider know that a patient has been added to the schedule? How will the record room be notified to send the patient record? How will the appropriate forms such as charge tickets be generated for this patient? All of these areas should be considered in the scheduling process. Because they are frequently the responsibilities of the scheduler, they can be established as part of the responsibilities of the scheduling system. As the first point of contact with the patient, this becomes the starting point for the care process, and careful consideration of these issues in the design of the scheduling process can significantly improve the information and patient flow.

Administrators' Needs

Finally, the needs and expectations of the practice's administrators must be considered. Although the scheduling system may not affect them directly on a day-to-day basis, it has the potential to serve as an invaluable source of information about how many patients are seen in a given period of time, what types of patients are seen, what time of day and what day of the week they are coming, how many patients show up for appointments, how many cancel, and how efficiently each provider's time is being used. The information obtained from the scheduling process can provide an accurate picture of what the patient volume and flow is throughout a practice.

The variations in demand for the practice's resources can be established through appointment history information collected during the appointment scheduling process. This information can then be used to project demand in the future and to match resources with this demand. The scheduling system then becomes an important tool in planning adequate resources to meet the need.

If an appointment scheduling system addresses all of the needs identified above, then it will also be able to effectively address the needs of the patients. The next step in the establishment of such a system is the actual design.

Schedule Design

Once the needs of the providers have been identified and compiled, the challenge is to establish schedules that will meet these needs. The simplest way to accomplish this is to use a standard calendar type of schedule that divides the day into 10- or 15-minute segments and to simply block out the times as appointments are made. This simple method, although straightforward, quickly becomes inadequate in the complex process of scheduling appointments and maximizing the use of a provider's time. It is not usually flexible enough to truly meet the needs of the providers, schedulers, or patients.

As much as possible it is important to design schedules that meet the needs of the providers, rather than trying to redesign the providers' needs to match rigid schedules. This will increase the providers' satisfaction with the system and will also help to support the most efficient use of their time.

Many options can be incorporated into the schedule design which are limited only by the system in place or by the imagination of its designer. Creative solutions using the tools available must be found to address the complex problems of appointment scheduling. For instance, a flexible schedule should contain blocks of time for the providers to attend meetings and seminars or to perform other nonappointment tasks. Some types of visits can be scheduled only at certain times during the day because of the availability of a fixed resource, such as a piece of equipment or a specific room. Time for walk-in or same-day appointments must also be considered. The structure of the schedule must be built around situations historically encountered for each specific provider and department. Situations such as high rates of no-show appointments, if expected to continue, must be considered in the schedule design if the efficient use of a provider's time is to be maximized.

Schedule Design Techniques

Several techniques can be used in schedule design. The first is *wave booking*, which allows for overlapping appointment times for one provider. For example, a provider may require 30 minutes to see a new patient and 30 minutes to see a return patient; however, the schedule might be set up to accommodate one patient every 15 minutes.

This design is useful if a provider has access to two examination rooms. While one patient is being seen, the next patient can be shown to the other examination room to change into a gown. This type of schedule reduces the time between patients and accommodates the time a patient takes to get ready.

As discussed earlier, this type of schedule design can also be used to reduce the impact of no-show appointments. If a provider is scheduled to see patients whose appointment times overlap and one does not show up, then the time spent by the provider waiting for the next patient will be minimized. Although this is of benefit to the provider, the drawback of this design is that the patients may spend longer times in the waiting room. This is especially true if wave booking is used for a situation in which the provider has access to only one examination room, rather than two.

Another design used in many schedules is *flex scheduling*. In this design, a block of appointment times is set aside and used for either one type of appointment or another but not both. This might be used for a 30-minute block of time in which a provider would like to see either a new patient for whom 30 minutes is required or two follow-up patients for whom only 15 minutes each is required. A design that provides this type of flexibility can be very useful when the types of patients expected are not entirely predictable.

The concept of *scheduling by exception* is used quite effectively by many providers. This design simply designates the times during which certain types of appointments should not be scheduled. This provides for greater flexibility and is extremely easy to learn. However, as with a calendar type of schedule, the varying appointment duration is not taken into consideration in the design process and the potential for time gaps between scheduled appointments is relatively high.

Finally, one more style that is frequently of use in designing a schedule is *block scheduling*. This designates a block of time in which multiple appointments will be scheduled and can be useful for situations in which a provider will see a group of patients at the same time, such as for group therapy. This style can also be useful for situations in which patients are not expected to come at an exact time, such as for lab tests.

No matter what single design or mix of styles is incorporated into the schedules, it is extremely important to create a system that can be flexible. Each office must have schedules that can be modified or added to whenever necessary to meet the changing environment. The importance of this will become apparent as the providers' needs are compiled and as the schedulers begin to use the system. Flexibility allows the schedules to be a tool that enhances the process and does not hinder it.

Centralized or Decentralized

To design an appointment scheduling system that meets the identified needs of the practice and providers and maximizes the efficient use of resources, weigh the pros and cons of a centralized or a decentralized system. To establish an effective system, the responsibilities of the schedulers as well as the general profile of the providers who work in the practice must be considered. It may also be important to consider the physical layout of the office space and how this affects patient flow.

When centralized scheduling is used, a pool of people is responsible for the scheduling system. The people in this group set up and modify the schedules, maintain patient appointments, and provide any information from the system that is needed by the practice (eg, daily schedules for the providers, lists of appointments for the reception areas). In this type of system, the manager of the scheduling process can maintain a great deal of control over how things are done. It is possible to establish procedures for schedule and appointment maintenance. Because communication among the schedulers is maximized, minimal time is needed to train a new employee on the scheduling process. If a new scheduler has difficulty remembering how to proceed with a particular situation, there are potentially many resources to which to turn.

This form of scheduling also has some advantages for the patients. They can call one number and make many appointments. Also, because this system requires established standards to function, the patients will encounter the same procedure for making an appointment no matter which department they are trying to access.

Because this system allows for maximum control over the process, it tends to work well in a practice where there is a high fluctuation of providers on staff to see patients. For example, this system has worked very well in facilities with a large number of residents. When providers change every year, it can be difficult to maintain consistency and control over the scheduling process. A centralized system can help to alleviate this situation.

Although a centralized system has many advantages and in many cases can be the best choice, it has a number of disadvantages that should be considered. Because control of the system rests with a small group of people who service many providers and the entire patient population, a centralized system can become highly impersonal. Schedulers are not directly involved with the providers and are therefore not as attuned to the likes and dislikes of each one. This can cause some dissatisfaction on the providers' part, because they do not have direct control and supervision over a system that determines the way they spend their time. This is not to say that the providers do not have any input into the system. As was emphasized earlier, it is extremely important to set up a system that truly meets providers' needs, so they do have some influence over how the schedules are set up and what types of patients are scheduled. However, a centralized system does not give providers constant contact with schedulers; direct supervision and decision-making lies with the scheduling manager.

An impersonal centralized system also affects patient contact. Schedulers take calls from the entire patient population, so they cannot be familiar with everyone who calls. This can have a negative effect on patients who desire personalized service where their health is concerned.

However, if the system provides the scheduler with quick and easy access to patient-specific information, such as address and phone number, these interactions can be more personal. Personalization can be increased even further if there is other patient information kept with the appointment information. For instance, a patient calls to schedule an annual physical and does not have to state the name of the primary care physician or that he or she prefers morning appointments, then that patient is likely to be favorably impressed. Access to information such as this can go a long way toward improving the patient's satisfaction with the scheduling process.

The final factor that should be considered when designing a centralized scheduling system is that it requires a smaller staff for making appointments than does a decentralized system. Because their sole responsibility is with the scheduling process and they are not working in multiple locations, schedulers can be extremely efficient and focused. At the same time, this may have implications for the staff required in other areas of the facility. Other staff members must be responsible for collecting full registration and insurance information as the patient arrives and perform any other arrival or exit processing.

Advantages of a Decentralized System

In a decentralized system, each group of providers has its own schedulers, who work at an appointment desk located in the same area as the examining rooms for those providers. The schedulers are thus in constant, close contact with the providers and are familiar with each provider's preferences with regard to the scheduling of patient appointments.

A decentralized system allows much more personalized service. The schedules and the scheduling process can be tailored to individual providers' needs. Since the schedulers see only patients who come to their providers, they can become familiar with each patient's needs, preferences, and manner and can, as a consequence, make more appropriate scheduling decisions. For example, if a provider always needs 15 minutes longer for an appointment with a particular patient, the scheduler can take this into account when making that appointment. A scheduler in a centralized system, on the other hand, is not likely to ever know a patient-provider relationship well enough to make such a decision. The scheduler's familiarity with both the patients and providers can greatly enhance everyone's satisfaction with the appointment process.

One result of the proximity of the scheduler and providers is that providers have much more direct control over the process. This creates a system with more flexibility and fewer rules. In a centralized system, where only a few schedulers are trying to meet the needs of several providers, relatively strict rules must be established to make the system work. In a decentralized situation, all providers do not have to conform to the same process, so the rules involved in the management of the system are greatly reduced.

Another characteristic of a decentralized system is that the schedulers usually have other responsibilities associated with the practice. They are sometimes responsible for the arrival processing and for collecting patients' demographic and insurance information. They are frequently involved in acquiring the patient's medical record, ensuring that the appropriate paperwork accompanies the chart, and making sure that the chart is returned to the record room. They may remind patients of other appointments they have on the same day within the same facility or of follow-up appointments. They are also, as a result of their face-to-face contact with the patients, frequently involved in providing other information to the patients, such as directions to another department or the laboratory. These tasks greatly change the definition of a scheduler's job in a decentralized environment. They handle tasks for which other people could be responsible in a centralized system. Although it is necessary to hire more scheduling personnel for a decentralized system, those personnel cover a wider range of responsibilities.

A decentralized system works very well for many situations. It allows for maximum flexibility and high satisfaction because of its more personalized approach for patients and providers. However, it does present challenges for effectively managing it. The most obvious challenge is that the personnel involved with the scheduling system are located throughout the facility rather than in one central place. This can become problematic if there is anything that needs to be communicated to all of these people at once, such as a new clinic-wide policy that applies to appointment scheduling.

Establishing a decentralized system does not necessarily mean that all other associated tasks must also be decentralized. For instance, if the physical layout of a facility dictates that all patients come and go through one main entrance, then it might be appropriate and most efficient to have a central arrivals desk where all patients can be checked in and directed to the correct location.

Security

Whatever type of system is designed, the security of the appointment information must be considered, because it is inappropriate to allow general access to it. If a facility is using a paper system and scheduling out of books, then it is necessary to ensure that only the appropriate people have access to the books. This is usually accomplished by keeping each book in a designated location and locked, if necessary.

The issue of confidentiality becomes more complex if a computer-automated scheduling system is used. The information about the providers' schedules and the patient appointments contained in the system could potentially be accessible to anyone. A good computerized system should have built-in access codes to control who has access to appointment and schedule information, as well as who can make appointments or modify schedules. A system must be sensitive to all of the security needs of an organization. Many people may have access to the system. Although this may enhance flexibility, the access to specific information within the system should be carefully controlled.

Patient Relations and Marketing

If an appointment scheduling system is designed well and implemented properly it can be a strong marketing and patient relations tool. As the patient's first point of contact with the health-care environment, the appointment scheduling system can have an important impact on the patient's initial satisfaction with the facility. If, in time, a patient requires more care, the scheduling system remains the primary point of access to the providers in the facility. The scheduling process must be designed to be as efficient, flexible, and informative as possible.

To accomplish this, first consider the scheduler's access to information about the provider, the types of visits to be scheduled, their duration, and the hours the provider works. This is the basic information that the patient should expect to receive from the system. The scheduler needs other information so that it can be passed on to the patient, such as instructions about preparation for the visit (fasting for a particular test or bringing insurance forms) or clear directions to the facility. The more information available to the scheduler, the more pleased the patients are going to be with the process, and the more likely they are to want to return to that facility.

When scheduling appointments, the scheduler must have access to information about the patient. This is especially important when scheduling return visits. Specific information can help patients to feel they are receiving personalized service. Other information will help ensure that the policies of the practice are being enforced.

The first type of patient information required is the demographic data. If the scheduler verifies patients' addresses over the phone, this information can then be used to update the demographic data being used by the billing office. This, in turn, will improve written communications with the patients. This may affect the billing for previous appointments as well as the delivery of appointment reminder letters.

Which patient-specific information is available to the scheduler at the time an appointment is made varies with each facility, depending on the office policies and the structure of the information system. Many items can be included in an attempt to improve the practice's business procedures. A patient is not likely to call the billing office to make a new appointment, so it is frequently helpful to have some basic financial and insurance information available to the scheduler. This can greatly improve the enforcement of policies regarding patients with credit problems and the collection of payments due. Depending on the policies in place, the scheduler may simply have access to a note that is attached to the patient's demographic information which indicates that the patient should be connected with the billing office when he or she calls. In other systems, it may be desirable to allow the scheduler access to more specific information, such as the actual current balance for this patient's account. The way in which this information is handled, however, must be based on internal policies.

In addition to demographic, insurance, and financial information, it is helpful to have access to information that directly affects the scheduling process. This might include such things as appointment history, whether or not this person should be treated as a VIP, and his or her physician's name. Appointment history information can facilitate a proactive approach to appointment problems, improve the relationship with the patient, and reduce the effect these problems may have on the efficient use of a provider's time. Indicating that a patient is a VIP or that a patient's appointments have been frequently canceled by the provider can be used in the appointment scheduling process to prevent the future canceling of an appointment by the provider. If a patient's primary care provider is known, then the scheduling process becomes more personalized and efficient.

The more patient-specific information that can be accessed by the scheduler, the more informative and accurate the scheduling process can be. However, careful decisions must be made regarding this information. If financial and/or insurance information is made available to the schedulers, then their responsibilities are expanded beyond the scheduling of appointments. Frequently this is appropriate for the practice and it can be the most efficient method for maintaining this information and using it effectively. However, the extra responsibility must be recognized and taken into consideration in hiring and staffing the facility.

The best way to use this information is to have it automatically available when accessing a patient's file. The sheer bulk of this information must therefore be considered in the design process. The appointment scheduling process has to be efficient. Patients will not be satisfied with the service if they must wait for 10 minutes while schedulers read through their files each time they request new appointments. One way to reduce this review time is to simply use notes or indicators in a patient's file which quickly let schedulers know whether or not they need to do anything special with this patient. Another option is to have this information available when the patient arrives rather than while an appointment is being made. Obviously, this would not be appropriate for information that directly affects the scheduling of the appointment. It may actually be a more effective means, though, to deal with situations such as credit problems.

Good Patient Relations

With the growing competition in the health-care field and the need to encourage and increase the flow of patients, all systems that affect the process of bringing patients into a facility have the potential to act as marketing and patient relations tools. The appointment scheduling process is one of these systems. As the keeper of the patient appointment data base, a scheduling system contains much information that can be used effectively as a business tool for a group practice.

The files containing upcoming appointments can be used to either send reminder letters or to call the patients. A friendly card or call to remind a patient of a scheduled appointment can be an easy and cost-effective way to reduce the no-show rate. The appointment scheduling system can also be used to maintain files regarding dates for annual visits. In an effort to improve patient care, this sort of file can be used to remind patients when it is time to make an appointment. A similar file can also be maintained to list patients who are waiting for appointments in case of cancellations. In the interest of maximizing the use of a provider's time as well as improving the relations with the patients, there must be a procedure in the scheduling process to fill any time periods freed by cancellations.

The appointment scheduling system can be an ideal catalyst for communicating with outside physicians as well as with patients. If the appointment system is designed with this in mind, then the appropriate information can be collected at the time the initial appointment is made. This information should include the name of the physician or agency that referred the patient as well as the address and/or phone number. There should then be a procedure established to ensure that a letter of acknowledgement will be sent to the referring party each time an appointment is made. A letter of acknowledgement, thank you, and follow-up to a referring physician will encourage him or her to send more patients in the future. In a specialty practice, this form of communication can become an essential marketing tool for the business.

Information Source

In the appointment scheduling process, a wealth of information is collected and centralized for the medical practice. This includes patient-specific information, provider information, and resource utilization information. In the continuing effort to maximize the use of all resources and productivity, health-care administrators, providers, and scheduling managers should have easy access to all of this information and then utilize it to analyze, evaluate, and improve the health-care process.

The information available from an appointment scheduling system can assist in the management of day-to-day activities through the production of daily schedules, lists for the registration/arrival desk, schedules for the laboratory, pull lists for the medical records department to ensure that the record is conveyed to the provider, encounter forms, test tube labels, registration forms, and any other items that need to be produced prior to the patient's arrival.

Each appointment must be filled using enough information to help each staff member within the process to accomplish his or her job. At a minimum, the provider needs the patient's name, appointment time, and the reason for the visit. All of this information should be available to the provider from the appointment scheduling process. The medical records personnel need the patient's name, the date and time of the appointment, the medical record number, and the name of provider being seen in order to ensure that the patient's chart will be delivered to the provider in time for the appointment. This information should be available to the medical records staff at least one day before the appointment date. To direct patients appropriately, the staff at a central registration/arrivals desk needs the names of the patients expected each day, their appointment times, the provider, and the department they will be visiting.

The appointment scheduling system collects a significant amount of information that can be used to examine the appointment volume, patient flow, and how efficiently each provider's time is being used. This information can be an invaluable tool to the administrators of a practice. By virtue of the basic purpose of the appointment process, all systems—whether using books or computers—collect the information needed by the administrator. It is therefore important to consider the administrator's access to this information. The system supplies information on patient demand and the percentage of a provider's schedule that is either unbooked or consistently overbooked within the month. The sooner an administrator can have access to this information after the close of a period, the more effectively it can be used to make staff adjustments in a timely fashion.

There should also be information available that indicates the no-show rate and the cancellation rate for each provider and department. Such information can be used to establish new policies to help reduce these rates as well as to examine the design of the providers' schedules to be sure that the impact on each provider's time is minimized.

The scheduling system can also play a role in improving the billing process. Information about which patients showed up for their appointment and which did not needs to be communicated to the billing office. A good billing system can be enhanced only by close communication with the appointment process, given that the effective management of a health-care facility requires not only that patients are seen but also that they are billed.

Summary

One of the necessary tools for an effective group practice is an effective scheduling system. To establish such a system, the needs of the providers, schedulers, administrators, and patients must be carefully considered and incorporated into the design. To meet all of these needs, an appointment system must be flexible and dynamic. As a practice grows, its needs will change. The appointment system must be able to change to meet any new requirements.

It is also important to remember that the appointment scheduling process affects much more than whether or not a patient and a provider meet. It is the entry point for the patient into the practice, and as such it becomes a powerful marketing tool. Finally, appointment scheduling is the source of valuable information that needs to be used in making effective management decisions for any practice.

29 | Record Keeping for Salaries and Payroll Taxes

TIMOTHY C. SHAMROY

By now, you have probably received numerous payroll checks, and at the end of the year a W2 form, but you have never had the responsibility or the knowledge to prepare payroll checks for your employees and/or report payroll taxes to the federal, state, and local governments.

The lack of knowledge when beginning the payroll process can be very frustrating and time consuming. Be prepared to be confronted with terms, words, and forms you have never seen before.

The purpose of this chapter is not to provide all the details and knowledge required, but rather to present a general overview so that the process is better organized and understood.

Why is Record Keeping for Salaries and Payroll Taxes Important?

This is a good question because once the process is mastered and understood, it might tend to become rote and boring but no less important. Some very important things must be remembered about payroll and related taxes: for example, unlike some other expenses, salaries must be paid on time, every time. Without this there will be constant turmoil among the staff. Complaints to the Department of Labor, Internal Revenue Service, or other governmental agencies might ensue. Salaries and payroll taxes will make up a large part of a business's expenditures—perhaps the largest. Pension, profit sharing, 401K, and other deferred compensation plans are tied to compensation information. The timely and accurate reporting of salaries and payroll taxes is required by federal, state, and local laws; failure to comply will result in very stiff and costly penalties. Individual salaries are the bases for workers' compensation insurance. Finally, accurate payroll information can be used as a management tool to measure productivity.

Do I Qualify as an Employer and Do I Have Employees?

If you are an employer and have employees you are responsible for the payment of wages, the collection and deposit of related taxes, and the reporting of this information. Generally an employer, as defined by the IRS in *Circular E: Employer's Tax Guide*, is a person or organization for whom a worker performs a service as an employee. The employer usually gives the worker the tools and place to work and has a right to fire the worker. A person or organization paying wages to a former employee after the work ends is also considered an employer.

Determining who are employees may be more difficult. Employees are defined under common law or special statutes depending on the situation. The *Employer's Tax Guide* presents a general definition:

> Anyone who performs services is an employee if you, as employer, can control what will be done and how it will be done. This is so even when you give the employee freedom of action. What matters is that you have the legal right to control the method and result of the services.

For the purposes of this chapter I will assume that all readers are employers with employees. IRS publication 539 offers examples of various employer-employee relationships; if it does not clarify a difficult situation for you, consult an accountant or file Form SS-8 with the IRS for a specific decision.

How Should Employees Be Paid?

This seems a simple enough question, but it should be answered early. Decide exactly how the system is to work before you have numerous employees. There are four basic methods of determining employees' pay: an hourly rate, a weekly rate, a monthly salary, and a yearly salary. Also, what is the impact of overtime? If there is overtime, does it apply in excess of eight hours a day, or in excess of 40 hours a week?

Consider if the use of employee time cards and a time clock is appropriate. At a minimum, a time card or some similar document such as a time sheet should be used. These are especially important when paying hourly rates and computing overtime, sick leave, and vacation pay.

Whether an hourly, weekly, monthly, or yearly method is selected, be as consistent throughout the staff as possible. This does not mean there cannot be both hourly employees and yearly salaried people; however, consistency will lead to easier record keeping.

How Often Should There Be a Payroll?

Once you decide how to pay your employees, determine how often to pay them. The three most common methods are weekly, every two weeks, and twice a month. I prefer every two weeks (this breaks down the year into 26 equal pay periods) or twice a month. Paying weekly requires too much paper work, processing, and reporting.

Whatever the method, again, be consistent, as switching is very difficult. Also, consider holding back one or two weeks as it helps the cash flow. For example, assuming a two-week pay period—the 1st through the 14th—pay this at the end of the third week, thus holding back one week.

Payroll Taxes and Reporting

Two or three basic taxing agencies are responsible for the administration of payroll taxes and reporting. Each of these agencies handles one or more of the payroll taxes:

Federal: the Internal Revenue Service is responsible for the federal payroll taxes: federal withholding (income tax), social security tax (FICA), and federal unemployment (FUTA).

State: the agency varies from state to state. For example, in California the Employment Development Department is responsible for state personal income tax (PIT), state disability insurance (SDI), and state unemployment insurance (SUI).

Local: the local agency commonly responsible for city or county taxes, if any apply.

Each agency has its own reporting forms and requirements but all use similar information—wages and salaries paid to employees. Variations in forms and taxes will occur from state to state and local authority to local authority. For example, Nevada has no state income tax but California does. Become familiar with your area's requirements.

Federal Withholding

The federal withholding (income) tax varies from employee to employee based on the total amount of the employee's salary paid for that particular pay period, the employee's marital status, and the number of income tax allowances the employee requested. This information comes from the employee's W4, a federal form that should be completed on commencement of employment. Remember, it is mandatory that every employee complete a W4 and that it be maintained in the employee's record. It shows the employee's full name, social security number, home address, marital status, number of allowances claimed, any additional employee tax withholding desired, the employee's signature, and the date the form was completed. It is very important to have the new employee complete one when he or she begins employment. This record will stay in force until the employee desires a change, at which time he or she should complete a new W4.

FICA (Social Security Taxes)

The 1990 social security tax and wage base was as follows: For the employer, 7.65%, and for the employee, 7.65% (totaling 15.30%) applied to the first $51,300 in wages paid to an individual in a calendar year. This tax differs from federal withholding in that the amount of tax does not vary based on the number of dependents or marital status; it is applied uniformly. FICA is the first of a series of taxes to be discussed where the employer bears a portion of the expense, rather than the tax being deducted solely from the employee's pay. With FICA, the employee pays half the tax and the employer contributes a like amount.

Both of these federal taxes are deposited regularly to the Internal Revenue Service and are reported quarterly to the IRS on Form 941. These amounts will appear on annual W2 statement information to employees.

FUTA: Federal Unemployment Tax

The FUTA tax differs from both social security and income tax in that it is never deducted from the employee's pay and is solely the responsibility of the employer. This tax, like social security, is a fixed percentage of the employee's wages, with the percentage being applied to a maximum amount of compensation for each individual employee. For 1990, the percentage was applied to the first $7000 an employer paid to an employee during the calendar year.

This tax also differs in that it is reported annually, not quarterly. It is reported on Form 940.

Federal Tax Deposits

Once employees' payroll checks are written, it is time to consider when to make the payroll tax deposit. Be aware that the employees are going to take home only the net check—that is, the gross salary less the appropriate payroll taxes and other deductions. The employer is responsible for depositing all taxes in a timely manner to the various tax authorities. In the case of federal taxes—withholding and FICA—the depositing requirements are the same.

As a general rule, depositing all the payroll taxes right after the pay period avoids trouble and possible penalties, which amount to 10% of the tax. However, sometimes cash flow may not permit this procedure.

There are stiff penalties if deposits are late or incorrect, so it is wise to become very familiar with the tax depositing requirements. The requirements between federal and state taxes may vary; this is not true in California, but may be so in other states. A brief outline of the depositing rules for federal withholding and FICA is shown in Table 29.1.

Depositing Federal Unemployment (FUTA) Taxes

The deposit requirement for FUTA tax differs from that for income taxes and social security taxes. Deposits are made the month following the end of any calendar quarter. The calendar quarters end March 31, June 30, September 30, and December 31. The basic rule to remember is if undeposited taxes at the end of a quarter exceed $100, you need to make a deposit during the first month following quarter end.

Table 29.1 Summary of Deposit Rules for Social Security Taxes and Withheld Income Tax

Deposit Rule	Due
1. If at the end of the quarter your total undeposited taxes for the quarter are less than $500:	You may pay the tax to the IRS with Form 941 (or 941E) or you may deposit them by the due date of the return.
2. If at the end of any month your total undeposited taxes are less than $500:	No deposit is required. You may carry the taxes over to the following month.
3. If at the end of any month your total undeposited taxes are $500 or more but less than $3000:	You must deposit them within 15 days after the end of the month. No deposit is required if you were required to make a deposit for an eighth-monthly period during the month under Rule 4. However, if you were required to make a deposit under Rule 4 in the last month of the quarter, deposit any balance due of less than $3000 by the due date of the return.
4. If at the end of any eighth-monthly period (the 3rd, 7th, 11th 15th, 19th, 22nd, 25th, and last day of each month) your total undeposited taxes are $3000 or more:	You must deposit them within three banking days after the end of that eighth-monthly period.

Source: Circular E: Employer's Tax Guide.

Filing Quarterly Tax Returns for Withheld Income Tax and Social Security Tax

Generally speaking, all employers who are subject to income taxes, withholding, or social security must file a Form 941. Failure to file this form in a timely manner can result in large penalties, and in some cases the penalty will equal 100%. This 100% penalty would apply in cases where income and social security taxes that should be withheld are not withheld and not paid to the IRS. It is extremely important that the filing be done accurately and in a timely manner. Table 29.2 shows when Form 941 tax returns are due.

For filing the federal unemployment tax return (FUTA) use Form 940. Unlike the previously discussed taxes, this filing is done once a year and is due by January 31 for the prior 12-month period.

At the end of a calendar year, additional reporting is required. Employees receive W2s for both state and federal taxes, and other annual reporting is required. Table 29.3 is a brief calendar for federal purposes that will assist in reporting activities. By January 31 all employees should receive an accurate and complete W2 form and the federal unemployment tax return, FUTA, should be filed. By February 28, a summary of federal income tax and social security taxes is filed with the Internal Revenue Service on Form W3. This summarizes all employees' W2 activity for the last calendar year.

Table 29.2 Form 941 Due Dates

Calendar Quarters	Ending	Due Date
1st Quarter: January, February, and March	March 31	April 30
2nd Quarter: April, May, and June	June 30	July 31
3rd Quarter: July, August, and September	September 30	October 31
4th Quarter: October, November, and December	December 31	January 31

The employer is required, under penalties of perjury, to sign each of the tax returns.

State and Local Taxes

Each state and local (city or county) authority may also impose similar tax requirements on the employer. The employer is responsible for being familiar with each of these requirements. Although separate and distinct from the federal requirements, you can bet that the process will be similar.

For example, in California there is personal income tax (PIT) that requires withholding from employees. There is no state social security tax. There is a state disability tax (SDI), which is solely the expense of the employee, but it is the responsibility of the employer to calculate, withhold, and report to the Employment Development Department. SDI, like social security taxes, is calculated based on a fixed percentage applied to a predetermined amount of compensation per employee.

California has an unemployment tax. This tax is the employer's cost and no deduction is made from the employee's pay (similar to the FUTA tax). Like federal agencies, states and cities may require quarterly and annual tax reporting. Federal W2s show the state income tax and local taxes. Even though the taxes are somewhat different, the general concept of the employer's responsibility to collect, report, and deposit payroll taxes applies.

The Selection of a Payroll System

This leads to the next step—how to manage the task of payroll preparation and reporting. The key is selecting a proper payroll system.

Payroll may be processed by hand, but in today's world the use of a computerized system or an outside agency is suggested. For a small expenditure, one can select an internal automated system or an external agency such as the bank to have the payroll calculated and all the related returns prepared. Either choice will take most of the burden off the employer's shoulders. Where there are more than four or five employees, an outside

Table 29.3 Summary of Federal Tax Forms

Form	Description
W4: Employee's Withholding Certificate	This form is completed by each employee at the start of employment. It identifies the number of employee allowances for personal income tax withholding. If the number of allowances differs between federal and state, have the employee complete two forms. This form is part of the employee's individual payroll file and may be changed by the employee to alter the amount of tax withheld by the employer.
W2: Wage and Tax Statement	This form is completed by the employer annually. It summarizes the employee's wages, tips, and other compensation plus the related federal, state, and local taxes withheld.
W3: Transmittal of Income Tax Statements	This form is completed by the employer annually and is due by February 28 for the prior calendar year. This is a summary of the W2 information and should reconcile with the quarterly payroll tax returns filed during the year. A different form may be required for state and local reporting.
941: Employer's Quarterly Federal Tax Return	This form is completed by the employer quarterly and is due by the end of the month following the close of the quarter. Key information reported includes total wages subject to withholding, social security wages (FICA), payroll taxes, tax deposits, and tax liability by pay period.
940: Employer's Annual Federal Unemployment Tax Return	This form is completed by the employer annually and is due by January 31 for the prior calendar year. Key information includes total payments to employees, quarterly tax liability and employer's tax deposits. The FUTA tax is dependent on the unemployment contribution required by your particular state.

agency is recommended. Time is better spent in practice management than in keeping track of the payroll tax elements and the numerous changes that take place each year.

The selection of a proper payroll system or outside service is not difficult if approached properly. Decisions need to be made as to the system's requirements. For example, the key element of any payroll system is the ability of the system to capture employee-specific data: employee's name, address, phone number, social security number, hours worked, start date, current salary, termination date, amounts withheld, changes in status, and the like. This information should be available in an individual employee's master file.

The system should be able to keep track of information related to vacation, holiday, and sick time pay, in addition to other important features. Accounting for the contributions to pension plans may be useful. The ability to automate other deductions from wages (medical or life insurance premiums, employee advances) may be necessary. Once captured, the information can be summarized into monthly, quarterly, and yearly reports. Will the system produce payroll checks, W2s, and information for all the quarterly and yearly tax returns plus various management reports? Does the system meet the requirements of your accountant?

Record Retention

The IRS requires that employers keep all records related to employment taxes for at least four years, but seven years is preferable, to be on the safe side. These records should be easily accessible in case the IRS or another agency wishes to review them. The records to maintain should include at least the following:

Your federal employer identification number

Amounts and dates of all wages, annuity, and pension payments, if any

The names, addresses, social security numbers, and occupations of the employees and the recipients of money

The dates the employees were employed

Periods for which employees were paid while absent from work because of sickness or injury, the amount paid, and the weekly rate of payment you or your third-party payors made to them

Copies of employees' and recipients' income tax withholding allowance certificates (W4s)

Dates and amounts of tax deposits you made

Copies of tax returns filed by you or your corporation

Records of fringe benefits provided, including substantiation required under Code section 274 and related regulation

Summary

If the preceding paragraphs make the accounting for salaries, payroll taxes, and their related record keeping appear to be overwhelming, it should not. The key is getting off to the right start.

Keep in mind, it is important from the beginning to gather the necessary information for each individual employee. This can be done by questionnaire, W4 form, or other such document which can be obtained at any office supply store.

A system should be in place for processing periodic routine information to generate payroll checks. It should handle the summarization of this information in a fashion that provides accurate monthly management reports plus quarterly and yearly information to be reported to the appropriate federal, state, and local authorities.

Finally, and perhaps most important, is that this information may be used for better practice management. For example, it may be advantageous to keep track of and note on a regular basis the average hourly wage per employee or the average hourly increase per employee. Other questions can be answered through use of accurate payroll and salary data. These might ask, What is my labor cost per patient visit? or What is my labor cost as a percentage of revenue? Do I have an employee attendance problem? What are the productive hours per employee? and What is my labor cost as a percentage of my total expenses?

The foregoing is a brief overview of record keeping for salaries and related payroll taxes. Seek the guidance of outside authorities (eg, your accountant) or read the federal *Circular E: Employers' Tax Guide.* This is published annually and contains changes that are mandated by law. State agencies publish similar materials that should also be read.

Do not let the task become overwhelming. Be organized and understand what is required. Keep in mind that the actual record keeping can be maintained by an outside agency such as a bank and the services provided are good. It is important, however, to have a feel for the responsibility of both the employer and the employee.

Suggested Reading

Commerce Clearing House, *Payroll Management Guide.* Chicago, IL: CCC.

Internal Revenue Service, *Circular E: Employer's Tax Guide* (Publication 15). Washington, DC: U.S. Government Printing Office (current year).

State of California, Employment Development Department, *California Personal Income Tax Withholding Guide.* Sacramento, CA: current year.

State of California, Employment Development Department, *Employer's Guide* (DE4525). Sacramento, CA: current year.

30 | Security Measures and Avoiding Theft and Embezzlement

MICHAEL W. MURPHY, CPA AND
DREW J. SUTTER, CPA

Every organization, from a single physician to a large group practice, must protect its assets from theft and embezzlement. The primary way an organization does so is by establishing a system of internal control. In addition to safeguarding assets, a system of internal control serves to check the accuracy and reliability of accounting data, promotes operational efficiency, and encourages adherence to prescribed managerial policies.

A system of internal control may be simple or complex, depending on the size and complexity of the organization and the cost the organization is willing to incur relative to the benefits expected. Regardless of the complexity of the system, it cannot provide absolute security; it can only provide reasonable safeguards to protect the organization's assets and ensure the accurate and timely reporting of financial information.

Characteristics of Effective Internal Control Systems

A reliable system of internal control has certain characteristics that promote the objectives stated above. Those characteristics are as follows:

Proper authorization of transactions and activities

Adequate segregation of duties

Adequate record keeping

Adequate physical safeguards over access to and use of assets and records

Independent checks on performance

Competent, trustworthy personnel

Each of these characteristics is discussed in more detail in this chapter.

Proper Authorization of Transactions and Activities

In order to maintain control over assets, every transaction must be properly authorized. In many cases, management establishes policies that provide for general authorization of transactions. An example of this is a charge master, which details the fee to be charged for each procedure performed.

For some transactions, authorization should be made only on a case-by-case basis. For example, the acquisition of capital equipment over a predetermined dollar amount should occur only upon the specific approval of an authorized individual (the physician-owner) or group (the finance committee of a large group practice).

Adequate Segregation of Duties

"Segregation of duties" means that the responsibilities of maintaining custody of assets, authorizing transactions, and record keeping are separated among employees. One person should not be in a position to both perpetrate and conceal irregularities. For example, if the cashier receives cash from patients and also maintains the accounts receivable records, it may be possible to divert the cash received and manipulate the records to conceal the diversion.

Similarly, the authorization of transactions should be segregated from access to related assets. For example, the person who authorizes the addition of an employee to the payroll should not be responsible for distributing paychecks to the employees because it may be possible for that individual to add a fictitious employee to the payroll and divert the paycheck.

Obviously, adequate segregation of duties is difficult in a small entity with few employees. In such a situation, the involvement of the physician-owner becomes extremely important; the system of internal control can be improved significantly if the physician-owner performs such duties as reviewing supporting documentation before signing checks and approving all write-offs of bad debts.

Adequate Record Keeping

Every entity, regardless of size, must have an accounting system and records that identify, classify, record, and summarize transactions. The level of complexity of the accounting system is dictated by the entity's size and the diversity and complexity of its operations. For example, a small entity with effective day-to-day involvement by a physician-owner will not need the extensive accounting procedures, sophisticated records, or formal control procedures of a large, multilocation group practice. On the other hand, even the smallest physician practice cannot operate efficiently and effectively using "shoebox" accounting methods.

Adequate Physical Safeguards over Access to and Use of Assets and Records

Assets such as currency and supplies must be physically protected from theft by such means as safes and locked storerooms. Additionally, documents and records must be protected from unauthorized access and accidental or intentional destruction. Consider the accidental destruction of a master patient accounts receivable file. At a minimum, in the absence of effective backup records and procedures, it would be extremely costly and time-consuming to re-create such records. It might well be impossible.

Independent Checks on Performance

Regardless of the extent of controls and the level of compliance with them, intentional irregularities and unintentional errors are possible. Consequently, the need exists for an individual—not the person who originally performs the function—to review and check the work. Examples of such checks include a periodic surprise count of the petty cash fund by an individual with no access to it, and reconciliation of the bank accounts by an individual who is not involved in the handling of cash or the related record keeping.

In large organizations, the system of internal checks on performance usually includes one or more internal auditors who are independent of the accounting function and report directly to top management. Internal auditors' duties include studying, evaluating, and testing the entity's system of internal control to make sure it is effective and operating as planned.

Competent, Trustworthy Personnel

This is probably the most important characteristic of any system of internal control and often is the most overlooked. If an organization employs honest personnel who know and understand their duties, the characteristics of internal control discussed previously tend to take care of themselves. On the other hand, incompetent and dishonest employees can make a well-designed system of internal control relatively useless.

Making a judgment on the integrity of employees is a difficult task. Many embezzlements that come to light turn out to have been perpetrated by long-time, trusted employees. Consequently, the other characteristics of internal control cannot be ignored, regardless of how much faith is placed in employees.

All employees should be required to take annual vacations, during which another employee performs the vacationing employee's duties. In this way, temporary concealment of fraud may be detected. Additionally, all employees handling cash should be covered by a fidelity bond.

Examples of Basic Internal Control Procedures

Listed below are examples of internal control procedures relating to cash, receipts, disbursements, and other functions relevant to the business of medicine. This listing is not intended to describe a complete system of internal control, but rather is intended to illustrate some basic controls and the reasons for them.

Cash

Petty cash funds should be counted and reconciled periodically on a surprise basis by an employee with no access to them.

Each petty cash fund should be the responsibility of *one* individual and kept under lock and key so only that individual has access to it. Expenditures from petty cash should be limited to a relatively small amount, say $20, so that all significant purchases are handled through the normal purchases and disbursements system.

Bank accounts should be reconciled promptly on a monthly basis by an individual independent of the handling or recording of receipts and disbursements. The objective here is to separate the bank reconciliation process from anyone who would have the opportunity to originate fraudulent transactions in either receipts or disbursements. Such a reconciliation should include the following:

Deposits in transit, outstanding checks, and other reconciling items should be investigated as to their nature and the reasonableness of the delay in clearing the bank account.

Paid checks should be compared with entries in disbursements records and tested for unusual features, such as altered payee or amount, unauthorized signatures, and questionable endorsements.

Total deposits shown by bank statements should be reconciled with total receipts shown in related general ledger cash accounts.

Unless some other independent control exists, an employee should not be allowed to prepare the bank reconciliation for the account on which his or her own payroll check is drawn. This prevents that employee from raising the amount on the check and concealing it in the bank reconciliation.

Receipts

The majority of embezzlements relate to the diversion of receipts to the personal use of the embezzler. In a common scheme called *lapping,* the theft of the collection of a patient's account is temporarily concealed by crediting the account with a payment subsequently received from another patient. This scheme requires continued lapping until the embezzler eventually replaces the stolen funds or permanently conceals the theft by writing off some patient accounts. Another common fraud is to divert cash payments made at the time services are provided and conceal this by never entering the revenue into the system. Examples of controls over receipts are listed in the following paragraphs.

An employee who opens mail containing patients' payments should not be responsible for updating patient receivables records or even have access to the records. Otherwise, a diversion of receipts might be concealed by manipulating the patient receivables records.

To the extent practicable, receipt of over-the-counter payments should be limited to a centralized location at the facility. Such payments received directly from patients should be recorded by a cash register or evidenced by a prenumbered receipt, and cash register tapes or carbon copies of the receipts should be reconciled to recorded revenues by an employee independent of the cash receipts function. Blank copies of receipts should be safeguarded.

An individual who does not handle receipts should review receipts records and compare them with bank deposit records to determine that all receipts were deposited.

Monthly statements should be sent to all patients with outstanding balances. Such statements should be prepared and mailed by an employee who does not handle receipts. Additionally, patient billing complaints should be investigated by an individual independent of the receipts function.

Incoming patient checks should be restrictively endorsed immediately.

Receipts should be deposited daily; they should not be kept on the premises overnight.

All write-offs of receivables should be approved by supervisory personnel based on examination of supporting documentation. The individual approving the write-offs should not have access to patient payments received.

Disbursements

Payments to vendors and other disbursements should be approved based on examination of supporting documents (eg, a check request and/or a vendor's invoice) by authorized personnel.

Checks above a stated limit (eg, $500) should require dual signatures.

Employees who prepare or sign checks (or have access to signature plates or operate check-signing equipment) should not also maintain or have access to accounting records relating to disbursements.

Signed checks should be stuffed for mailing by an individual independent of the function of accounting for disbursements. A secretary with no accounting responsibilities is a good candidate for this job.

Vendors' invoices, check requests, and other documents supporting disbursements should be canceled (eg, stamped "PAID") to prevent their accidental or fraudulent reuse.

Payroll

The ideal situation for payroll is one in which a separate personnel department handles all matters relating to employment, changes in pay rates, and terminations. In small organizations where this is not practical, information regarding employees and their pay rates should be maintained and controlled by personnel outside of and without access to the cash functions, and these records should periodically be compared with detailed payroll records (eg, payroll ledger). Additional controls are as follows:

Payroll checks should be delivered by an employee independent of the payroll function (ie, the employee should have no other duties relating to payroll record keeping or preparation of payroll checks), preferably someone who knows most (if not all) employees by sight.

Any individual with the authority to add an employee to the payroll should not have access to signed payroll checks. This prevents the individual from adding a fictitious employee to the payroll and diverting the paycheck.

The organization should have procedures in place to ensure that terminated employees are deleted from the payroll.

Supervisory personnel should periodically review payroll records to look for fictitious employees, dual payments, or unusual pay rates.

Other Control Considerations

In addition to the specific controls discussed above, certain high-level controls should be implemented. These types of controls will vary by organization but might include:

comparison of financial data to independent, nonfinancial information (eg, comparing revenues to statistics such as the number of x-rays performed by a clinic's radiology department)

preparation of a monthly financial report to be reviewed by the board of directors, finance committee, or owner

annual preparation of a budget and monthly comparisons with actual results, with explanation of all significant variances

Electronic Data Processing Systems

In today's environment most, if not all, physician practices utilize some form of electronic data processing equipment to perform the required accounting functions. Although the controls previously described are equally applicable to a data processing (DP) environment, these systems will require additional levels of controls to properly safeguard the organization's assets. Numerous books cover internal controls in data processing environments, so only certain high-level issues are highlighted in this chapter.

DP controls generally are divided into two major categories: general controls and application controls. General controls are usually performed by employees of the DP department and include controls over (a) information security; (b) system acquisition, development, and maintenance; (c) computer operations; and (d) information system support. Application controls relate to the procedures and controls within specific applications (eg, payroll, cash receipts, accounts receivable, cash disbursements) and center around numerous manual and software procedures required to perform a transaction and verify its accuracy.

Critical to a successful DP system is locating a system that meets your organization's needs, is supported by a reputable vendor, and can be easily maintained by capable personnel.

In closing, we emphasize that an effective internal control system cannot succeed simply through lip service. The system must be documented, periodically reviewed, updated to address the changing environment, and continuously monitored for adherence. Remember, the best internal control system is developed to safeguard your assets by preventing or detecting, on a timely basis, errors or fraud that might cause the financial statements to be misstated or your assets to be lost or stolen. If the system is not monitored appropriately, the timely detection of problems may not occur.

Suggested Reading

Arens, Alvin A., and Loebbecke, James K., *Auditing: An Integrated Approach* (4th ed.). Englewood Cliffs, NJ: Prentice-Hall, 1988.

Sullivan, Jerry D., Gnospelius, Richard A., Defliese, Philip L., and Jaenicke, Henry R., *Montgomery's Auditing* (10th ed.). New York: John Wiley and Sons, 1985.

31 | Maintaining an Effective Risk Management Program: Malpractice and Other Considerations

DON HARPER MILLS, MD, JD,
ORLEY H. LINDGREN, PHD, AND
DIANE G. BROWN, RN, JD

Risk management embodies various functions that identify, manage, and prevent risks of liability and devise means to fund those risks. Physicians and health services managers are becoming increasingly aware that effective risk management can improve the quality of care and protect provider assets. Therefore, whether your practice is primarily office- or hospital-based, you need to understand and become active in risk management.

Risk management was originally developed to promote safety and control liability costs in industry. It was first applied in health care in the early 1970s. It was spurred on by increases in jury awards for medical malpractice and out-of-court settlements against hospitals and physicians, which in turn were caused by a national trend of increased consumer activism and the proliferation of high-technology medicine with attendant benefits and risks.

In the malpractice insurance crisis of the mid-1970s, many companies began charging sharply higher rates. Some refused to renew longstanding accounts, or they withdrew entirely from the medical malpractice market, leaving their customers at risk. This spurred hospitals and physicians to organize innovative insurance arrangements. It also stimulated them to implement risk management programs, in the belief that they could help control liability risks and financial losses. The concept of risk management also appealed to patient groups and the general public because it was equated with improved patient safety and hence better health care. The concept and practice of risk management gained widespread acceptance as a means to protect both hospitals and physicians from costly malpractice claims and to improve the quality of medical care.

Approximately 80% of malpractice liability claims over the past decade involved physicians and arose from events that occurred in hospital settings. For this reason it is not surprising that doctors and hospitals have been the primary locus of modern clinical risk management programs. However, this is changing somewhat as office practice and ambulatory medicine grows. Increasingly the diagnosis and treatment of serious ailments occurs not only in hospitals but also in clinics and doctors' offices, where a variety of high-risk medical technology is being utilized. As an office-based physician you also probably maintain hospital privileges and perform a portion of your work in a hospital setting. Risk management and quality assurance are in place in one form or another in almost all hospitals in the United States, and their activities will affect your practice in that setting and will warrant your attention and active involvement.

Risk management has a number of functions. It is concerned with the orderly and cost-effective transfer of risk through various insurance arrangements. It is concerned with the reduction of risk through the identification of sources of liability, particularly those stemming from personal injury to patients. It facilitates and carries out actions to reduce the extent of patient injury after it has occurred to an individual. It also provides information about prior risks so that system changes may be implemented to prevent future risks of injury and consequent liability. Risk management is concerned with effective communication and documentation among providers and patients. It seeks to help providers optimize their handling of problem situations and problem patients. Risk management, in order to be successful, requires physicians' active participation.

Protection of Assets through Insurance Mechanisms

Protection of assets, a basic element of risk management, is accomplished primarily through professional liability insurance, in which the risk of loss of assets is transferred to a third party. Malpractice litigation is so ubiquitous these days that practicing physicians must have an asset protection plan in place. A few have concluded, for personal reasons, that they will not or cannot purchase professional liability insurance, thereby exposing their personal assets to potential loss. The means by which these assets may be protected from litigation loss varies from state to state. Those who intend to practice with or without professional liability insurance protection should consult experts in their communities to determine what collateral protection they need and what may be available.

Occurrence Coverage

Different types of professional liability insurance are available to physicians through insurance companies and various self-insurance organizations. The oldest and safest form is the *occurrence* type of coverage, which protects the policyholder (you) for the particular patient's injury regardless of the date when that injury precipitated a lawsuit. For example, if you had occurrence coverage for the year 1991, any adverse event that took place in 1991 that leads to litigation at any later time is covered by that policy. Even a lapse between the event in 1991 and a lawsuit in 2010 is still covered by that policy. This is the best form of professional liability coverage, but it is no longer routinely available and is usually more expensive than other types of coverage. If you can afford it, and it is available, the occurrence insurance policy is the type you should obtain.

Claims-Made Coverage

Claims-made policies are the type presently available to most physicians in North America. Physician-controlled insurance organizations, for example, provide claims-made policies at beginning rates that are substantially less than those required for occurrence policies. In succeeding years, however, the premiums increase until about the fifth year, when the premium for the claims-made policy is approximately the same as that required for the occurrence policy. So, although claims-made coverage is more affordable for the beginning practitioner, ultimately it will cost the same as occurrence policies.

Costs aside, this type of coverage may pose significant problems for the unwary physician consumer. Insurance carriers must be notified of the potential of a claim in the policy year of coverage under a claims-made policy. For the policy year of 1991, all occurrences within that year that give rise to claims need to be reported to the insurance carrier while the insurance is still in force. That is, notification must be made during the policy year, or, if not, during any subsequent policy year when insured by the *same* carrier. If you purchase claims-made insurance for the year 1991 and switch to another carrier in 1995 and thereafter, a claim arising for the first time to your knowledge in 1996 from an event that occurred in 1991 may *not* be covered by the pre-1995 policy, unless you bought "tail" coverage for the pre-1995 policy. As of 1996, the pre-1995 policy would no longer be in force, and the new 1995 policy with a new carrier would not cover pre-1995 events.

Tail Coverage

In effect, a claims-made insurance policy weds the policy holder (you) to the insurer. The only way to break that relationship and maintain subsequent protection is to buy what is called *tail coverage* from the insurer. This policy is sold to you for a specific price to cover you for subsequent claims arising from events in the years you purchased claims-made coverage from that company, even though you have terminated that policy. Because not all potential claims are clearly identifiable at the time of occurrence, it is generally advisable to purchase tail coverage. However, depending upon the vagaries of the insurance market at any particular point in time, tail coverage can be expensive and difficult to obtain.

Other Mechanisms of Insurance Coverage

Risk retention groups, cooperatives, and self-insurance programs of larger group practices are other means to protect your assets. These may provide you with coverage at a premium substantially below that quoted by regular insurance companies and offer other advantages and disadvantages. In most states insurance organizations are subjected to review by state insurance agencies and are backed up by that state's guarantee law requiring that claims against a bankrupt insurance agency be paid by other insurance companies doing business in that state. These alternative forms of coverage may also be completely assessable—that is, you may be responsible for ultimate losses that exceed the company's premium structure. If the premium quoted to you seems unusually low, you need to determine the question of assessability and the extent to which the company comes under the jurisdiction of the state's guarantee laws. You should also inquire as to the financial strength of the company and the extent to which you would receive any protection through reinsurance or excess insurance coverage that they purchase.

The attraction of risk retention groups is that they often write coverage for a number of states in a region. This means that if you go from one state to another, you may not need to seek new means of professional liability coverage. This is a definite advantage over doctor-controlled companies that are restricted to one state and write only claims-made policies. It is not a simple matter to terminate a claims-made policy in one state and start a new one in another state, because you may need to purchase tail coverage from your first state. If you do not, the company in the new state may require that you pay an additional premium for *nose* coverage, which would protect you from previous injuries that have not been reported.

Communication and Documentation

Creating the medical records of patients in your office is as important as creating similar records in the hospital. You may not need to communicate with other physicians through these records if you are a solo practitioner, but most American physicians will ultimately be in some type of group practice, and the records will be required reading for other physicians in the practice. Also, the medical record may be required by another physician who may be called upon to diagnose and treat your patient for a variety of reasons. Therefore for medical reasons it is imperative that you create records that communicate adequately with your colleagues. Charting protocols should be developed for the nurses, physician's assistants, and nurse practitioners involved in your office practice as well. Often these professionals spend more time with the patients than you do, and it is important that they document their assessments, observations, and instructions.

For medicolegal purposes it is imperative that you create records that will allow a re-creation of the findings, decisions, and medical management you provided. These records are mandatory for your own credibility in the event your patient disagrees with your findings, recommendations, or treatments. For instance, assume you gave a penicillin injection to a patient who developed an anaphylactic reaction with severe sequelae. In retrospect the patient alleges he told you of a prior reaction he experienced to penicillin, but you assert that you asked about any prior reactions and were told there had been none. Your written record should, if properly done, be able to resolve this communication conflict. In the absence of written records juries tend to believe patients at least as often as they believe physicians, which means that you would have a 50-50 chance of convincing a jury that your recollection is the correct one. If your records document that the question was asked and answered negatively, and this documentation appears logically in the sequence of the chart you maintained for this patient, the jury will probably find in your favor on this pivotal issue.

Another reason to create and maintain a complete patient record is reimbursement. Increasingly, both government and private payors are basing payment on the level of care (LOC) and intensity of service reflected in the office chart.

Record Ownership

In most states you will have both the right and the duty to retain possession of your original patient records, including x-rays, lab slips, and diagnostic tracings. Occasionally you may be subpoenaed by a court to produce the originals in litigation; if this happens, remember that originals can go astray, so be sure to make and retain copies. Except in this case, originals should never be let out of your possession. Patients have the right to information contained in your records about them, but you should release copies only. Any release of records must be accompanied by an authorization addressed to you and signed by the patient to disclose that information to a third party. The most common avenues of disclosure will be third-party payors and subsequent treating physicians who have taken over the management of your patient. When either of these sources requests information, send copies of records as authorized directly rather than giving them to the patient for transmittal. Under no circumstances should you refuse to send copies of records to a subsequent treating physician, even if the patient has not paid your bill, but never give patients their original records or x-rays for transmittal. Protection of your files and records is of paramount importance for the protection of your practice. A lost or missing medical record usually signals a lost liability case.

Original records in your office should be retained as long as practicable. For patients under current management, old records must be retained indefinitely. For patients who have left your practice, records should be retained at least 10 years; in some highly litigious regions in the country they should be retained indefinitely. If space is limited or too costly, records may be placed in lower-cost, long-term physical storage or captured on microfilm or electronically. Your state's medical society is usually a reliable source for record retention guidelines.

Telephone Documentation

A telephone conversation between you and a patient may be just as critical as a face-to-face communication in your office. In both instances, the crux of the information conveyed should be documented. Develop a telephone memorandum system and carry it with you at all times, even on trips; when at home, keep it at your bedside. Make brief notes of your conversations with patients, staff, and consultants and make particular note of the management you recommend. Give such notes to your secretary or office clerk daily for insertion into the chart. Increasingly, office and professional staff (nurses, physician's assistants, and nurse practitioners) have responsibilities for telephone contacts with patients, so a system should be in place for documentation of these contacts as well.

Diagnostic Instrument Logging

You will receive laboratory and radiologic reports of procedures performed on your patients at your request, and you need a system that brings these results to your attention when they arrive. Do not allow office personnel to insert the information into the patient's chart without your review. You are on "constructive notice" of everything that is in your patient's chart, even if you have no actual knowledge of it. Therefore if you delay diagnosing a serious disease that showed up in a report that was inserted into your patient's chart without your review, you will have a difficult—if not impossible—time explaining this during a deposition or in front of a jury.

Attention should also be given to reports not received. It is your responsibility to determine the results when tests or procedures are ordered for patients. Thus a system should be in place whereby the office staff monitors receipt of reports and follows up on those not received on a timely basis.

Constructive notice also pertains to pieces of information you insert in the patient's chart but subsequently forget. For instance, if a patient tells you he is allergic to penicillin and you enter that information in the chart on that day, you may forget about that communication a year later when you decide he needs penicillin for an acute streptococcal pharyngitis. If you fail to question him again about the allergy and the penicillin you give him results in an anaphylactic reaction, you will be held legally accountable for failing to take note of the prior information in your chart. That is, you are on constructive notice of everything that is in your patient's chart. If something as important as a specific allergic history is given to you, not only should it be documented at the time of communication, but the front of the chart should be tagged so that the history is brought to your attention at every subsequent office visit. Hospitals tag their charts routinely; you should, too.

Records Alteration

Occasionally when you look at old charts and remember something that was not documented, you will be tempted to alter the record to make it more complete. Avoid that temptation. If you want to correct or augment an existing record, do so on a separate sheet of paper, and make a reference note in your old chart at the date that you wanted changed or augmented. If you err by writing improper words or thoughts when you are creating the original record, you need not start over. You may cross through what was written incorrectly and write the correction immediately thereafter. Do not erase or obliterate incorrect words or phrases—this creates the impression of a coverup. Once your original page has been created and a day or two passes, do not go back and correct the original page. Leave the original page in place and create a new page noting alteration or augmentation.

Many states have statutes or regulations pertaining to the creation of false medical documents. These documents include birth certificates, death certificates, insurance forms, and even your own office notes. You will be asked to fill out cause-of-death sections on death certificates for your patients at times when you are busy doing other things. Take time to think about what you are writing in that cause-of-death section. Make sure that the cause-and-effect sequence is correct and medically reasonable.

Do not succumb to a patient's request to submit a fraudulent insurance report for a procedure his or her insurance policy does not cover. That is, do not perform a hemorrhoidectomy and bill the insurance company for a tonsillectomy when the former procedure is not covered by that patient's insurance. Although this may be a sympathetic act on your part, it is nevertheless a fraudulent act that could jeopardize your practice.

Written Outpatient Instructions

No patient should leave your office with instructions for home care that are not in writing. Patients are invariably anxious when being seen in your office and more likely than not will forget your recommendations for home care. Providing these instructions in written form therefore will improve outpatient management and compliance. Hospitals already do this and you should, too, in your office practice. With the increasing emphasis on ambulatory care and outpatient, rather than inpatient, treatment, this is especially important.

Instructions should include activity level, medications, diet, and condition-specific instructions on when to contact your office should there be problems or complications.

Of course, keep copies of all outpatient instructions in your office chart. USP now publishes drug information documents that can be given to patients when you prescribe specific drugs for them. These information sheets identify the drug, briefly state the purpose of the drug, indicate the more likely possible complications, and the circumstances under which you should be contacted if they occur. These information sheets are not for purposes of consent but for outpatient management—to help the patient comply with your recommendations. You should obtain information sheets on all drugs used in your office and get in the habit of distributing these sheets to patients when specific drugs are prescribed or dispensed. You should note in your original office chart whenever one of these information sheets is given. When office or nursing staff perform the outpatient instruction function, they should document this as well. It is advisable to note who provided the information and have the patient or patient's caretaker indicate by signature that written instructions were explained.

Special Communications to Patients: Warnings

Because your knowledge of medicine and health care is superior to that of most of your patients, you are required to exercise protective management for your patients, specifically in providing information and warnings.

There are times when you will be required to warn your patients to avoid possible future harm. For instance, you have a duty to warn your patients about the sedative effects of prescription drugs. Failure to give such a warning may leave you vulnerable to lawsuit by your patients or by people you have never seen before. An example is that of a drowsy patient who injures another person in an automobile accident. In all states but Michigan the third party may sue the physician for his or her injuries. In *every* state you are responsible to your patients for their injuries if you fail to warn them about drugs and driving. Do not rely upon the pharmacist to provide a warning; it may not be forthcoming or it may be inadequate to absolve you from responsibility in the eyes of the jury. Do it yourself and then document that warning has been given. Even a stamp with your initials in the patient's chart on the date of visit could constitute enough evidence for a jury to believe that a warning was actually given to the patient at that time.

Warnings about driving are just as important for patients with diseases that could imperil driving ability. For example, seizure disorders, acute and chronic alcoholism, and any other metabolic or neurologic impairment could imperil your patient's driving ability. Whether or not your state has reporting requirements for some of these diseases, you can be liable to your patient or to some third party for injuries suffered because of failure to warn.

If a patient refuses your recommendations for specific therapy, your responsibility extends beyond merely accepting that refusal. You need to go one step further by informing the patient of the potential adverse medical consequences of that refusal. For instance, if the foot ulcer of a diabetic patient becomes bad enough, you may feel that intravenous antibiotics and hospitalization are required for aggressive wound care to avoid losing the leg. If the patient refuses on the basis of lack of money or some other reason, you ought to warn the patient about the potential of losing the leg in the absence of aggressive management available in the hospital. Of course, any time such a warning is given, it should be documented. If the patient ultimately loses the leg because of progression of the ulcer and sues you, he probably will complain that you never told him about the seriousness of the consequences of his refusal. Only the written documentation of the warning will lead the jury to accept your version of the facts.

Warning a potential victim who has been identified as being at risk of harm by your patient is a duty you acquired as an outgrowth of California's *Tarasoff* case. If a patient you are seeing communicates a threat concerning a third party to you, you should consider the seriousness of the threat and the likelihood that it will be carried out in deciding whether or not you should contact the potential victim and the police.

Informed consent is nearly as important in office practice as it is in hospital practice. You should be sure that patients you treat are old enough to give consent—usually 18 years of age—and are mentally competent to understand that to which they are consenting. If the procedures you perform in the office are relatively benign, you need not engage in an extended discussion of them. Consent will be implied by the fact that the patient cooperates. However, if you perform complex surgical procedures in your office, such as cosmetic surgery, you should undertake as formal and elaborate a consent approach as you would in a hospital. You should discuss with the patient the procedures to be performed, including their purposes and dangers, alternatives, and the consequences of refusing, and document this conversation in the patient's chart. If you prescribe highly dangerous drugs—those with significant risk of adverse effects—special disclosures about need and risk should be made to the patients and documented in their charts. Antineoplastic drugs and corticosteroids are examples.

There are times when you must be your patient's advocate against a third party, such as an insurance carrier or state or federal health program. As the patient's doctor you have the primary obligation to the patient for clinical management—a principle established in the California case *Wickline v. State of California*. If the third party payor decides to limit that clinical management by cutting off funds, it is the obligation of the physician to alert the patient to seek an appeal process to avoid getting injured by a cutoff of medical management. If the third party payor acts unreasonably it might also have direct liability to the patient. Whenever such a warning is given to the patient that funds are being cut off, be sure to document that warning in the appropriate spot on the patient's chart.

Prepare for Emergencies

Drugs that you administer in the office will be capable of causing severe, immediate adverse reactions; anesthetics you administer and procedures you perform may induce a variety of reactions. Your office therefore should be prepared by possessing all the necessary equipment to treat these reactions. This equipment should be concentrated in a labeled area in your office so that personnel do not need to scurry around trying to find syringes, drugs, and oxygen bottles while a patient is becoming more hypoxic. You and your office personnel need to be trained to use this equipment correctly. Practice drills on emergency response should be arranged for you and your office staff several times a year.

If you perform surgery under general or intravenous anesthesia in your office, you should possess resuscitative equipment similar to that found in hospital operating rooms. When you send people home from your office after general or intravenous anesthesia, be sure that they are accompanied and that written instructions for monitoring for reactions are given to the companion. There is a tendency to discharge patients for office post-anesthetic monitoring earlier than they would be discharged from the hospital setting. This places an increased burden on you to see that proper outpatient monitoring is continued for critical periods of time, to ensure that a major catastrophe does not go unnoticed, and that complete discharge instructions are given to and understood by the patient or companion.

Office Equipment and Procedures

Equipment used for patient care should be maintained in good operating condition and inspected at appropriate intervals. The manufacturer's manual and guidelines should be followed scrupulously. If you decide to use devices in ways other than those recommended by the manufacturer, create a protocol outlining your intended use, supported by literature references, if any. Such a recommendation is particularly useful for drugs that you wish to prescribe for purposes beyond the indications covered in the package insert or in dosages that differ from the recommendations in the package insert. The manufacturer's drug brochure is not intended to be *the* standard of practice for the use of the drug; however, in most states that package insert is admissable into evidence against you for a reaction to the drug, provided you failed to comply with the recommendations found in it. If you were unaware of the information in the package insert and had no scientific support for your deviation, the chances of defending you successfully are materially damaged. You should be aware of the manufacturer's comments in its insert for all drugs you regularly use, and you should create your own protocol in instances where you feel a deviation from such usage is appropriate on a regular basis. These protocols can be created and kept in a separate file in your office. In individual instances, deviation from the manufacturer's recommendations can be noted in the patient's chart with a statement of scientific rationale.

Drawing arterial or venous blood in the office requires special protective measures to protect patients from hurting themselves should they faint or become dizzy. These patients should be lying down, at best. If they are sitting up, the chair needs to support the patient on three sides, at least.

Intramuscular injections in your office must be given by those who know how to do it. Injury to the radial or sciatic nerve following an intramuscular injection is rarely successfully defended. It is important, therefore, for someone in your office to be appointed to monitor the injection technique of those who will do the injections. Such monitoring should be periodic throughout the year and should be documented, particularly in offices that have rapid turnover of office personnel.

Sterilization procedures in your office are more important than you think. A patient who alleges acquiring an infectious disease through your office will point first to your sterilization procedures. Did you utilize appropriate sterilization technique? Did you follow the manufacturer's recommendation? Did you document monitoring sterilization procedures in your office? Failing to answer these questions places many office-based physicians at an unacceptable risk of losing a lawsuit alleging transmittal of diseases. Disposable needles are now used and of course should never be reused. But what about instruments for minor surgical procedures? Look at what you do in your office to see if an HIV or hepatitis infection could be transmitted because of sterilization techniques that are improperly carried out or monitored. Hepatitis transmittal in dental offices from patient to patient is frequently difficult to defend when there are monitoring shortcomings. This problem may also exist if you do surgical procedures and needs to be a focus of your own risk management efforts.

Terminating Patient Care

Patients can terminate your management at will without notice. However, you need to determine whether a patient who fails to return has terminated your management as opposed to merely being noncompliant. For this reason, you need to establish a system in your office that will allow you to notify patients who should be closely monitored on an outpatient basis. For instance, management of an infected foot with outpatient wound care and antibiotics requires subsequent office evaluations to determine therapeutic progress. The patient who fails to return should be contacted and warned about the necessity for continued evaluation. To be able to carry out such a recall, your appointment log book should be color coded for those patients who need to be seen and who will be contacted if they fail to show up. It may be that the patient intends to go elsewhere and has terminated your care. That is the patient's right. But if the patient has expressed no such intention, injury from his or her noncompliance may be avoided by proper follow-up by your office. Remember, you have knowledge superior to the patient's concerning the need for management. His or her noncompliance may not necessarily eliminate your legal responsibility to follow up.

You may not unilaterally terminate a patient's management without notice to the patient or without giving that patient adequate time to seek a replacement physician. In the usual outpatient management setting, you should discuss terminating the patient's management during an office visit and then write a memorandum to the patient confirming the office discussion. You should provide several names of other physicians in the same specialty or clinics. It is to your benefit as well as to the patient's for you to state that the patient's welfare would be better protected if he or she sought care from another physician. In metropolitan settings a week or two weeks may be required for a patient to seek and secure replacement management. In that interval, you will continue to respond to any requests by the patient for emergency management. That will be discussed by your terminating conversation in the office and confirmed by the letter to the patient thereafter. The follow-up letter should be certified with return receipt requested, if only to establish the date when the letter was sent. Terminating the management of a patient unilaterally is difficult in a hospital setting, but this process can be assisted by the hospital risk manager or administrator. The patient will not be able to seek your replacement; therefore, you will probably have to assist in finding a replacement who will take over your management while the patient is still in the hospital. This must be discussed with the patient and documented in the hospital chart. The physician who will replace you must also document his or her intention in the hospital chart so that the nursing staff knows whom to contact in the future. Usually either the medical staff bylaws or hospital policy will spell out the procedures for transfer of care. Development of similar procedures for physician offices is also recommended.

Local Assistance

Most states and county medical associations have programs to assist physicians in office management development, both for medicolegal issues and for economic problems. Do not hesitate to use these resources in your community to answer specific questions.

Your professional liability insurance carrier or risk retention group will also be able to answer specific questions dealing with potential liability claims. Be sure to notify your insurance carrier promptly of any claim or suit, or any expression of significant dissatisfaction by a patient, or of any significant adverse outcome in your office practice that may be the basis for a lawsuit. The same principle holds true for the portion of your practice that occurs in hospitals: hospital risk management and your professional liability carrier should be notified promptly. If a patient suffers a fatal anaphylactic reaction, this should be the subject of notification even though you may be convinced at the outset that your action was appropriate and that the adverse event was a risk of the procedure or was caused by something other than your actions. Legal responsibility determination requires that the many aspects of the matter be examined. If you fail to notify your insurance carrier of the adverse outcome, valuable evidence may be lost by the time a law suit is filed; also you may find yourself uninsured if the claim arises a year or two later and you are now with another carrier with a claims-made policy.

Early warning of potential liability claims can be achieved if you and your staff adopt an attitude of alertness and take an active role in reporting and tracking adverse occurrence or potential liability claims. Early warning provides you and your liability carrier the opportunity to carry out a timely review, to sequester pertinent evidence, and to make intelligent decisions as to what management action to take, if any.

If your risk manager/insurance carrier has been notified promptly, you can receive immediate professional advice on what to do and what not to do, and you can receive other professional assistance designed to help the patient correct the problem and prevent the likelihood of a liability claim. Possible early actions may include (1) explaining to the patient and carefully documenting in the patient's medical record what happened and why; (2) making arrangements with the patient and his or her family for corrective action to be taken, usually at no cost to the patient (sometimes the patient's share of these costs will be picked up by the hospital risk management department or your insurance program); (3) providing referrals and facilitating the arrangement of social and/or medical resources in the community (these costs may be picked up by public and private agencies and by your insurance company); and (4) planning and implementing changes in procedures, staffing, and equipment to make sure the problem does not happen to the next patient.

Appropriate risk management can reduce the negative emotional, physical, and economic effects of a patient's injury and may reduce the chances that the patient will pursue formal litigation. Moreover, it provides an opportunity for true prevention. A near-miss or minor injury can provide the information to bring about positive, constructive changes in your office or hospital practice that will reduce the risk of serious injuries and liability in the future.

Suggested Reading

Morlock, L., Lindgren, O., and Mills, D. H., "Malpractice, Clinical Risk Management and Quality Assessment." In Goldfield, N., and Nash, D. B., (Eds.), *Providing Quality Care: The Challenge to Clinicians* (pp. 225–257). Philadelphia: American College of Physicians, 1989.

"Tarasoff v. Regents of University of California." 131 *California Reporter* 14 (1976).

"Wickline v. State of California." 228 *California Reporter* 661 (1986).

United States General Accounting Office. *Initiatives in Hospital Risk Management.* Washington, DC: GAO, 1989.

32 Marketing Strategies for the 1990s: How to Obtain and Increase Referrals to Your Practice

SHARON NOVAKOFF, MHSM
AND MARSHA ANDERSEN

Among the many changes that medicine has experienced in the last few years is the acceptance of health-care "marketing" as part of the business of running a medical practice. Although marketing is more accepted, it is not necessarily better understood. For many people marketing and advertising are synonymous, and the distrust for marketing is really an objection to tacky advertising, which can demean the profession. Marketing is a process that follows the course of analyzing a situation, determining the proper course of action, and implementing a plan of action to correct the problems. The plan may or may not include some form of advertising.

The purpose of this chapter is to help a physician market his or her practice. The marketing plan template presented in Appendix 32.1 is a tool to help a physician make the marketing process operational and establish a direction for growth. The main text of the chapter will address the detail behind each section of a standard marketing plan. Implicit throughout the chapter is the need for the physician to write the plan and, most important, to discipline himself or herself to keep track of the results in a systematic fashion.

Situational Assessment

Marketing a practice is not advertising—it is understanding the environment and the impact of the practice on that environment. It is knowing what the needs are in the community and developing the practice to meet those needs.

To market a practice you must begin with an assessment of the community and of the practice itself.

Demographics

What are the demographics of the community? Do particular ethnic groups in the community require special attention? If so, the physician may want to become familiar with that population by joining particular service groups, learning the language, or employing office personnel who are members of that group.

The demographics of the community also include the ages, income, or life-styles of people who live in the area. If a new residential community is developing near the practice, the physician will want to know the ages of individuals moving into that community, their income levels, and the type of health-care issues they are likely to experience. A community of older adults may be concerned about issues relating to medication interactions, whereas a young family community would be more concerned with the availability of well-child care.

Similarly, the physician will want to assess whether the location of the practice is consistent with the type of patients with whom he or she wishes to work. If the practice is located in an area that is shifting from residential to industrial, the physician will want to examine his or her interest in treating industrial injuries or relocating the practice to a more residential part of town.

The chamber of commerce in most towns has a report that describes the ethnic mix and income levels of its residents. These reports are generally available at little or no cost and usually provide a considerable amount of information.

Target Markets

A *target market* is the group of patients the physician is most interested in reaching. It is important for the physician to determine the target market, as the strategies will differ accordingly. If the physician is interested in treating sports medicine problems and the area is heavily saturated with managed care plans (preferred provider organizations [PPOs] or Health Maintenance Organizations [HMOs]) utilized by the younger, active members of the community, then the physician will need to become involved with managed care plans. If, on the other hand, the physician is interested in treating nursing home patients, then an appropriate strategy might be to sponsor educational classes for the nursing staff of local nursing homes. The physician can target multiple populations simultaneously but will need to approach each target market separately.

Competition

Who are the other providers in the area? The physician attempting to market a practice will need to assess the strengths and weaknesses of the other providers in the area. This will enable the physician to capitalize on the business opportunities that are available and to recognize the threats that exist.

Unique Features

Does the practice have special features that are not readily available in the area? These features could include the advantage of being a female physician in a community where there are few women in practice. It can also include the reputation of the senior partner or partners. It would certainly include any special training or ability on which the physician could capitalize to secure speaking engagements or participate in community lectures.

Practice Trends

Physicians often do not take the time to analyze their own practice trends, yet there is a tremendous amount of valuable information to be learned from this. Who is the physician actually seeing in the practice? A healthy medical practice will have a core of patients that have been with the practice for years and are experiencing more need for health care as they get older. It may appear that the practice is busy, but if the physician determines that there is not a regular influx of new patients to the practice then the practice may be in a vulnerable position.

Trends in payor categories can also indicate strengths and weaknesses in the practice. For example, Medicare payments are becoming increasingly restrictive and the paperwork requirements more costly to process. Medicaid payments are traditionally low and are expected to remain low. The number of private paying patients continues to decrease as managed care plans (PPOs or HMOs) increase. The physician will need to be careful of the practice's reliance on any one payor.

Putting all of this information together can help determine if, in fact, the practice is attracting the patients the physician is most interested in treating. Improving the mix of patients takes time, but it is unlikely that it will happen at all if the physician is not actively assessing the situation and taking steps for change.

Physical Environment

Does the office have a special advantage or deficit in its physical layout? Issues related to parking or wheelchair access can be very important to patients. The physician should walk through the front door of the practice on a regular basis. Does the lobby feel comfortable? Are the magazines current? Does the office staff attire represent the physician well?

There are numerous elements to assessing the practice; each is important and each will have an effect on the success of the practice. The following pages will highlight key areas that are basic to the marketing of almost all practices.

"Marcus Welby, M.D."

Patients watch physicians very carefully and often make decisions regarding the "quality" of a physician's service based on the physician's personal interactions. It is unusual to find a patient who can objectively judge actual quality of care, but most patients can usually make a judgment about the treatment received from the doctor and office staff. Each physician has an individual bedside manner, but the following sections describe who is watching and what they are looking for.

Image

Hospital nurses are probably the most frequently asked source for a physician referral. Community members seek out nurses (and other hospital professionals) to inquire about the "best physician" for certain types of problems. That occurs largely because people know that nurses have many opportunities to observe the personalities and work of physicians. Although it is important to be courteous and friendly with the nursing staff of your hospital, that is only a small part of what is important. Nursing is often called the "caring profession," and that is what they are watching for: do you care about, as well as care for, the patient?

If a physician has a difficult patient in the ICU, then it is assumed that the physician will be readily available if that patient gets into trouble at any point during the stay. The physician may be perfectly comfortable handling the situation by phone, but if the physician's response to the problem sounds uncaring or too casual, he or she is soon likely to lose the respect of the nursing staff. Also, if a member of the nursing staff has an idea to make the patient more comfortable or has performed some special service for the patient, the physician would do well to recognize that effort. After all, if the well-being of the patient is of foremost importance to the physician, then clearly that physician would be grateful for all efforts on behalf of the patient. The examples are endless but the theory is the same: nursing staff will be very sensitive to signals from physicians that they care about their patients. The physician starting or building a practice may want to take a serious look at the signals he or she is sending.

Bedside Manner

Caring is as elusive to define as quality, but the same saying applies: "I know it when I see it." In medicine it has always been called bedside manner, and it consists of well-known actions that can be easily overlooked. Eye contact is probably the most basic element. A patient or a patient's family may not believe that the physician is really recognizing them or their health problems if the physician does not make eye contact. There are also times when it is appropriate to touch a patient, to lend support at a time when the patient needs it. Physicians who can recognize these moments and respond accordingly have tremendously loyal patient populations. If a physician is wise enough to know when a patient needs a little extra support, then the patient can trust that the physician is truly in touch with problems at hand; and remember, try never to forget a patient's allergy—aside from being dangerous, it is perceived as impersonal or even insulting.

Patient Perceptions

Courtesy is also an element of caring. Listening to patients and their families is part and parcel of being a physician. This takes time. There is also ample room in any record-keeping system for the physician to jot down the names of the patient's relatives or important events that the physician can mention at a later visit. Because patients have relatively little knowledge about the full scope of care, they are more likely to attach great importance to the elements with which they are familiar.

People generally want to be taken seriously, but never so seriously as when their health is in question. Although it is expected that the physician will immediately diagnose the problem and begin treatment, if patients have not had an opportunity to give input they will rarely have confidence in the resolution. A physician can easily employ some very helpful practices. The physician should never look rushed. If the office staff needs to speed up the schedule, there are a number of ways they can alert the physician in code that will not be detected by the patient. A comment such as "Doctor, Mrs. Jones' lab tests are ready" can be used to tell the physician to move along.

Physicians are besieged with phone calls. If physicians are to return any calls in a timely manner, it must be the calls from their patients. Many times the office staff can make the calls, but if the patient feels the need to speak to the physician directly, then the physician should respond. It is also extremely powerful for a physician to call a patient to find out how he or she is responding following a traumatic episode. Patients are likely to say that they are fine but unlikely to ever forget that the physician called them.

Patients can be voracious readers, and the volume of medically related literature available in the supermarket is staggering. Patients like to be knowledgeable but they are rarely happy about knowing more than their doctor. The physician needs to stay abreast of current trends. *Ladies' Home Journal* and *Reader's Digest* may not strike a physician as particularly reliable sources for current health-care knowledge, but these publications are well respected by the public. The physician may not be particularly impressed with the advice these publications give and may need to tell the patient that the information is not relevant to the current situation. However, it is the manner in which the physician rejects these ideas that is important. If the patient considers the information important enough to share with the physician, then it will not help the relationship for the physician to dismiss it as nonsense.

Appearance

Dress and grooming do count with patients. A clearly avant-garde or disheveled appearance will not inspire confidence in a patient. It does not particularly matter what fashion style a physician chooses, but it is important to make a professional statement.

Patient Relations

The relationship between the patient and the physician is complicated, but it often boils down to the issue of trust. Patients constantly evaluate whether the physician "cares" for them and knows how to provide the proper medical care. Physicians who have completed their training on how to diagnose and treat a patient have often spent little time learning how to "care" for them.

Patient relations begins with the telephone. Often the telephone provides the first contact a patient will have with a medical office. Most of the time, the person on the other end of the phone is someone other than the physician. In fact, in most offices the least-trained member of the staff is assigned to answer the phone.

In assessing patient relations in the office, the physician should consider the issues addressed in the following sections.

Telephone

Why are people calling the office? What is the response to each category of call? If the practice has a lot of new patients calling, how are the calls being handled? Does your staff know the answers to the most simple questions, such as hours of operation, what the charges for visits are, and what insurance you take? If not, do they tell the patient they will find the answer? If the patients are being asked to immediately schedule an appointment without being able to engage in a dialogue, the physician might encounter a lot of "no-show" first appointments. If a patient asks questions regarding a medical problem, how is that call handled? Often a lot of unnecessary negative connotations are inserted into these conversations. Statements such as, "The doctor is very busy now, would you like to speak to the nurse?" may make the patient feel relatively unimportant. The statement, "The nurse will definitely want to talk with you, why don't we start there?" is a better, more positive way to communicate. Being nice is important, but there is more to it than that. It is also important to listen carefully to what people are saying. How are insurance issues being handled? Do new patients know that the physician understands insurance and will work with their insurance company on their behalf? Or do patients feel that they will have to do this on their own?

Scheduling

The ease of scheduling and the expectation of a reasonable waiting time are also meaningful to patients. Is the appointment time predictable to patients? Or do patients assume that they will wait a long time before being seen? There are numerous unavoidable reasons a schedule can get off track. There are also numerous ways to reduce the occurrence. The office staff can help you by analyzing the main reasons for delays. Are they overscheduling? Are they leaving enough time for emergencies? Are they effective at developing signals that let the physician know the schedule is running behind? In any case, it is important to let the patient know that the office respects their time and tries to minimize waiting times.

Billing

Just as billing is a complicated business for physicians, it is also complicated for the patient. Medicare is becoming increasingly prolific with their letters to patients regarding charging and billing practices. Office billing practices need to be clear and patients need to feel confident that they can talk with their physician and the office staff regarding any problems they might be having, either with the doctor's billing or the content of insurer correspondence. It is also crucial that the office staff provides a reasonably private area for these discussions to take place. Talking through a sliding glass window in the patient lobby area simply will not do. The physician also needs to establish clear policies with the office staff and then permit them to do the work assigned to them. If a physician wants to handle payment conversations, it should be done in a way that does not undercut the office staff.

Education

Patients have consistently shown a high degree of interest in learning more about medical issues. Because it is unlikely that the physician will have enough time to impart all the knowledge the patient would like to have, it makes sense to take a hard look at alternatives to patient education. The easiest way is to have pamphlets available in the office on common problems seen in the practice, but generally, patients are interested in more than this.

If any space is available, the physician might consider setting up a VCR and having selected patient education tapes available. This is also a good way to compensate for the times when the physician is running late.

The physician may have the opportunity to sponsor classes in the lobby of the office in the evening. Many hospitals have nurses or other professionals available to participate in classes with physicians on issues of interest to the community. Also, remember that patients have a great deal of interest in their own health. Physicians can provide patients with checklists that record items of interest, such as blood pressure, cholesterol level, height, and weight.

Environment

The office environment is also worth examining. It is not unusual to find physicians who have not walked through the front door of their offices in years. Having a clean and attractive lobby is the practice's equivalent of a first impression, and it is well noted by patients. The physician needs to assess whether the personality of the physical space is consistent with the office image the physician wants to portray.

Doctor to Doctor Relations

Professional etiquette and courtesy between physicians is understood as a given. However, taking a moment to review these suggestions may be one of the most important things a physician can do to establish a practice.

Referrals

The golden rule of referrals is an age-old one: Always return the patient to the referring physician after seeing or treating him or her. If you are referred a patient for consultation, follow up immediately with a thank-you letter and a report of your findings. Send along copies of test results for his or her records.

If the patient must be hospitalized, research the hospital's policy about which physician's name(s) can be listed on the medical record. Referring physicians should be listed whenever possible, as this allows them access to test results and progress reports. Many hospitals have computerized systems, and it can be very frustrating for a physician to attempt to call up his or her patient list and not be able to locate patients because their names have not been entered on the record. It also reinforces the feeling that they are part of the treatment team and are knowledgeable about the patient's condition.

Contacts

Get to know the emergency department medical staff. Make your availability known, and respond quickly when given your first referrals. Investigate their on-call system, and work your way into it, if possible.

Be a "lounge rat." The medical staff lounge at the hospital is a great place to pick up referrals and get to know your colleagues.

Keep your social ear to the ground. Socializing after hours and on weekends with other physicians and their spouses is an important part of the give and take in a medical community. Try always to remember how uneasy you felt when you were new in town and did not know anyone. Inviting newcomers—as well as established physicians—into your home or to meet others is always appreciated and remembered.

How to Use Your Hospital

Hospitals are generally set up to work with the medical staff as a whole, not with individual physicians. It is frequently frustrating for the physician to correlate hospital activities with individual needs. There can, however, be great benefit to the physician in understanding and then using a hospital's services. The hospital may have valuable programs to maximize the success of their physicians. A physician has no reason to hesitate taking advantage of available assistance. Some of the services to look for in a hospital are discussed in the following sections.

Hospital Marketing

Physician referral programs are fairly common in most hospitals now. However, the sophistication of these programs differs greatly. In general, the more information that the program has, the better it can serve the physician. Equally important is the reception that the referred caller receives from the physician's office staff. If the office staff demonstrates that the program is important to the practice and that they are working hard to schedule the referred patients, then the physician referral program representatives will work harder to assist the physician. It is also valuable for physicians to let the hospital administration know that the help they receive in acquiring new patients is important and appreciated. A hospital's administrative decision regarding the amount of funds allocated to staffing and advertising a physician referral program will more than likely be a direct reflection of how important it believes the program is to the physicians.

Hospital Programs

Hospitals advertise particular services according to their assessment of the marketplace and the financial return on the investment. Other more subtle factors are also considered, and high on the list is the medical staff's interest in certain services. If the hospital chooses to advertise a particular specialty and links the responses to the physician referral service, the physicians in that specialty stand to benefit from the advertising. A physician (or a clinical section) can request that the hospital assess a promotional campaign featuring his or her specialty area. Or, because there is clout in large numbers, it is wise to network with others in your specialty.

Hospitals often have a number of programs that are regularly promoted to the community, such as a senior citizens' program, a women's program, or an industrial medicine program. Learning about these programs—and knowing which elements of the programs have been most successful—will also help the physician make decisions about which element of his or her practice is most likely to attract new community members.

Hospital-Community Relations

Community groups frequently call hospitals to find speakers for their meetings. Physicians who volunteer their expertise as speakers will have the opportunity to meet many individuals in the community at one time. The hospital's public relations department will generally be the area most knowledgeable about the community and the topics in which groups are interested. Some hospitals will volunteer secretarial time and technical assistance to prepare presentation materials for physicians.

Managed Care

Most hospitals are active in the managed care (PPO, HMO) arena. This presents one of the most important opportunities for the physician to garner new patient volume. It is important to get to know as much as possible about the hospital's activities in managed care and how the physician can participate.

Medical Staff

Becoming part of the hospital community is helpful in a number of ways, and getting to know the medical staff office personnel is a good place to start. The committee structure of a hospital is a good way to get to know other members of the medical staff and begin developing referral practices. Not all committees are the same, and it makes good sense for a physician to spend time learning which committees are influential and which physicians are the "movers and shakers." The medical communities that surround hospitals generally have a number of ongoing social events, and it is important for physicians to attend some of these. All hospitals have call panels for certain areas, for instance, the emergency department. New physicians will need to become familiar with these call panels and with the formal and informal mechanisms by which they can be included in them.

Physicians' Services Department

Hospitals recognize the importance of physicians to the hospital's success. Many hospitals have set up departments that are specifically designed to assist physicians. The services of these departments will differ, but physicians' services departments exist to help physicians be successful and to develop a loyalty between the physician and the hospital. The types of services to look for in these departments include marketing services, practice management assistance, new physician start-up programs, assistance to recruit a partner, and services for physicians planning to retire. Because the success of these departments is, in part, measured by the number of physicians taking advantage of the services, a physician should not hesitate to use any or all of the services available.

Hospitals and physicians have theoretically been working together for many years, but in fact, they are just beginning to learn how to work together in today's environment. As with any situation, the key is to get to know people, begin to communicate, and be willing to try new ideas.

Managed Care Plans

"Managed care" has many variations but the phrase generally refers to any situation where the payor (insurance company or employer) has established contract rates and terms with the health-care providers. The contract rate typically represents a discount from the usual and customary charges in the geographic area. The terms generally include the payor's right to become involved in the utilization review or case management of its employees' health care.

Many variations exist in managed care plans and it is becoming increasingly difficult to distinguish one type of plan from another. In general, the preferred provider organizations (PPOs) are based on a reduced fee for service and are available to individual physicians. The health maintenance organizations (HMOs) have a more complicated payment scheme that is based on dividing the premium dollars among providers. The HMO approach requires an organized physician group to receive and disseminate the funds to physicians.

The number of people enrolled in managed care plans varies markedly across the nation, but it is clear that the numbers are significant and continuing to increase. In many areas, managed care plans have reached enrollment levels that exceed 30% of the surrounding population. Physicians interested in building their practices clearly need to participate in these plans.

Information

Although participating in managed care plans is important to developing a practice, physicians would be at a disadvantage if they simply responded to any contract that arrived in the mail. These contracts do not come without some risk—the payment terms and contract obligations can differ significantly by contract. It makes sense to plan your involvement in the often complex managed care contracting process by learning which contracts have done well in your community.

Your local hospital administrator or chief of the medical staff will be able to present you with an overview of contracting and can refer you to individuals who will have the detailed information. To help analyze the merits of available managed care plans, be sure to obtain the answers to these questions:

1. Which managed care plans have a large market share in your area? Which plans have contracts with the hospital? Can the hospital provide you with a list of its contracts and the name and number of a contact person for each plan?
2. Which managed care plans are available to individual physicians, and which plans operate through organized physician groups?
3. What organized physician groups exist, and who are the physicians who represent the elected leadership of those groups? What are the conditions for membership? What is the application process like?

Participation

When the physician has determined the impact of different managed care plans in the area it is relatively easy to compare the payment terms of the individual contracts. Most of the PPO contracts will be based on a relative value scale (RVS) schedule. The area standard for the RVS rates in your specialty will be easy to determine. The HMO plans are more complicated, and the physicians who represent the elected leadership of the physician groups will be the best source of information on how to compare the HMO payment scheme with fee-for-service charges.

There is a significant secondary value to joining the physicians involved in organized managed care contracting. The leadership of these groups tends to be very knowledgeable and aware of current health-care trends. These physicians have also had the experience of working in unison to achieve their individual goals and future opportunities, and they benefit from the professional camaraderie that tends to develop among the physician participants.

Please note, however, that the financial benefits of joining these plans may not be immediate. Businesses usually publish a provider directory for employees who participate in these plans. Depending on the printing schedule of the directory, a new physician's name may not be available to employees until months after the contract has been signed. To mitigate this circumstance, the physician can make certain that the office staff members are aware of all signed contracts so that they can inform patients who call that the physician is a participant in their plan. Also, many hospitals have a physician referral service that matches potential patients with physicians. Many callers to a referral service ask for the names of physicians who participate in their managed care plans. If your hospital has this service, make sure that they also have a current listing of your contracts.

How to Use Your Community

It would be advantageous to reside in the community in which you set up your practice. Getting to know—and be known by—your community is an excellent way to become established quickly. This can be accomplished by putting together a simple public relations plan that may involve one or many of the resources discussed below.

Community Groups

Join a service group such as the Lions, Rotary, or Soroptimist clubs. There is great value in the camaraderie generated by performing a community service, and this is a great opportunity to meet people outside the field of medicine. After joining, arrive at meetings early, and introduce yourself to those you do not know. Participate in the group's service projects as often as your time allows.

Join the chamber of commerce. Running a medical practice is a business, and this group of business owners can be a great source of referrals. Generally, they are eager to help new chamber members to become established in their business.

Professional Visibility

Offer your time to a speakers bureau. Most hospitals provide speakers as a free community service. Make yourself known to those who coordinate the scheduling of speakers. Also, service groups are always looking for interesting speakers to be guests at their meetings. Contact the group's program coordinator.

Provide information about a new medical service or one in which you have a special interest or expertise. Remember to present your information in terms the lay public can understand and will enjoy hearing. By carefully preparing a 15-minute presentation with some slides or a flip chart, you can influence perceptions and public opinions about your subject matter while building your own visibility and/or patient loyalty.

Community Participation

Volunteer your service to the local sports teams. Contact the local schools and offer your service as an on-site team doctor or during the preseason time when physicals are needed. Once established, loyalties built between these athletes, their parents, and the physician often last for decades.

Participate in health-care special events. Consider sponsorship and participation in such events as open houses, health fairs, or free screenings. This can be in conjunction with the hospital, local shopping malls, the American Red Cross, churches, and so on.

Communication Pieces

Communication pieces are a most valuable tool, and if used properly and consistently, can help promote your medical practice. With a targeted message, they can inform relevant audiences such as prospective patients, referring physicians, and third-party payors about the distinctive features of your service. They can also assist you in maintaining an existing patient base. Although "advertising" medicine has long been considered taboo in professional circles, the increased competitive environment requires one to maintain a special rapport and visibility with all of these audiences.

Options

Well-designed communication pieces contain your theme or message that is targeted to relevant audiences. Informational brochures introduce you, your credentials, and unique features to the community and other professions. Informal invitations can bring audiences into your practice to meet you and your staff. Patient brochures serve as instructions on how your office functions, containing information such as hours of operation, billing practices, services rendered, policies on phone calls, and emergency instructions. A doctor-to-patient newsletter maintains this valuable link and can serve as a vehicle for interesting health information. Appointment reminder or follow-up postcards are a quick and simple way to stay in touch with your patient. A "health record" is a take-home document of immunizations, medication administration, results of examination and tests, and diagnoses that your patient can keep on file. After a patient's visit, a patient satisfaction questionnaire will give him or her the opportunity to communicate opinions and provide valuable insight into the patient's perception of the office visit. Although all of these pieces perform a different function, not every physician will want to make the investment to produce all of them at one time. Patient brochures and appointment postcards are generally the most serviceable of the communication pieces.

Production

When communication pieces are designed and printed professionally, they send the message of a quality medical practice. With the assistance of a graphic artist, typesetter, or local print house, they can be produced at a reasonable cost. If the hospital has a physicians' services department, it should be able to recommend vendors for you to use. If not, try contacting the hospital's public relations office staff. They often work with vendors who are creative and reasonable in price.

Identity System

The general look of the pieces should be in keeping with the area of specialty you service. The message contained within should clearly state how you are prepared to meet the individual's needs. For example, if a pediatrician wants to attract working mothers, the graphic on the front should be "warm and fuzzy," and the message should emphasize extended hours, ease of access, and telephone "triage" to avoid unnecessary visits and lost work time. If a subspecialist wants to attract referring physicians, the graphic might be anatomical and communications should emphasize prompt consultation availability, timely feedback, involvement of the referring physician in decisions, and return of the patient to the referring physician. They should be typeset or word processed on a high-quality printer, and professionally laid out by an artist or printer. They should be printed on quality paper stock in a pleasant color.

Distribution

Distribution of the pieces can be via direct mail, handouts in your office, or a variety of community contacts such as the chamber of commerce, health fairs, or community events. For ease of mailing, they should be designed and folded to fit a standard envelope size and printed with your return address. If it is a postcard, it must conform to U.S. Postal Service size and weight regulations. A small investment of time and money at the outset will make a considerable difference in the visibility of your practice, patient acquisition, and patient loyalty.

Conclusion

Many of the elements of a marketing plan are simply common sense. As such, people often feel that it will not be necessary to actually write a plan; however, it *is* necessary. Given the multiple issues involved in starting a practice, it is easy to put aside some of the commonsense things that one intended to do. Writing the plan will help the physician to stay on track and remind the physician of where he or she stands in implementing the plan. The plan should serve as a reference point that the physician can update as often as needed.

Keeping track of which strategies were most successful in attracting new patients is equally important. Every physician should ask new patients how they came to the practice and should record the answers.

Creating a marketing plan is a great deal of work; however, if you have read this far in the chapter, you know that you can probably find people at your hospital to help write the plan and, most likely, to type the finished product.

Appendix 32.1

Marketing Plan

Objectives

Establish clear objectives for the practice that can be quantified. To achieve each objective, there needs to be a specific action or set of actions that the physician intends to implement.

Example: To increase new patient volume by 20%, one might:

Increase volume of patients from a desirable geographic area by 10%

Increase number of managed care contracts by 10

Increase return of patients for follow-up appointments by 30%

Establish new office practice with a patient base of 200 within the first six months

Situational Assessment

1. *Demographics:* Who are the people in the community?
2. *Target markets:* Who are the people in the community that the physician would most like to reach?
3. *Competition:* Who are the other health-care providers in the area? What are the strengths and weaknesses of the other providers?
4. *Unique features:* What is special about the practice that would be perceived as important by the members of the community?
5. *Practice trends:* What is happening in the practice? Is the practice strong in terms of reimbursement mix and balance of patients?
6. *Physical environment:* Do any changes in the office space need to be made?

Actions

What are the specific actions that the physician is planning to take in these areas to achieve the objectives?

"Marcus Welby"

1. *Image:* Who are the people with whom the physician interacts, and how do they perceive the physician?
2. *Bedside manner:* How does the physician respond to patients and families?
3. *Patient perceptions:* How effective is the physician's communication style with patients?

4. *Appearance:* What message is the physician's personal image and style communicating to the people with whom he works?

Actions

What are the specific actions that the physician is planning to take to improve his or her personal image?

Patient Relations

1. *Telephone:* How are telephone calls to the practice being handled?
2. *Scheduling:* Are the waiting times for patients acceptable?
3. *Billing:* Is the office responsive to patients' financial issues?
4. *Education:* Does the practice have sufficient educational materials available?
5. *Environment:* How does the physical environment appear to patients?

Actions

What changes is the physician planning to make to improve the patients' experience in the office?

Doctor to Doctor Relations

1. *Referrals:* Is the physician responsive to his or her referral sources?
2. *Contacts:* Is the physician developing professional contacts in the community?

Actions

What actions can the physician make to improve his or her relations with other professionals?

How to Use Your Hospital

1. *Hospital marketing:* Is the hospital's marketing program supporting the physician's activities?
2. *Hospital programs:* Does the hospital sponsor particular programs that can benefit physicians?
3. *Managed care:* What are the opportunities in managed care to develop the practice?
4. *Medical staff:* Does the physician know how the medical staff operates within the hospital?
5. *Physician services:* Does the hospital have a department specifically designed to assist physicians?

6. *Hospital-community relations:* Does the hospital sponsor community programs in which a physician can become involved?

Actions

In what programs or services is the physician planning to become involved?

Managed Care

1. *Information:* Does the physician have a clear understanding of the volume and trends in managed care in the area?
2. *Participation:* Is the physician participating in the right managed care plans? Are there organized groups of physicians in the community to deal with managed care contracts?

Actions

In which managed care plans or physician groups is the physician going to participate?

How To Use Your Community

1. *Community groups:* Are there important social groups that the physician should join?
2. *Professional visibility:* Are there opportunities for the community to hear the physician's message?
3. *Community participation:* Is there an opportunity to participate in community events?

Actions

In what group(s) is the physician going to participate?

Communication Pieces

1. *Options:* What are the communication pieces that the physician might want to have?
2. *Production:* How does the physician arrange to have these pieces created?
3. *Identity system:* What is the image and continuity of image that should exist?
4. *Distribution:* How will people receive the communication pieces?

Actions

What communication system is the physician going to create?

33 | Patient Satisfaction: Its Importance and How to Measure It

HAYA R. RUBIN, MD, PHD,
AND ALBERT W. WU, MD, MPH

Physicians put little store in patient satisfaction, perhaps because they are skeptical that it reflects the quality of care. Each recalls a patient whose satisfaction apparently hinged on a medically unnecessary procedure or has heard of patients who complained or even sued because of a bad outcome, despite exemplary care. In contrast, patients describe "wonderful" doctors whom colleagues think are incompetent hand holders, ignorant, and attached to dubious medical practices. Physicians and other providers then reason that little can be concluded from patient satisfaction and that there is no reason to measure it. For example, John R. Ball, M.D., Executive Vice President of the American College of Physicians, was recently quoted as saying, "The kindly physician may not be treating the patient optimally, but the patient may feel satisfied and rate him highly."

There are two important reasons to measure patient judgments of health care. First, they do give information about the quality of care, though not necessarily all its technical aspects. Secondly, patients use their judgments to make important decisions about their care which affect both themselves and their providers.

Defining Patient Satisfaction

This chapter uses the term *patient satisfaction* to denote patients' subjective evaluations of their health care. Historically, patients' opinions have been obtained by asking them how "satisfied" they are. Therefore, patient evaluations of care are often referred to as patient or consumer satisfaction with health care. This usage may be misleading, as *satisfaction* does not fully describe how patients evaluate their care. More accurate terms for this concept might be patient *judgments, evaluations,* or *ratings* of health care, but in deference to tradition, *patient satisfaction* is used here interchangeably with these terms.

Some patient satisfaction questionnaires and surveys contain other types of questions that could not be described as patient ratings of care. Some ask patients to report about events that occur, rather than asking for their opinions—for example: "On average, how long do you usually have to wait to get an appointment for an acute problem? Same day; 1–2 days; 2–4 days; 4–7 days; more than a week." Although such questions can help to explain patient judgments, the term *patient satisfaction* in this chapter does not include patient reports of care. Some patient outcome or follow-up questionnaires also include questions about health, rather than about the health care patients have received. *Patient satisfaction*, as used in this chapter, also does not include questions about health or functioning.

Patient Satisfaction: One Indicator of the Quality of Care

Few studies have compared patient satisfaction with other measures of the quality of care in a patient population. Although providers' anecdotal impressions suggest that patient satisfaction and other measures may not always agree, more systematic examination would be required to draw a conclusion about their general relationship.

The few studies comparing patient and expert judgments of care suggest that they are moderately related but that patients tend to be less critical than are experts. Linn noted that the number of deviations from an explicit algorithm for burn care correlated moderately well with patients' overall satisfaction with the emergency room visit. Ehrlich, Morehead, and Trusell also found a moderate relationship between physician auditors' and patients' ratings of hospital care. However, Ehrlich et al. also found that patients gave excellent ratings to 74% of cases rated fair or poor by physician auditors. The disagreement between patient and physician raters in Ehrlich's study, as in others, was partly because physicians were asked to review records for technical aspects of diagnosis and treatment whereas patients were asked to give overall ratings, which may consider many other aspects of care. Further study would be necessary to clarify the relationship of technical quality to patient satisfaction.

In contrast, an overwhelming body of literature suggests that patient satisfaction accurately represents the quality of interpersonal treatment. In the United States, much of the public expects high-quality medical care to include features in addition to technical competence—for instance, humaneness and compassion, informed consent, and respect for patients' values. We do not know if these properties influence health outcomes or survival, but they are essential components of high-quality care. Recent reviews have surveyed the features of care related to higher patient satisfaction with outpatient and inpatient care (Table 33.1).

There would be no point in measuring patient judgments if nothing could be done about them. A practical corollary of the fact that patient judgments reflect certain features of care is that they can be changed by altering provider behavior, the physical environment, or the organizational structure.

Table 33.1 Features of Care Related to Increased Patient Satisfaction

Outpatient Care by Physicians[1]
Overall features
Overall performance of resident M.D.s, rated by nurses
Overall performance of resident M.D.s, rated by supervising faculty
Technical competence
Physician asking for opinion or help
Technical ER care for burns, rated by clinical algorithm
Performance of an EKG in ER for chest pain
Interpersonal features
Better interpersonal skills, coded by trained observers
Better interpersonal manner, rated by trained simulated patients
More patient centeredness, coded from audiotape
More encouragement, coded from videotape
More physician tension, coded from audiotape
Less physician control, coded by trained observers
More physician courtesy, rated by trained observers
Better listening, rated by trained observers
Greater empathy, rated by trained observers
Information
Amount of information given, scored on videotape
Information giving, rated by trained observers
Time or attention to specific content
Amount of attention to psychosocial issues, coded from videotape
Time spent discussing prevention, scored on videotape
Miscellaneous
References to prior visits, coded from videotape
Continuity of care

Inpatient care[2]
Amount of patient education, controlled trial
Extra perioperative nursing visit (eliciting concerns, giving information and reassurance), controlled trial
Technical quality of medical care, judged from record by M.D. auditors
Quality of nursing care, rated by nurse auditors

[1] Based on information from Kaplan and Ware (1989) and Ware, Davies, and Rubin (1988).
[2] Based on information from Rubin (1990).

Patient Satisfaction: A Predictor of Patient Behavior

Patient ratings of medical care predict their subsequent behavior, including how they comply with medications prescribed, how well they follow providers' advice, whether they return or go elsewhere, whether they re-enroll in a health plan, whether they recommend us to others, whether they complain about their care, and perhaps whether they sue. As Kaplan and Ware pointed out, the RAND Health Insurance Experiment provided one dramatic example of the impact of patient satisfaction: patients were 10 times more likely to disenroll from plans with the lowest satisfaction ratings than from those with higher ratings. For these reasons also, apart from quality concerns, providers need to monitor how patients feel about their care. If providers fail to pay attention, others may not; professional societies, hospitals, third-party payors and provider organizations are beginning to incorporate these measures into accreditation and payment schemes.

How to Measure Patient Satisfaction

Before asking patients to judge their care, a provider, practice, health plan, or hospital must make several decisions. What is the goal of your survey? Who should you survey—potential or actual patients, enrollees or those who have been provided care, active or inactive (or ex-) patients, an entire practice or a random sample, patients or family members? When should you survey them—in the hospital or after discharge? At the time of a visit or at regular intervals? How should you collect information—by mailed questionnaire, telephone interview, or in person? Who should do the survey—the provider or hospital in question or an independent firm? What kinds of questions should be asked? What makes a good survey instrument? Can standard surveys be used or adapted?

The Survey Goal

To be meaningful, a patient satisfaction survey should have clearly defined goals.

First, what is the end result you care about most? For example, are you interested in patient satisfaction as one dimension of quality of care? In increasing patient compliance? In increasing the rate of return appointments? In improving your profit margin? In having patients recommend your hospital more? In improving its community reputation and market share?

Second, what features of your practice are you interested in examining? Do you want to compare different providers or hospital units to see which might need intervention? Do you want to find out which components of the process need the most improvement so you can allocate resources most productively? Do you want to compare patients with two different payment systems or insurance plans? Do you want to test the effect of a new service you plan to provide—such as evening hours or a new patient education program—or of something you plan to eliminate, such as part of your staff?

Who Should be Surveyed?

The choice of whom to survey depends on the desired goal. If the survey is being carried out to monitor the quality of care, a sample of patients who have received care within a defined period would be the appropriate choice. Alternatively, if one is most interested in finding out about access to a practice, hospital, or group plan, its general reputation, or potential markets, it would be appropriate to survey the community from which patients are generally drawn, if this can be identified. If attrition from the practice is an area of concern, a sample of ex-patients or inactive patients may be appropriate.

If one wishes to compare two groups of patients—for instance, those using different providers in a practice, or on different hospital wards, or at two points in time—the sample of patients should be chosen to ensure that enough patients are in each group to draw conclusions. As a rule of thumb, one should include at least 50 patients per subgroup being compared (eg, 50 for each provider or for each unit in a hospital). However, how many patients are necessary depends on the sensitivity of the survey scales and questions. Detailed sample size calculations are beyond the scope of this discussion and are best performed in consultation with a statistician.

There is a temptation to survey all patients in a practice, or all patients who have been hospitalized, so as not to miss anyone's input. Although this approach has intuitive appeal, in practice random sampling from groups one wishes to compare turns out to be more accurate and more efficient. Unless a practice is very small, a blanket survey will spend available resources on the initial contact, and little will be left for follow-up, resulting in a low response rate and inaccurate results. Vigorous follow-up of nonresponding patients is important to avoid such bias (see the section on Characteristics of a Good Survey, later in this chapter). It is better to concentrate available resources on achieving careful follow-up of a random sample than to survey the entire patient population.

A few patient characteristics may affect patients' judgments of providers. For example, older patients give slightly higher ratings and depressed patients give lower ratings. If two different practices, providers, hospitals, or organizational procedures are being compared, enough patients should be selected to compare responses within each of these patient categories (eg, patients under 40, 40–65, and over 65; patients with a diagnosis of depression and those without).

When to Survey

For information about ratings of general medical care, surveys can be conducted at any point in time. However, surveys designed to elicit information about a particular outpatient visit should be conducted just after the visit is completed for maximum recall.

To find out patients' judgments of hospital care, it might seem most convenient to survey patients in the hospital. However, such a survey will miss patients too sick to respond, creating an important selection bias. In addition, surveys performed prior to discharge cannot elicit information about the adequacy of discharge arrangements. On the other hand, although overall impressions of each aspect of care may remain stable for as long as a year, patients may have forgotten some of the details of their hospitalization by then. Therefore, detailed surveys will be most accurate if conducted within six weeks of discharge.

Depending on the survey's goal, it may be a one-time undertaking, a two-stage process (eg, before and after a change in practice), or part of an ongoing monitoring effort to improve the quality of care.

The amount of time that it takes to conduct one round of a survey depends on the number of respondents desired, the number served per unit of time, and the response rate. The number of respondents desired should be determined in consultation with a statistician, and it will depend on the amount of variation in responses to the questions and on how small a difference one wishes to detect.

Data Collection Methods

Successful surveys can be conducted using either self-administered questionnaires or telephone interviews. In-person interviews are labor intensive and costly. It may be appropriate to make this decision based on which is the lower-cost option. Two studies of response rates to mail and telephone patient surveys showed that higher response rates were obtained at lower cost in a mail survey with vigorous follow-up, compared with an identical telephone interview.

For small practices or provider organizations without in-house survey capabilities, survey research firms are available to collect data. As response rates to mailed surveys vary widely by community and survey firm technique, one should ask survey firms for references and previous clients, hire those with the best response rates, and choose the method that provides the highest response for the lowest cost.

Who is Doing the Survey?

The questionnaire or interview can be represented to patients as coming either from the provider or from a person or firm hired to perform it. For example, a questionnaire may say, "We are conducting a survey of our patients to find out your opinions about the care we deliver. Your opinions are very important to us," with a physician's signature. Alternatively, the questionnaire may say, "F & K is an independent research firm. We have been asked by your physician, Dr. B., to conduct a survey of patient satisfaction. Your opinions are anonymous and will only be shared with your doctor as part of a statistical report, without your name attached."

Studies suggest that higher ratings are likely to result using the more personal approach. This may skew survey results, so that most are very positive, and may hide differences among patients with different experiences of care and with different intentions toward the provider. Using a less personal approach may make different patients' judgments more evident.

However, response rates may be lower with a less personal approach, so more vigorous follow-up efforts should be planned.

An important implication of these "context" effects is that there should be a standard approach; one should not compare data from patients approached in different ways.

Characteristics of a Good Survey Instrument

Includes the important aspects of care. Patients distinguish among different dimensions of care and rate them separately, even if all contribute to their overall judgments of care. If a survey consists of only one overall question, important differences may be overlooked. For example, a patient may feel that a doctor does not appear especially knowledgeable or technically competent but that he or she does seem very caring and compassionate. Both dimensions will contribute to the overall rating, but the difference will show up only if separate ratings of competence and compassion were also obtained.

Tables 33.2 and 33.3 list dimensions of care that may contribute to patients' overall judgments of care or satisfaction, for general medical care, specific visits, and hospital stays.

Uses several questions for each aspect. Questionnaires that represent each aspect of care with multiple questions are more sensitive to differences and more reproducible than are those that use single items.

Long enough to be interesting, short enough to finish. Reading the last two sections, one might wonder if the resulting questionnaire might be so long that patients would not return it. One of the basic principles of survey research is to keep the questionnaire brief. However, patients are prone to discard very short questionnaires (e.g., five-item return postcards with no room for comments) because they seem trivial.

Table 33.2 Dimensions of Outpatient Care That May Influence Patient Judgments

Interpersonal treatment/humaneness
Technical skill
Information and education
Facilities
Access
Convenience
Appointment availability
Office waits
Cost
Continuity
Availability of hospital care

Based on information from Ware, Davies, and Rubin (1988).

Table 33.3 Components of Hospital Care That May Influence
Patient Judgments

Nursing Care
  Giving medications
  Responsiveness to call bell
  Information and responses to questions
  Bedpans and personal hygiene assistance
  Emotional support
  Communication with doctors and other nurses
  Treatment of visitors
Medical care
  Physicians
    Monitoring of patients and diagnostic testing
    Availability and response to symptoms
    Treatment and surgical procedures
    Giving information
    Involvement of family
  Other professional staff (pharmacists, social workers, physical, occupational, and
    respiratory therapists, dieticians)
  Technicians (IV, blood, x-ray)
  Other staff (transport, patient liaison/ombudsman, chaplain, volunteers)
Living arrangements and accommodations
  Noise
  Cleanliness and maintenance
  Room arrangements
  Scheduling of routine functions
  Visiting policies
  Activities and distractions
  Personal services (telephone, etc.)
  Food
Pre-admitting and admitting
(admitting office or emergency room)
  Reception (paperwork and payment arrangements)
  Testing
  Response to symptoms or pain
  Provision of information
  Communication with floor staff
Discharge
  Instructions about discharge procedure
  Instructions about self-care and expected course
  Provision of discharge medications
  Patient escort service
  Parking facilities for discharge
Billing

Based on information from Meterko and Rubin (1990).

However, beyond a certain length, the opposite effect occurs. Therefore, a survey should take no more than 15 minutes to fill out or half an hour to answer on the telephone, in order to achieve high response rates in an initial contact. In a self-administered survey, the average patient can fill out five closed-ended items per minute, and even more if all items have the same response scale.

A good strategy might be to devote several questions to each of a few areas important to the outcome of interest, rather than to attempt to devote questions to a comprehensive list of different aspects of care.

For example, patients' impressions of how caring the nurses were and how comfortable the hospital environment was are highly related to whether patients would return to that hospital if they needed to be hospitalized again. If a survey's goal is to find out how to influence more patients to return, it may be more valuable to devote additional space to evaluating these aspects than to ask many questions about doctors, preadmission procedures, food, billing, and parking. In contrast, patients' impressions of whether a hospital stay improved their health are highly related to ratings of both medical and nursing care. A survey aimed at improving this outcome should include more questions about physicians.

Uses appropriate response scales. The method used to elicit a patient's opinions of care can affect results dramatically. For example, when response scales employ the word *satisfied*, most respondents choose the best possible response category, even when open-ended questions elicit remarkably negative experiences. Reasons for this may include feeling obligated to express gratitude, feeling inadequate to judge health-care experts, and fear of being viewed negatively if dissatisfied.

Rating scales (eg, Excellent, Very Good, Good, Fair, Poor) result in a more normal distribution of responses than does a satisfaction scale, and they also better predict patient intentions to comply or to return to the same provider.

Great care should be taken with questionnaires that utilize Agree–Disagree response scales. Because some patients—particularly less-educated ones—tend to agree with any statement, items should be included stating both positive and negative thoughts about the same content (eg, "the doctor treated me courteously" and "the doctor was rude"). It is even better to put the judgment into the response scale (eg, "How would you rate the doctor's courtesy? Excellent, very good, good, fair, or poor."). It is best to use the same response scale for all items, as this allows different aspects of care to be compared with each other.

Pretested. Questionnaires should be pretested to make sure the questions elicit reproducible responses and to guard against bias resulting from the questionnaire itself. Good questions elicit similar responses when administered differently—for instance, at different times, or by mail or telephone. This makes it easier to include patients who can only be reached in different ways and to compare providers or sites with different survey techniques. Questions should be suitable to the diversity of patients being surveyed in terms of education, race, gender, and cultural background.

Predicts the outcome of interest. Survey scales are most meaningful when studies have been conducted to validate them against whatever outcome the survey is being conducted to predict. For example, if the survey is attempting to predict how many patients are dissatisfied enough that they would not return and which aspects of care are responsible, it is helpful to have studies that demonstrate how scores on particular scales are associated with the intent to return to the practice.

Available Instruments

Many commercial firms use patient satisfaction instruments they have developed and will offer to analyze the data and prepare a report for the provider. These services seem attractive because they save the provider from searching for the correct survey questionnaire and analyzing and interpreting the results.

Although a survey firm may collect the data, it may not be desirable to use the firm's own questionnaire, which might omit areas of care important to patients. For example, some hospital questionnaires do not ask patients about their medical care by the hospital.

A recent review by Kaplan and Ware lists published questionnaires for measuring satisfaction with general medical care or specific physician visits. Most widely used in research surveying satisfaction with general medical care have been the scale devised by Hulka et al., which was revised by Zyzanski et al., and versions of the Patient Satisfaction Questionnaire (PSQ) by Ware et al. Sample questions from each dimension of PSQ are provided in Table 33.4. Published and studied questionnaires used to examine patient satisfaction with specific outpatient visits include the Visit-Specific Questionnaire by Ware and Hays and the Medical Interview Satisfaction Scale by Wolf et al.

The published literature does not contain carefully developed, well-studied questionnaires for acute care screening or emergency visits, except one specifically for burn care, by Freudenheim.

For hospital care, Rubin has written a detailed review listing questionnaires about which information was published through 1987. One of these questionnaires, Patient Judgments of Hospital Quality, elicits reproducible and distinct patient judgments about a comprehensive range of dimensions important to patients, and has published mean ratings for 10 hospitals. Although many hospital systems contract with survey firms or perform in-house surveys for large numbers of hospitals, no others have published descriptive statistics from more than one hospital with information about reproducibility and accuracy.

Table 33.4 Sample Items from Each Dimension of the Patient Satisfaction Questionnaire[1]

Technical Competence
  Doctors are very careful to check everything when examining their patients.
Interpersonal Manner
  Doctors act like they are doing their patients a favor by treating them.
Access to Care
  People have to wait too long for emergency care.
Costs of Care
  The amount charged for medical care services is reasonable.

[1] Extracted from Ware, Snyder, and Wright (1976) with permission. Response scale for all items: Strongly Agree, Agree, Not Sure, Disagree, Strongly Disagree.

Analyzing and Interpreting the Results

If a practice or hospital has sufficiently skilled personnel, it may be best to perform in-house data analysis and to design one's own reports. Survey research firms may not present meaningfully the data they collect. For example, reports may not indicate statistical significance or confidence limits when comparing providers, time points, different aspects of care, or how much different aspects of care affect patients' overall judgments. If one contracts with a research firm for analytic services, the contract should specify the content of reports and statistical analyses desired.

Some companies specializing in patient satisfaction surveys claim to have accumulated large data bases of providers, patients, or hospitals, and offer to provide comparison data with others in their data base. At first, this may seem like a good reason to use their services and their questionnaires. However, a single survey firm is unlikely to have enough clients to form a good comparison group for practices with different specialties, services, sizes, and locations. Standards for patient satisfaction with each type of practice, or each type of episode of hospital care, have not yet been developed. At present, survey results will be most meaningful for questions that can be answered using data collected within the client's own practice, hospital or system, and does not depend on comparisons with other groups or populations.

Summary

Patient ratings of care reflect what they think is important about the quality of care, including the doctor-patient relationship and what they can judge of the adequacy of diagnosis and therapy. For patient rating surveys to be most useful, one should have specific goals in mind. For example, one may wish to compare providers or sites, to identify particular aspects of care that need improvement, to evaluate new programs, or to assess changes over time. These goals determine what questions should be included, who should be surveyed, and when they should be surveyed. Surveys are more likely to provide valid results when conducted using previously tested questionnaires and methods or when conducted by researchers with extensive experience in designing and analyzing patient satisfaction surveys.

Patient judgments are an important indicator of quality of care and should figure into how we evaluate ourselves and our colleagues. These evaluations can then be used to target areas where improvements will yield the greatest benefit.

Suggested Reading

Borgiel, A. E. M., Williams, J. I., Andersen, G. M., et al., "Assessing the quality of care in family physicians' practices." *Canadian Family Physician* 31(4, 1989):853.

Carey, R. G., and Posavec, E. J., "Using Patient Information to Identify Areas for Service Improvement." *Health Care Management Review* 7 (Spring 1982):43.

Ehrlich, J., Morehead, M. A., and Trusell, R. E., *The Quantity, Quality, and Costs of Medical and Hospital Care Secured by a Sample of Teamster Families in the New York Area.* New York: Columbia University School of Public Health and Administrative Medicine, 1961.

Freudenheim, M., "Patients' Grades Help to Set Pay for Health-Plan Doctors." *New York Times* (May 26, 1990).

Greenley, J. R., Schultz, R., Nam, S. H., and Peterson, R. W., "Patient Satisfaction with Psychiatric Inpatient Care: Issues in Measurement and Application." *Research in Community Mental Health* 4(1985):303.

Hulka, B. S., Zyzanski, S. H., Casssel, J. C., and Thompson, S. J., "Scale for the Measurement of Attitudes toward Physicians and Primary Medical Care." *Medical Care* 8(1970):429.

Kaplan, S. H., and Ware, J. E., "The Patient's Role in Health Care and Quality Assessment." In Goldfield, N., and Nash, D. (Eds.), *Providing Quality Care: The Challenge to Clinicians.* Philadelphia, PA: American College of Physicians, 1989.

Linn, B. S., "Burn Patients' Evaluation of Emergency Department Care." *Annals of Emergency Medicine* 11(1982):255.

Mauksch, H. O. "Patients View Their Roles." *Hospital Progress* (October 1962):136.

Meterko, M., Nelson, E. C., and Rubin, H. R. (Eds.), "Patient Judgments of Hospital Quality: Report of a Pilot Study" (Supplement). *Medical Care* 28(9, 1990).

Meterko, M., and Rubin, H. R., "Patient Judgments of Hospital Quality: A Taxonomy." *Medical Care* 28(9, 1990):510–514.

Rezler, A. G., and Flaherty, J. A., *The Interpersonal Dimension in Medical Education.* New York: Springer Publishing Co., 1985.

Rubin, H. R., "Can Patients Rate the Quality of Hospital Care?" *Medical Care Review* 47(3, 1990):267–326.

Rubin, H. R., Ware, J. E., Nelson, E. C., and Meterko, M., "The Patient Judgments of Hospital Quality (PJHQ) Questionnaire." *Medical Care* 28(9, 1990):517–518, 545–556.

Skipper, J. K., and Ellison, M. D., "Personal Contact as a Technique for Increasing Questionnaire Returns for Hospitalized Patients after Discharge." *Journal of Health and Human Behavior* 7 (1966):211.

Vaccarino, J. M., "Malpractice: The Problem in Perspective." *JAMA* 238(1977):861.

Walker, A. H., and Restuccia, J. D., "Obtaining Information on Patient Satisfaction with Health Care: Mail vs. Telephone." *Health Services Research* 19(1984):291.

Ware, J. E., "Effects of Acquiescent Response Set on Patient Satisfaction Ratings." *Medical Care* 16(1978):327.

Ware, J. E., and Hays, R. D., "Methods for Measuring Patient Satisfaction with Specific Medical Encounters." *Medical Care* 26(1988):393.

Ware, J. E., Davies, A. R., and Rubin, H. R., "Patient Assessments of Their Care." In U.S. Congress, Office of Technology Assessment (Eds.), *The Quality of Medical Care: Information for Consumers* (OTA-H-386). Washington, DC: U.S. Government Printing Office.

Ware, J. E., Snyder, M. K., Wright, W. R., and Davies, A. R., "Defining and Measuring Patient Satisfaction with Medical Care." *Evaluation and Program Planning* 6(3–4, 1981):291.

Ware, J. E., Snyder, M. K., and Wright, W. R., *Development and Validation of Scales to Measure Patient Satisfaction with Health Care Services: Volume I, Part B. Results Regarding Scales Constructed from the Patient Satisfaction Questionnaire and Measures of Other Health Perceptions.* Springfield, VA: National Technical Information Service, 1976.

Wolf, M. H., Putnam, S. M., James, S. A., and Stiles, W. B., "The Medical Interview Satisfaction Scale: Development of a Scale to Measure Patient Perceptions of Physician Behavior." *Journal of Behavioral Medicine* 1(1978):391.

Zyzanski, S. J., Hulka, B. S., and Cassel, J. C., "Scale for the Measurement of Satisfaction with Medical Care: Modifications in Content, Format, and Scoring." *Medical Care* 12(1974):611.

34 | PPOs: Definition and Background

MICHAEL JOHN TICHON, ESQ., JD

Increasing frustration with rising health-care costs has led to the development and growing dominance of managed health-care plans. Managed health care can mean many things and describe various organizations including health maintenance organizations (HMOs), preferred provider organizations (PPOs), and claim and utilization review programs. The purpose of this chapter is to describe and discuss generic forms of PPOs. A PPO, if properly organized, can avoid much of the adverse consumer and physician reaction that has hindered HMO development while preserving many of the advantages of both HMO and fee-for-service medical care.

Definition of a PPO

The PPO is primarily an organization of fee-for-service providers who have a contractual arrangement to provide health-care services, typically at a discount, to a defined pool of patients who have free choice of provider, but have an economic incentive to utilize PPO member providers. One of its primary characteristics is selectivity: providers are selected by the PPO sponsor. The sponsor may be a provider organization. In this case, selection may be based on membership or affiliation with the provider organization, be it a hospital or medical association. Often, the sponsor is a payor, such as Blue Cross or a commercial health insurance company. In this case, selectivity may be based on the perceived efficiency of providers or their willingness to accept the rates offered by the payor.

Providers joining or forming the PPO do not take insurance-type financial risks. In other words, the PPO does not sell to individuals and collect premiums. The PPO may take other forms of risk once there is a contract with a payor, but the payor collects the premiums and is responsible for providing all covered health benefits. For example, in one form of risk a provider-sponsored PPO and payor may agree to establish a fund to reward practitioners who meet or exceed the PPO's utilization standards. Typically, the fund is created by withholding an agreed percentage of earned fees.

Essential features of a PPO also include utilization review and, ideally, rapid payment of provider claims. The primary care physician's role of gatekeeper is often emphasized. Most PPO primary care physicians are general practitioners who will then refer patients, as needed, to the specialists in the system. The primary care physician is then viewed as the gatekeeper who will select the most efficient specialists.

PPO enrollees typically have freedom of choice of provider but also have a financial incentive to use the preferred providers rather than a noncontracting provider. Typically, the incentive is reduced copayments if the enrollee uses the preferred providers and substantially higher copayments if the enrollee uses nonpreferred providers. A generic PPO is illustrated on Figure 34.1.

To summarize, characteristics of a PPO typically include the following:

providers selected by payor or self-appointed on the basis of both quality and efficiency

formation of a panel of providers: hospitals and/or physicians

negotiated or discounted fee schedules

providers do not take insurance-type financial risks

utilization review

Figure 34.1. The generic PPO structure.

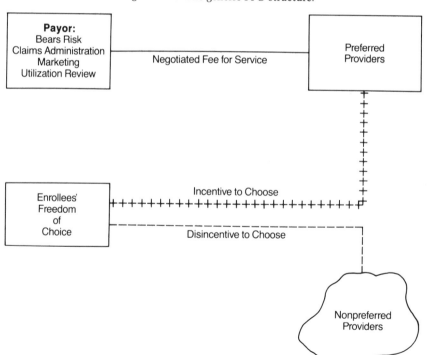

rapid payment of provider claims

emphasis on primary care physician as the gatekeeper

enrollee flexibility in choice of provider with financial incentive to use the preferred option

The attraction of the PPO for payors is the payor's ability to extract financial savings in exchange for sending a higher volume of patients to the selected providers. The payor can be a self-funded employer, a multiemployer trust or union trust fund, an insurance company, or a Blue Cross plan. The PPO does *not* collect premiums or market to individuals, but does market to and negotiate with the payors. Payors bear the financial risk in the insurance sense and perform the claims administration, marketing, and utilization review. The preferred provider organization may perform all, or a portion, of the utilization review function and may do some marketing to the payor.

Utilization review by the preferred provider organization may include computerized profile analyses based on diagnostic related group (DRG) or type of illness to determine which physicians use more services than other physicians and who are the "outliers," as they are known in DRG parlance. Then the PPO must decide what to do about outlier providers. Does it put them on probation? Does it terminate their existence in the PPO?

What does a PPO offer the enrollee? Freedom of choice, but with a monetary disincentive. If a consumer wants to maintain a family physician, he or she may have to pay all or a large part of the bill if the family physician is not part of the PPO. If the patient wants to go to a local hospital rather than the PPO preferred hospital selected by the employer, he or she may have to pay 60% of the bill, rather than, for example, a $100 deductible and a nominal copayment. To be competitive, however, premiums and benefits must be comparable to those of a traditional Blue Cross or other benefit package or those of the competing HMO.

Organizational Models

A Comparative View

In the traditional insurance system, individual providers, be they physicians, hospitals, or other facilities, are not integrated into any specific delivery system. There is no contract between providers and payors, but usually fee-for-service payments. Payors perform the functions of risk taking, claims administration, marketing, and, perhaps, utilization review. No contract exists with providers, but there is an insurance contract with the enrollee. There is no selectivity of providers, and minimal regulation is enforced by the state insurance commissioner. Please refer to Figure 34.2.

A traditional Blue Cross plan is slightly different from the foregoing insurance arrangement and from a PPO. Although there are member providers, there is usually little or no provider organization. There is little

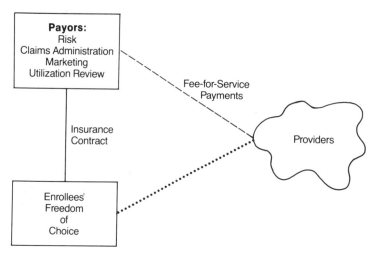

Figure 34.2. How the PPO differs from traditional insurance: no contract with providers, no selectivity of providers, minimal regulation.

selectivity, but there is a contract calling for the hospitals to perform utilization review, follow certificate of need provisions, and so on. The Blue Cross payment formulas have ranged from cost to a cost-plus to a fee-for-service payment. Blue Cross plans do have a subscriber agreement, and the subscribers have freedom of choice so long as a subscriber goes to a member provider. Please refer to Figure 34.3.

On the other end of the spectrum from the traditional, unmanaged, unorganized insurance arrangement is the HMO. Unlike a PPO, an HMO bears financial risk. The HMO also does its own claims administration, marketing, and centralized administration. It has a direct financial relationship with its subscribers. It collects premiums. Subscribers may have a vote on the board or be part of the actual HMO plan itself, unlike PPO enrollees. HMO physician providers are highly organized. They can be employees, belong to an independent practice association (IPA), or be part of a group practice. Utilization review is emphasized. Hospital rates are usually negotiated. The HMO subscribers, unlike PPO subscribers, have little freedom of choice: they *must* use HMO providers. The HMO providers bear financial risk in the form of responsibility for care in return for capitation payments. Usually the HMO is highly regulated, whereas PPOs are virtually unregulated. Please refer to Figure 34.4.

One irony in health care today is that an individual subscriber or enrollee may find a PPO, a Blue Cross plan, an HMO, and self-insured employer plan all offering the same benefits. To a subscriber they are alike, but each program would be organized and regulated differently. The HMO would be subject to relatively stringent regulation, whereas the PPO would be subject to none. The self-insured employer and the insurance company

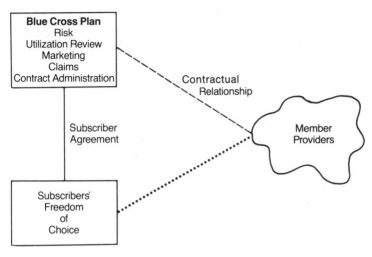

Figure 34.3. How PPOs differ from the Blue Cross plan: contract with providers, no selectivity of providers, varying degrees of regulation.

Figure 34.4. How PPOs differ from HMOs: subscriber/member has little or no choice of provider, providers are organized, providers bear financial risk, usually highly regulated.

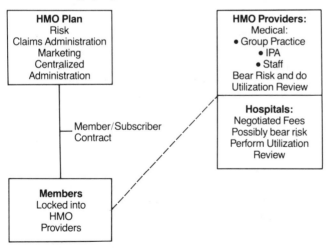

- Subscriber/Member has little or no choice of provider
- providers are organized
- providers bear financial risk
- usually highly regulated

would experience some regulation. The Blue Cross plan, depending on the jurisdiction, would be subject to either extensive or minimal regulation. Yet all these arrangements are doing the same thing! It is one of the anomalies that currently exist in the system.

Sponsorship

PPOs may be sponsored by employers, other payors, entrepreneurs, or providers. Most PPOs today are either provider sponsored or payor sponsored. However, there is a small but increasing number of employer-sponsored PPOs.

The entrepreneurial PPO typically consists of a claims administrator or an insurance broker seeking specific providers and marketing those providers to his health insurance accounts. A profit results from the fee for accessing the preferred network and the administration fee for processing claims. Although it is a very simple concept and allows PPOs to form quickly, it is one variant that contains some substantial risks for the providers. The entrepreneurial PPO, unless backed by an insurance company or other regulated payor, contains little or no protection for the providers or beneficiaries against payor insolvency or financial misconduct on the part of those administering the plan. These entrepreneurial plans typically take the form of multiple employer trusts (METs), which, until the passage of P.L. 97-473, were generally immune from state regulation. In California the experience with METs is checkered. Many did not maintain adequate reserves and became insolvent, leaving subscribers and contracting providers to obtain whatever relief they could from the bankruptcy courts. Since 1977 46 plans have collapsed, and only 20 of these have paid all outstanding claims.

PPOs are also evolving into two different types of structures: a true PPO with freedom of choice and a financial incentive to use the preferred providers, and an exclusive provider organization (EPO) which is analogous to an HMO provider structure. In California, insurance regulations govern EPOs. These regulations borrow heavily from HMO-type regulations.

EPOs tend to blend HMOs and PPOs together. EPOs may pay providers capitation or other forms of payment that achieve the same effect as HMO capitation: namely, putting providers at risk beyond a certain expected level of utilization. Today there are also several point-of-service HMO plans that provide limited benefits if enrollees go to providers who are not part of the HMO's panel. In the future, this hybrid may become a major form of managed care. At this time, however, the hybrid is technically still a form of HMO and is, or should be, regulated as such.

Hospital-Physician Relationships

Several possible models exist for establishing joint hospital-medical staff PPOs. Please refer to Figure 34.5. In the first variant, the hospital contracts directly with the PPO payor. In California, under its Prudent Buyer Plan,

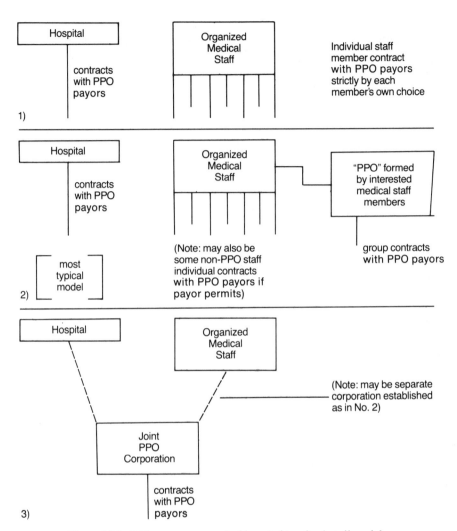

Figure 34.5. PPO structures: typical hospital/medical staff models.

Blue Cross contracts directly with each hospital and also contracts directly with the individual members of the hospital's medical staff. Blue Cross, in effect, deals with each physician directly by furnishing a prepared contract and area-specific relative value scale (RVS) schedule for medicine, surgery, and several specialties. The physicians are offered the contract eventually on a "take it or leave it" basis. Individual medical staff members contract separately from the hospital.

In the second variant, the hospital again contracts directly with the payor, but the medical staff may contract with the payor as an organization. If the physicians form an organization to negotiate collectively, their organization will play the role of a PPO in terms of negotiating a contract. The organization may sign a contract with payors on behalf of its member physicians. Potential antitrust and other legal concerns are associated with this model, and this physician PPO must be organized and operated carefully to avoid legal difficulty.

Physicians typically form one of two kinds of organizations. In the first model, the physicians act as a single entity, usually a professional corporation. Once a physician joins the entity, he or she must abide by its collective decisions as to what contracts are accepted. A second approach is called the "messenger boy" approach. In either model, the physicians generally do not attempt to integrate their practices. They unite only for the purpose of soliciting offers. Because of restrictions imposed by the antitrust laws, the "messenger boy" model does not negotiate on behalf of individual physicians, but plays a sophisticated game of cat and mouse. A presentation by this type of group might include the following solicitation:

> We cannot, as competing physicians, go to you and negotiate a contract because we may violate the antitrust laws. We will, however, listen to your offer and communicate it to our membership. Each member will then consider your offer and individually accept or reject it. . . . Is that your offer? Because we're generally representative of our medical staff, we can tell you that your offer is too low. You may wish to present another offer, but we will take your offer back because we cannot negotiate with you under the antitrust laws.

Such conversations are somewhat artificial and are giving rise to a third variant in the form of an integrated (physician-hospital) PPO corporation. Physicians form their own (professional) corporation composed of members of the medical staff. That corporation then enters into a joint venture with the hospital. The joint venture then markets the combined package of hospital and medical services to payors. Obviously, there are a variety of ways in which this joint venture can occur. For example, the hospital may form a separate subsidiary corporation to engage in PPO activities and that subsidiary would in turn enter into arrangements with the medical staff or a medical staff-sponsored entity.

Capitalizing on their joint ventures, hospitals and their medical staffs may begin to compete directly with insurance companies and Blue Cross and Blue Shield plans. They may compete at several levels. At the simplest level, such a joint venture could drop its sole reliance upon insurance companies for contracts and align itself with a benefits administrator, or otherwise acquire benefit administration expertise. Once the joint venture acquires benefit administration expertise, it then has all the necessary elements to compete with insurance companies. It could then directly market to major self-insured employers and convince other employers to self-insure to gain cash flow and cost advantages.

At a more sophisticated level, such a joint venture could form its own insurance company or HMO. However, both these evolutionary steps require substantial capital and involve new political and regulatory issues for hospitals. Therefore, although competition—especially from HMOs—may force these joint ventures to consider forming their own HMOs, some time will elapse before PPOs actually evolve into HMOs.

Marketing

PPOs have marketing problems similar to those faced by HMOs. PPOs, like HMOs, will usually be limited to a certain service area. If employers are located at one place, hospitals in another place, and the people who use the hospitals and doctors in a third place, geographic coverage becomes an issue. Networking has developed, and freestanding PPOs are forming networks that, on a nonexclusive basis, can market area-wide contracts and allow the local providers to market to their local employer groups. Networks are being formed not only by freestanding hospitals but also by for-profit and nonprofit hospital chains. Please refer to Figure 34.6.

A form of franchise network also exists. One provider group will form a statewide franchise network and will franchise local areas to a selected provider, allowing local providers to form their own local networks.

Legal Issues

Legal issues in PPO formation and operation abound. Perhaps the initial issue is whether PPOs should be regulated, and if so, by whom? PPO constituents—the physician, the hospital, the self-insured employer group, and the benefit administrator—all are currently regulated to some extent. The significance of this issue depends on the form of PPO. For example, a simple provider-spawned PPO that contracts with payors is less likely to raise regulatory issues than is a PPO that is formed as an EPO and puts providers at risk, as do HMOs.

A second critical issue is whether PPOs will run afoul of the antitrust laws. The PPO concept of selectivity gives rise not only to potential antitrust violations, but also to due process concerns. When a provider is not selected or appointed for PPO membership, will that individual have a right to due process? If so, what rights? Many PPOs use short-term participation contracts. The theory is that once the contract terminates and is not renewed, no due process is required. This may be effective, but the Health Care Quality Improvement Act and state law may require due process when a contract is terminated or not renewed. In addition provider-sponsored PPOs must be careful to avoid price-fixing issues when negotiating rates on behalf of members.

Confidentiality of medical records is another major legal issue. To the extent that the physician component of a PPO gathers qualitative information about its peers (how good a doctor is, or whether he or she is an outlier), there is little or no protection for that information. Unlike a peer-reviewed organization (PRO), hospital-organized utilization review committee, tissue or other committee of a hospital medical staff or medical society, PPOs

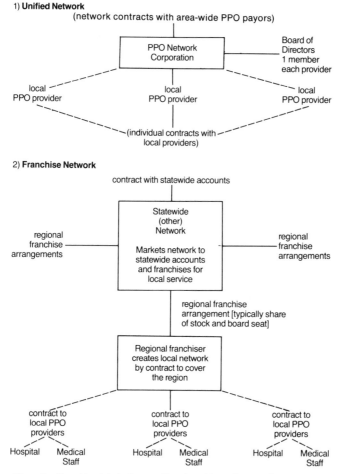

Figure 34.6. Networks in PPO structures. *Unified network:* The local PPO providers each own a share in the network and have a seat on the network board. Providers are selected based on quality and cost considerations. Usually the local PPO providers include both hospitals and their medical staff, and shares in the network are held 50-50 by hospitals and their medical staff; that is, if there are 10 local providers, there will be 20 board seats and 20 shares: one share and board seat for each hospital and its local medical staff PPO. There will be both local marketing by the local provider and network marketing to large regional accounts. Network membership is usually nonexclusive. *Franchise network:* The regional franchiser is typically a provider selected for quality and efficiency, which in turn creates and controls its local network. The franchiser may be a hospital, medical group, or joint venture of a hospital and its staff. The franchise network is not an exclusive arrangement, and it could be used to create a national PPO.

do not as yet have general statutory protection for the confidentiality of their records. Thus these records may be open for discovery in malpractice cases, unless common-law privileges apply. If common-law privileges are not adequate, PPOs must seek protective legislation; otherwise, they will not be able to conduct peer review in an effective manner.

A number of other legal issues arise when establishing PPOs. For example, franchise laws, HMO regulatory laws, laws regulating the corporate practice of medicine, and laws prohibiting rebates for the referral of patients may be applicable to PPOs.

Conclusion

From this overview, it is obvious that PPOs have great potential because they are a mechanism that providers may use to address current competitive and fiscal problems in the health-care field. It should be just as obvious, however, that these financial problems will not be easily resolved and that, of necessity, there is no one superior PPO organizational format. PPOs will evolve as society's response to the conflict between demand and expenditures changes over time. Finally, because of their novelty and their nontraditional role for providers, PPOs raise a number of interesting and challenging legal issues. Great care must be exercised in establishing PPOs.

35 | Getting Involved in the HMO Marketplace

NOAH D. ROSENBERG, ESQ., PAC, MPH

Numerous individual physicians and physician groups are being approached by a diversity of prepaid health plans that desire to contract either with the individual physician or the physician group to provide or arrange for the provision of medical and ancillary health-care services to health plan enrollees. These health plans routinely request either the individual physician or the physician group to accept financial responsibility for providing or arranging for the provision of covered services in return for a negotiated fixed monthly payment.

Health Plan Models

The individual physician or physician group may be approached by one of four different types of health plan organizational models.

Staff Model Health Plan

In this organizational model the health plan employs those physicians who provide or arrange for the provision of covered services to health plan enrollees. In certain instances this type of health plan will subcontract with an individual physician or physician group to provide services that employed physicians cannot provide or are unavailable to provide.

Group Model Health Plan

In this organizational model the health plan contracts with an economically integrated group of physicians who agree to provide or arrange for the provision of covered services to health plan enrollees in return for a negotiated fixed monthly payment or, in certain instances, a negotiated discounted fee arrangement.

Network Model Health Plan

In this organizational model the health plan contracts with two or more economically integrated groups of physicians that agree to provide or arrange for the provision of covered services to health plan enrollees in return for a negotiated fixed monthly payment or, in certain instances, a negotiated discounted fee arrangement.

Independent Practice Association (IPA) Model Health Plan

In this organizational model the health plan contracts with physicians in independent practices, one or more associations of physicians in independent practice, and/or one or more economically integrated groups of physicians.

Reviewing and Negotiating Prepaid Health Plan Agreements

Myriad financial, administrative, and legal issues must be thoroughly reviewed by an individual physician or physician group prior to assuming financial responsibility for providing or arranging for the provision of covered services to health plan enrollees. Although this chapter will identify some of the more important issues that must be reviewed prior to contracting with a health plan, each interested individual physician or physician group should also retain the services of an individual or entity that has substantial experience in reviewing and negotiating agreements with health plans. This has become particularly important in recent years because of the increasing number of health plan insolvencies and also because of the growing complexity of health plan compensation proposals. The individual physician should seriously consider affiliating with a physician group (eg, integrated physician group, independent practice association) in his or her efforts to provide or arrange for the provision of covered services to health plan enrollees. The physician group will frequently be able to negotiate a more viable economic relationship with a health plan and may further insulate the individual physician from exposure to economic and professional liability. The balance of this chapter will therefore use the term *physician group* in its discussion of evaluating and negotiating agreements with health plans.

Financial Viability of Health Plan

1. Request and review information pertinent to financial status.
2. Request and review information pertinent to billing process and experience.
3. Request and review information pertinent to insurance coverage and experience.
4. Request and review information pertinent to reinsurance coverage and experience (particularly relevant to self-funded purchasers).
5. Request and review plans to contract with competing provider systems.
6. Request and review benefit plan construction and targeted purchasing groups.

Administrative Viability of Health Plan

1. Request and review résumés of key administrative and management staff.

2. Request and review references from other contracting providers.
3. Request and review information pertinent to eligibility process and experience.
4. Request and review strategic and business plans (eg, introduction of new product lines).
5. Request and review marketing and sales program information.

Viability of Health Plan Agreement

This section will provide a summary of the author's recommendations for modification of a health plan agreement and for language that should, if possible, be included in a health plan agreement. These recommended modifications will be presented in the order in which they normally appear in a health plan agreement. It is essential to note, however, when reviewing these proposed modifications, that although many health plans agree to include the majority of these revisions in health plan agreements, in some situations health plans will not agree to certain provisions. It is also essential to note that certain language presented below must be included in a health plan agreement in accordance with applicable sections of local, state, and federal law.

Definitions

The following definitions should be included in each health plan agreement to clarify the meaning of each contractual term discussed in it and to avoid potential disputes regarding the meaning of contractual terms. It is essential that each defined term in a health plan agreement be used consistently throughout the agreement.

Capitation payment. Suggested language: " 'Capitation payment' means that payment made to Physician Group by Health Plan on a prepaid basis for the covered services to be provided or arranged for by Physician Group hereunder."

Copayment. Suggested language: " 'Copayment' means an additional fee charged to a subscriber or an enrollee which is approved by the department of corporations [or department of insurance, if applicable] provided for in the health plan agreement and disclosed in the evidence of coverage or the disclosure form used as the evidence of coverage."

Covered services. Suggested language: " 'Covered services' means those health care services and supplies that Physician Group is required to provide or arrange for the provision of the capitation payment described hereunder."

Emergency. Suggested language: " 'Emergency' means the sudden onset of a symptom, illness, or injury requiring immediate diagnosis and/or treatment in the judgment of Physician Group."

Enrollee. Suggested language: " 'Enrollee' means a person who is enrolled in Health Plan, including enrolled dependents, and who is entitled to receive covered services."

Evidence of coverage. Suggested language: " 'Evidence of coverage' means the document issued by Health Plan to an enrollee that describes those health-care services that an enrollee is entitled to receive."

Medically necessary. Suggested language: " 'Medically necessary' means medical or surgical treatment that an enrollee requires as determined by Physician Group, in accordance with accepted medical and surgical practices and standards prevailing in the service area at the time of treatment, and in conformity with the professional and technical standards adopted by the utilization review committee of Physician Group and Health Plan."

Out of area. Suggested language: " 'Out of area' means that geographical area which is greater than 30 miles from the principal business office of Physician Group."

Primary care physician. Suggested language: " 'Primary care physician' means a physician who has the responsibility for providing initial and primary care to patients, for maintaining the continuity of patient care, or for initiating referrals for specialist care. A 'primary care physician' may be a general practitioner, internist, pediatrician, or family practitioner."

Service area. Suggested language: " 'Service area' means the geographical area which is within a 30 mile radius of the principal business office of Physician Group."

Specialist physician. Suggested language: " 'Specialist physician' means a physician who is not a primary care physician and who is professionally qualified to practice his or her designated specialty."

Surcharge. Suggested language: " 'Surcharge' means an additional fee that is charged to a subscriber or an enrollee for covered services but which is not approved by the department of corporations [or department of insurance, if applicable] provided for in a health plan agreement or disclosed in an evidence of coverage or the disclosure form used as the evidence of coverage."

Obligations of the Physician

Provision of covered services. In each health plan agreement, a physician group should agree to provide or arrange for the provision of covered services on a 24-hour-per-day, seven-day-per-week, 365-day-per-year basis.

The covered services for which the physician group assumes responsibility should be specifically detailed in an exhibit to a health plan agreement.

Nondiscrimination. A physician group should agree not to discriminate against enrollees. Suggested language: "Physician Group agrees: (1) not to differentiate or discriminate in its provision of covered services to enrollees because of race, color, national origin, ancestry, religion, sex, marital status, sexual orientation, or age; and (2) to render covered services to enrollees in the same manner, in accordance with the same standards, and within the same time availability as said services are offered to non-health-plan patients consistent with existing medical ethical/legal requirements for providing continuity of care to any patient in the service area."

Representations and warranties. A physician group should represent and warrant that it is appropriately licensed, appropriately incorporated, and in good standing with pertinent local, state, and federal authorities.

Standards. A physician group should agree to provide medical care in accordance with generally accepted standards of medical practice in the service area. Suggested language: "All covered services provided by or arranged for by Physician Group shall be provided by professional personnel and facilities that comply with generally accepted standards of medical practice in the service area. Physician Group further agrees to provide or arrange for those consultants and specialists practicing medicine as are necessary and appropriate, and who comply with generally accepted standards of medical practice in the service area, to maintain the quality of covered services provided by or arranged for by Physician Group."

Administrative procedure. A physician group is usually required to comply with certain health plan administrative procedures. A physician group should agree to comply with only those administrative procedures that it has reviewed prior to execution of a health plan agreement. In the event that the health plan desires to amend these administrative procedures, it should be required to provide the physician group with written notice of any such proposed amendments a minimum of 30 days prior to the effective date of their implementation and provide the physician group with the ability to review and approve or disapprove of these amendments. The physician group should be given an opportunity to terminate the health plan agreement in the event it is unable or unwilling to comply with any amendment to the health plan's administrative procedures. Suggested language: "Prior to amending health plan administrative policies and procedures, Health Plan shall provide Physician Group with said amendment a minimum of 30 days prior to the effective date of implementation of said amendment to the administrative policies and procedures for Physician Group to review and approve or disapprove."

Use of physician group and physician group participating physician name(s) for marketing purposes. It is essential for a physician group to review and approve of all health plan use of its name prior to permitting the health plan to use its name in any media advertising. Suggested language: "Health plan shall have the right to list the name, address, and telephone number of Physician Group and each Physician Group participating physician in its list of participating providers distributed to enrollees. Notwithstanding the foregoing, Health Plan shall not have the right to list the name of Physician Group or a Physician Group participating physician in any newspaper, radio, or television advertising without receiving the prior written consent of Physician Group and/or a Physician Group participating physician."

Obligations of the Health Plan

Administration. Each health plan should agree to perform all necessary administrative, accounting, enrollment, and other functions including, but not limited to, eligibility determination, claims adjudication, data collection and evaluation, and maintenance of hospital and physician group risk pools.

Benefit information. Each health plan should agree to apprise its enrollees and physician group concerning the type, scope, and duration of benefits and services to which enrollees are entitled pursuant to an evidence of coverage.

Assistance to the physician group. Each health plan should agree to assist and cooperate with the physician group in the development and initial implementation of procedures necessary to carry out the terms of the health plan agreement (eg, utilization review procedures, quality assurance procedures, and billing procedures).

Statistical information and provision of data. Each health plan should agree to provide the physician group with detailed management information and data necessary to carry out the terms and conditions of the health plan agreement. In addition, the health plan should provide the physician group with monthly reports reflecting the status of any hospital physician group or health plan/physician group risk-sharing programs and use of professional and institutional services by all providers of care.

Identification and eligibility. Each health plan should provide a system by which its enrollees can identify themselves to the physician group and by which the physician group and/or the physician group participating physician can verify patient eligibility. Suggested language: "Health Plan shall supply enrollees with a means of identifying themselves to Physician

Group and/or a Physician Group participating physician (e.g., an identification card) which indicates the eligibility and coverage under a health plan evidence of coverage. Physician Group and each Physician Group participating physician shall make a good faith effort to confirm that the individual presenting a health plan identification card is in fact the individual whose name appears on the health plan identification card. Health Plan shall pay Physician Group at Physician Group's usual and customary charges for those covered services provided to an individual in the event Health Plan incorrectly identifies and/or verifies an individual to be eligible for benefits under an applicable evidence of coverage prior to the provision of covered services to said individual."

Marketing plan. Each health plan should provide the physician group with a detailed marketing plan that describes the health plan's marketing efforts in the physician group's service area (eg, nature of marketing programs, use of salespersons and compensation of said salespersons, use of media advertising, use of and examples of marketing materials, dollar amount of marketing budget).

Compensation

It is essential to recognize that there are different types of health plans, including (1) health plans that are licensed by local and state departments of corporations or of insurance and (2) health plans that are licensed by local and state departments of corporations or of insurance *and* which are federally qualified as health maintenance organizations (HMOs) pursuant to Section 1310 of the Public Health Service Act. Those health plans that are licensed by local departments of corporations or of insurance may establish their premiums based upon the actual health-care experience of the enrollees in a particular subscriber group ("experience rating"). Those health plans that are federally qualified HMOs are required in most, but not all, situations to establish their premiums based upon the actual health-care experience of their community (defined as all of the enrollees enrolled in a health plan, as opposed to just one particular enrollee group: "community rating"). Premiums that are based upon experience rating are often lower than premiums based upon community rating. Therefore, if a physician group enters into a health plan agreement that compensates the physician group based upon a percentage of premium, and the contracting health plan is an organization that utilizes experience rating, the dollar amount to be paid to the physician group will most likely be less than the dollar amount paid pursuant to an agreement with an HMO that utilizes community rating, even though the percentage of premium is equivalent in both agreements.

Capitation payments. In the event a physician group is paid on a capitation basis, language should be included in the health plan agreement that requires the health plan to pay the physician group no later than the 10th day of the month for each enrollee who chooses or is assigned to a physician group for that month. It is essential that a health plan agreement specifically identifies those covered services that a physician group is required to provide for the capitation payment. The health plan agreement should further specify that the capitation payment represents payment in full to the physician group except for applicable enrollee copayments and deductibles, coordination of benefit revenues, stop-loss payments, and any additional payment made to the physician group pursuant to the health plan's risk-sharing program.

Fee-for-service payment. In the event a physician group is compensated based upon a discounted fee-for-service schedule, the health plan agreement should require the health plan to compensate the physician group within 30 working days of the physician group's submission of a complete bill to the health plan.

Penalty. A physician group should negotiate an interest penalty to be paid by the health plan to the physician group in the event the health plan's payments to the physician group are not made on a timely basis.

Low-enrollment guarantee. In those instances where a health plan compensates the physician group on a capitation basis, the physician group should negotiate a low-enrollment guarantee. This low-enrollment guarantee may take several different forms, but the concept is one of a physician group being compensated on a discounted fee-for-service basis until the health plan's enrollment with the physician group reaches a certain minimum number.

Billing

Description of the billing process. It is essential that a health plan agreement specifically describes the method that the physician group must follow for purposes of submitting billing statements to the health plan and, also, that it identifies the types of reports that the health plan must provide to the physician group based on those billing statements.

Coordination of benefits. A physician group should have the right to coordinate benefits where dual insurance coverage exists and to retain coordination of benefit payments up to 100% of its usual and customary charges for those covered services rendered.

Stop Loss

Each health plan agreement that reimburses a physician group on a capitation basis should provide for a limitation on the physician group's financial liability in the event charges for covered services provided to an enrollee exceed a certain dollar amount. Each health plan agreement should contain, at a minimum, the following information regarding stop loss:

1. Identification of the stop-loss deductible
2. Identification of the method for valuing covered services to be applied against the stop-loss deductible (eg, physician group's charge schedules).
3. Identification of the stop-loss year (eg, calendar year, contract term) including a statement regarding whether the health plan will allow the physician group to credit the value of services commenced but not completed by the end of the stop-loss year to the subsequent stop-loss year deductible.
4. Date at which stop loss payment will be made.

In addition to reviewing the stop-loss provisions in a health plan agreement, it is essential for the physician group to review the stop-loss provisions in the agreement between the health plan and the physician group's affiliated hospital. The hospital's stop-loss deductible will undoubtedly affect the physician group's potential risk-sharing distribution as set forth in the next section.

Risk Sharing

Each health plan utilizes a different mechanism for hospital/physician group or health plan/physician group risk sharing. Although it is difficult to provide a complete summary of the items that must be included in a health plan agreement regarding risk sharing, it is essential that the following be included:

1. Identification of the amount allocated by the health plan for noncovered services ("hospital budget") including, but not limited to, the figure used for measuring hospital inpatient days per 1000 enrollees assigned to the physician group and applicable hospital per diem(s) or capitation payment(s)
2. Identification of those services that will be charged against the hospital budget (e.g., hospital inpatient and outpatient care, ambulance services, home health services, durable medical equipment)
3. Identification of capitation payment withholding, if any, as the physician group's contribution to the hospital budget
4. Requirement that the health plan provide the physician group with a monthly report regarding current charges made against the hospital budget
5. Identification of the amount of hospital budget surplus to which the physician group will be entitled in the event utilization of institutional services is favorable and the downside risk to the physician group in the event utilization of institutional services is excessive

It is essential for a physician group to carefully review the proposed health plan risk-sharing arrangements among the physician group, its hospital partner, and the health plan in a health plan agreement covering Medicare or Medicaid beneficiaries. Section 9313(c) of the Omnibus Budget Reconciliation Act of 1986 (OBRA) provides that, effective April 21, 1987, a hospital that knowingly makes a payment, directly or indirectly, to a physician as an incentive to reduce or limit services to a Medicare beneficiary is subject to a civil penalty of up to $2000 for each individual with respect to whom the payment is made and other penalties as prescribed by law (including expulsion from the Medicare program).

In addition, Section 9313(c) provides that any physician who knowingly accepts receipt of a payment from a hospital as an inducement to reduce or limit services to a Medicare beneficiary is subject to a civil penalty of up to $2000 for each individual with respect to whom the payment is made and other penalties as prescribed by law (including expulsion from the Medicare program).

The intent of Section 9313(c) was to correct perceived abuses under the Medicare prospective payment system. Congress wanted to preclude hospitals from developing and implementing financial incentive arrangements that would reward physicians for limiting services to Medicare beneficiaries in a medically inappropriate manner in order to control utilization of hospital services. Because of the broad scope of the language of Section 9313(c), however, it may be argued that Section 9313(c) is applicable to payments made to physicians by hospitals pursuant to a hospital/physician incentive/risk pool established by a hospital or an HMO based upon hospital utilization goals for Medicare beneficiaries. Therefore it is essential that the physician group carefully scrutinizes all risk-sharing arrangements to ensure that it cannot be construed that a hospital partner is making a payment to a physician group as an inducement to reduce or limit services to a Medicare beneficiary.

Utilization Review/Quality Assurance

Copy of utilization review/quality assurance plan. Each health plan agreement should identify who (i.e., physician group or health plan) is responsible for utilization review/quality assurance (UR/QA). Where possible, the physician group should retain control of UR/QA subject to monitoring of the UR/QA plan by the health plan as required by local, state, and federal law; if the health plan is responsible for UR/QA, a copy of the UR/QA plan must be attached to the health plan agreement and thoroughly reviewed by the physician group prior to executing the agreement.

Indemnification for UR. In the event a health plan is responsible for UR/QA, the health plan should hold the physician group and its participating physicians harmless from any liability or expense they incur which is directly or indirectly related to the utilization review activities of the health plan.

Suggested language: "Notwithstanding anything to the contrary in this agreement, Health Plan shall indemnify and hold Physician Group and Physician Group participating physicians harmless from and against any and all liability and additional expense incurred by Physician Group and Physician Group participating physicians which are directly or indirectly related to the utilization review activities of Health Plan and its respective agents, employees, contractors, and designees."

It is essential to note, however, that a physician group should never agree to indemnify a health plan for physician group UR/QA activities or for anything else. Liability incurred by a physician group pursuant to an indemnification provision will not be covered by most physician group risk carriers.

Attendance at UR/QA committee meetings. A physician group should refuse to allow outsiders (eg, representatives of a health plan) to attend its UR/QA meetings. The physician group may agree to provide the health plan with summaries of these meetings.

Insurance

All health plan agreements should include insurance requirements pertaining to both the physician group and the health plan.

Suggested language for the physician group and health plan: "_____ shall, at its sole cost and expense, maintain such professional liability insurance with coverage in the minimum amount of _____ Dollars ($_____) per claim and _____ Dollars ($_____) in the annual aggregate to insure it and its employees against liability for damages directly or indirectly related to the performance of any service provided hereunder, the use of any property and facilities provided by _____, and activities performed by _____ hereunder. _____ shall be entitled to receive not less than 30 calendar days' written notice of any proposed reduction or cancellation of such insurance coverage by _____. Evidence of the above-described insurance policies shall be provided to _____ upon _____'s receipt of five (5) business days' prior written notice of _____'s request for such information."

Term

Each health plan agreement should provide for a term of not more than one year. In addition, it is recommended that a health plan agreement *not* be automatically renewable. Finally, a provision should be included requiring the health plan to agree to renegotiate the compensation terms of the health plan agreement no later than 90 days prior to the end of the anniversary date of a health plan agreement and that any increase in compensation that is agreed upon between the parties after the commencement of the new agreement term be retroactive to the anniversary date of the health plan agreement.

Termination without Cause

Every health plan agreement should include a provision for termination *without* cause. Suggested language: "Either party to this health plan agreement shall have the right to terminate this agreement, at any time, without cause, by providing the other party with a minimum of _____ (___) days' prior written notice of termination. Termination shall take effect automatically upon the expiration of the _____ (___) day notice period."

The notice period for termination without cause should not exceed 90 days.

Termination with Cause

A physician group should have the right to terminate its health plan agreement with cause. Preferably, the notice period for termination with cause will be on an immediate basis; however, in most cases the health plan will require a notice period preceding termination. The notice period should not exceed 10 days. Grounds for a physician group's termination of a health plan agreement with cause should include, but not be limited to, the following:

1. Failure of a health plan to pay the physician group on a timely basis (eg, in the event the health plan does not pay the physician group within 10 days of the date agreed to in the health plan agreement, the physician group should have the right to immediately terminate the agreement)
2. A health plan's license is suspended or revoked
3. A health plan no longer maintains the insurance coverage required pursuant to the health plan agreement
4. A health plan breaches a material term, covenant, or condition of a health plan agreement without curing said breach within a designated time period

A health plan will also want the right to terminate a health plan agreement with cause. Under these circumstances, the physician group will want to negotiate as lengthy a notice period as it can. Grounds for a health plan's termination of a health plan agreement with cause may include, but not be limited to, the following:

1. The physician group no longer maintains the insurance coverage required pursuant to a health plan agreement.
2. The physician group breaches a material term, covenant, or condition of the agreement without curing said breach within a designated time period.
3. The physician group is not in good standing with local, state, and federal authorities.

Payment by Health Plan to Physician Group upon Termination

Many local, state, and federal laws require health-care providers to provide services to enrollees after the effective termination date of their health plan agreement to ensure continuity of care to enrollees. It is essential for the physician group to require the health plan to reimburse it at its usual and customary charges for all covered services provided after the effective date of termination of the health plan agreement.

Suggested language: "Physician group agrees to provide covered services to enrollees of health plan after the effective date of termination of this agreement until the earlier of (1) the date the enrollee is transferred to another physician group or (2) the enrollee's treatment is completed, provided, however, that health plan compensates physician group for all covered services provided to an enrollee after the effective date of termination of this agreement at physician group's usual and customary rate for said covered services."

Medical Records

All health plan agreements should include provisions regarding the ownership, review, and release of medical records.

Suggested language: "Physician Group shall maintain, with respect to each enrollee receiving covered services, a medical record containing such information and preserved for such time periods as required under applicable state and federal law. Said records shall remain the property of Physician Group. To the extent permitted by law, in accordance with procedures required by law and upon receipt of seventy-two (72) hours' prior written notice from Health Plan, Physician Group shall permit Health Plan to inspect and make copies of medical records during normal business hours, and shall provide copies of such records to Health Plan upon request. Health Plan shall reimburse Physician Group for all reasonable costs incurred by Physician Group as a result of said record inspection and duplication. Health Plan shall warrant that prior to requesting an enrollee's medical records, it shall obtain a valid written release from the enrollee (or his or her legal representative) authorizing Health Plan to obtain his or her medical records and shall hold harmless, indemnify, and defend Physician Group from any liability incurred by Physician Group as a result of such medical record release. Physician Group shall have no obligation to release medical records until it is presented with said medical record release."

Regulatory Requirements

Each health plan licensed by a department of corporations or of insurance is required to include the following language in its health plan agreements:

Suggested language: *"No surcharges.* In no event, including but not limited to nonpayment by Physician Group or Health Plan, Physician Group's or Health Plan's insolvency, or breach of this health plan agreement shall any enrollee be liable for any sums owed to Physician Group by Health Plan, and Physician Group shall not bill, charge, or collect a deposit or other sum or seek compensation, remuneration, or reimbursement from, or maintain any action or have any recourse against, or make any surcharge upon, an enrollee or other person acting on an enrollee's behalf. This provision shall not prohibit collection of copayments or coordination of benefit revenues from secondary carriers by which the enrollee is covered. If Health Plan receives notice of any surcharge upon an enrollee, it shall be empowered to take appropriate action.

"The obligations set forth in this section _____ shall survive the termination of this health plan agreement regardless of the cause giving rise to such termination and shall be construed for the benefit of an enrollee, and the provisions of this section _____ shall supersede any oral or written agreement to the contrary now existing or hereafter entered into between Physician Group and an enrollee or persons acting on behalf of either of them.

"Obligations following termination. Upon any termination of this agreement, Health Plan shall be liable in accordance with the terms hereof to pay for covered services rendered to any enrollee who retains eligibility under an applicable agreement with a subscriber group or by operation of law, and who is under the care of Physician Group at the time of such termination, and Physician Group shall continue to provide such services to any such enrollee until the services being rendered by Physician Group to the enrollee are completed, unless Health Plan makes reasonable and medically appropriate provision for the assumption of those services by another provider.

"Records. Physician Group shall maintain such records and provide such information to Health Plan or the commissioner of the department of corporations or of insurance ("Commissioner") as may be necessary for compliance with pertinent provisions of local, state, and federal law, as amended from time to time, and the rules and regulations promulgated thereunder (the "Regulations"), and Physician Group's obligations to retain records and provide information hereunder shall not terminate upon the termination of this agreement, whether by rescission or otherwise.

"Access to information. Health Plan and the Commissioner shall have access at reasonable times, upon demand, to the books, records, and papers of Physician Group relating to covered services provided to enrollees, to the cost thereof, to payments received from enrollees (or from others on their behalf), and, unless Physician Group is compensated hereunder, on a fee-for-service basis, to the financial condition of Physician Group."

Arbitration

If a health plan requires a physician group to participate in arbitration proceedings in the event of either a health plan agreement dispute or as a requirement of its enrollee grievance procedure, language should be added to the health plan agreement specifying that the physician group will not be required to arbitrate a dispute in the event its risk carrier(s) does not agree to said arbitration proceedings.

Suggested language: "Notwithstanding anything to the contrary in this agreement, any and all arbitration proceedings initiated pursuant to this agreement shall be approved by Physician Group's risk carrier(s) prior to the initiation of said proceedings."

In the event a health plan refuses to add the suggested language described above, the physician group should require the health plan to specifically exclude malpractice actions from the arbitration requirement.

General Provisions

All health plan agreements should include, at a minimum, the following general provisions.

Notices. Suggested language: "All notices required to be given hereunder shall be in writing and shall be deemed delivered if personally delivered or dispatched by certified or registered mail, return receipt requested, postage prepaid, addressed to the parties as follows:

Health Plan: _____

_____

Attn: _____

Physician Group: _____

_____

Attn: _____

"Notice shall be deemed given on the date it is deposited in the mail in accordance with the foregoing. Any party may change the address to which to send notices by notifying the other party of such change of address in writing in accordance with the foregoing."

Severability. Suggested language: "Any terms or provisions of this agreement which shall prove to be invalid, void, or illegal shall in no way affect, impair, or invalidate any other term or provisions herein and such remaining terms and provisions shall remain in full force and effect."

Governing law. Suggested language: "The existence, validity and construction of this agreement shall be governed by the laws of the State of _____."

Assignment. Suggested language: "Neither party shall assign this agreement without the prior written consent of the other party. This agreement shall be binding on the parties and their respective successors and assigns."

Waiver. Suggested language: "The waiver by either party to this agreement of any one or more defaults, if any, on the part of the other, shall not be construed to operate as a waiver of any other or future defaults, under the same or different terms, conditions, or covenants contained in this Agreement."

Independent Contractor. Suggested language: "In the performance of the work, duties, and obligations described hereunder, it is mutually understood and agreed that each party is at all times acting and performing as an independent contractor with respect to the other and that no relationship of partnership, joint venture, or employment is created by this health plan agreement."

Entire agreement: Amendment. Suggested language: "This health plan agreement states the entire contract between the parties in respect to the subject matter of this health plan Agreement and supersedes any oral or written proposals, statements, discussions, negotiations, or other agreements before or contemporaneous to this health plan agreement. The parties acknowledge that they have not been induced to enter into this health plan agreement by any oral or written representations or statements not expressly contained in this health plan agreement. This health plan agreement may be modified only by mutual agreement of the parties provided that, before any modification shall be operative or valid, it is reduced to writing and signed by both parties."

Service Exhibit

Prior to entering into capitation agreements with a health plan, a physician group should sit down with representatives of its affiliated hospital to establish a service matrix to be used in negotiating all health plan agreements structured on a capitation payment basis. Upon receipt of a health plan agreement, it will be essential for the physician group to carefully review the nature and scope of the covered services it will be required to provide. Hospital-based physician services, chemotherapeutic medications, pharmaceuticals not dispensed by the physician group, allergy injections and allergens, lithotripsy, ambulance services, durable medical equipment, home health care, and dialysis are examples of services that should be the financial responsibility of an affiliated hospital or the health plan.

In addition to defining what constitutes covered services, language should be added to specify that in the event local, state, or federal law requires the health plan to provide additional services and the health plan desires the physician group to provide those services, the health plan must agree to meet with the physician group to establish whether the physician group desires to provide these services and, if it does, that additional compensation will be paid for the physician group's provision of the additional services.

Preexisting pregnancy. A physician group should require each health plan to reimburse it for preexisting pregnancies.

Suggested language: "Health Plan shall pay Physician Group _____ Dollars ($_____) for each enrollee who is pregnant at the time of assignment to Physician Group. Said _____ Dollars ($_____) payment shall be in addition to any and all other monies due and owing Physician Group by Health Plan hereunder."

Pools for certain identified services. A health plan agreement should require the health plan to establish pools for payment for certain services including, but not limited to, AIDS, organ transplants, cardiovascular surgery, neonatal intensive care, and out-of-area coverage.

Summary

It is extremely important for each individual physician or physician group that is interested in contracting with a health plan to provide or arrange for the provision of covered services to health plan enrollees to carefully examine the financial, administrative, and legal viability of each health plan and its contract proposal. The individual physician should carefully review the viability of an individual contracting with a health plan on a risk basis, as opposed to an individual choosing to join a group of physicians which will represent the individual's interests in negotiating agreements with health plans. The author believes that the viable physician group is much more capable of ensuring the individual physician financial success in his or her participation in a health plan contractual relationship.

V | THE LATER YEARS

36 | Pension Plans and Tax Considerations

BARRY A. LITZER

Introduction

Although the income tax laws have severely restricted the ability of owners of small businesses to design pension plans to suit their own individual needs, such programs are still an important part of your overall business plan. These plans can provide both the owner and his or her employees with a way to both shelter current income from income taxes, and to assure the employee of significant assets upon retirement.

This chapter will review the various pension program alternatives and describe the requirements and benefits of each.

Why Establish a Qualified Plan

- The main benefit of qualified plans (those that qualify under IRS regulations) for both the employer and the employee is favorable tax treatment.
- The company receives a current tax deduction for contributions. Current year contributions may not have to be paid until the due date or, in many cases, the extended due date of the tax return.
- Employees are not taxed on contributions and earnings until they receive the funds.
- The employee's distribution may qualify for beneficial tax treatment.
- Qualified plans do more than save money: they can also make the company more competitive in hiring and retaining the best workers.
- A plan may increase the employee's incentive to boost productivity, especially if contributions are geared to profitability.
- Plan assets are protected from creditors.
- The plan can provide secure retirement funds for employees.

How beneficial the plan will be to the employee depends on how much the employer contributes to it. How much the employer can or must contribute depends on the type of plan the employer selects.

Qualified plans are either *defined contribution* plans (such as profit sharing, money purchase, or 401[k]) or *defined benefit* plans (commonly known as pension plans).

Defined Contribution Plan

In a defined contribution plan, the plan defines the contribution the company will make on behalf of the participant. Usually the contribution is expressed as a percentage of the participant's compensation. The maximum addition to the participant's account for one year is the lesser of $30,000 or 25% of his or her compensation. Defined contribution plans can be very flexible when it comes to contributions. The minimum contribution may be zero in some years or some percentage of earnings in other years. It all depends on the type of plan that is adopted. The actual annual contribution percentage will be the same for all employees but will vary each year based on the financial performance of the company, salaries drawn by the owners and other possibly subjective factors.

Defined Benefit Plan

This is a more complicated plan that defines the benefit (payments) participants will receive at retirement. The company's yearly contributions are determined actuarially based on the amounts needed to provide the promised benefit.

This benefit cannot exceed the lesser of $102,582 in 1990 (indexed for inflation) or 100% of the average of the employee's three highest consecutive years of compensation. Despite discrimination rules, these plans tend to provide greater benefits to owners and other highly compensated employees. Owners tend to be among the oldest and best-paid employees. Because benefits are determined actuarially based on compensation and must be available by retirement age, contributions are usually much higher for owners approaching retirement age.

Annual contributions must, however, continue no matter how the company performs. The plan's investment performance also affects the employer's contributions. The plan must maintain a pool of assets large enough to pay the promised benefits. If a plan's investments do well by adding income or asset appreciation to the available pool of assets, the annual contribution will be less. If the investments do poorly, the annual contribution will be increased.

Defined Contribution vs. Defined Benefit

Now that we have covered the two general types of plans available, let us look at some specific plan options for a company. As we examine each type of plan, the following questions will be answered: How flexible is the plan? How much will it cost to administer? What are the minimum and maximum contributions? What type of company should consider this plan?

We will first look at the most popular types of defined contribution plans.

Profit Sharing Plans

Many companies find profit sharing plans attractive because they offer considerable flexibility and low administrative costs. Plan contributions can be discretionary. Based on each year's results, the company can decide how much, or how little, to contribute to the plan. High contributions can be made in good years and low contributions in bad years.

The minimum contribution is zero. The maximum contribution is 15% of compensation paid to eligible employees. The easiest way to allocate contributions to the plan is pro rata so that each participant gets a contribution in proportion to his or her salary. For example, an individual earning $50,000 would receive a $5000 contribution. Only the first $209,200 (in 1990 adjusted for inflation) in compensation can be counted when determining the maximum contribution.

An owner with a salary of $300,000 will only receive $20,920 (10% of $209,200) as a contribution, even though 10% of his or her compensation would equal $30,000. Owners can make disproportionate contributions to key employees by using Social Security integration. Although all qualified plans are required to make allocations on a generally equivalent basis to all participants, some disparity is allowed to make up for the relatively less favorable treatment highly compensated employees receive under Social Security. Employees earning $150,000 receive no more Social Security benefits than employees earning $60,000.

Key Points Regarding Profit Sharing Plans

- Very flexible
- Low administrative costs
- Contributions can be completely discretionary
- Maximum contribution is 15% of total compensation of eligible employees
- No minimum contributions
- Best suited for companies that want maximum flexibility

Money Purchase Pension Plans

These are similar to profit sharing plans, but they allow the employer to make contributions beyond those permitted to profit sharing plans. They are, however, not as flexible as profit sharing plans. In a money purchase pension, the employer is required to make an annual contribution to the plan based on a fixed percentage of eligible compensation.

The set contribution can be as high as 25% of compensation. Once decided, the employer must make the same contribution every year no matter how the company does. The advantage of a money purchase plan over a profit sharing plan is the higher maximum contribution. The disadvantage is that the same contribution must be made each year.

To combine the best of both plans the company can establish two plans. The company then can set a low contribution for the money purchase plan, usually 10% or less, and retain the option of contributing more to the profit sharing plan if the company's annual performance warrants it.

Example: An employer establishes a 10% money purchase plan and a profit sharing plan. In bad years, the employer makes only the 10% contribution to the money purchase plan. In good years, the employer also contributes up to 15% to the profit sharing plan. Thus the employer has the advantage of a 25% contribution in good times while limiting the contribution to 10% in bad times.

The employer can also use Social Security integration to ensure that higher-paid employees will receive a proportionately larger contribution every year. However, if the employer has more than one plan, Social Security integration can be used in only one plan.

An employer must ask him- or herself the following questions in considering the establishment of a money purchase plan: Am I consistently profitable? Do I usually make or have the ability to make large profit sharing contributions? and Do I want to contribute more than 15% of compensation?

Summarizing Money Purchase Plans

- Not as flexible as profit sharing plans
- Low administrative costs
- Set contributions required each year
- Maximum contribution is 25% of eligible company compensation
- Minimum contribution can be set as low as employer wishes
- Best suited for consistently profitable companies that want to contribute more than 15% of compensation

401(k) Plans

This is probably the only section of the tax code that most people know by number, and for good reason. Never before have employees had such flexibility coupled with a tax-advantaged way to save for retirement. Since their introduction, 401(k) plans have become the most popular of the qualified plans.

A 401(k) plan allows employees to choose between receiving all their compensation now or deferring some until retirement. Deferred amounts are deposited into the plan, where they grow tax-free until distribution. Because the funds belong to the employees, the employees' account balances are always 100% vested.

Participation is voluntary during the calendar year. An employee can contribute up to the lesser of $7979 in 1990 (indexed for inflation) or a percentage of earnings specified in the plan (up to 25%).

Most employees can contribute the maximum if they so choose, but each employee decides how much to contribute within limits. An employee can elect to contribute nothing. However, there are some limitations to this flexibility, and mathematical tests are done to ensure that there is not too great a difference between the contribution of highly and nonhighly compensated employees. If the plan fails these tests, the contributions of highly compensated employees could be limited or even returned.

Employees also have the ability to make hardship withdrawals. Whereas funds in qualified plans are normally available only at the participant's death, disability, or separation from service, a participant with an immediate financial need and no other recourse can take a withdrawal. The money must be used to pay deductible medical expenses, purchase a principal residence, prevent eviction or foreclosure on a principal residence, or pay tuition for post-secondary education for the participant or his or her dependents.

A hardship withdrawal is taxable when taken and may also be subject to an additional 10% early distribution tax unless it is used for deductible medical expenses. The 401(k) also affords the employer great flexibility because the employer does not need to make a contribution to the participants' accounts. The employer does, however, have the option of making matching contributions.

The employer can establish a set formula for making contributions, and match 50% of the employee contributions (up to 6% of compensation). Alternatively, the employer may simply make a discretionary contribution each year. The first alternative is a good way to increase employee participation in the plan. After all, how often do employees have the chance to give themselves a raise?

The second option gives the same flexibility as a profit-sharing plan and couples the contribution to the company's performance, which could in turn increase productivity. Contributions for highly-compensated employees face the same discrimination test previously discussed.

Adding a 401(k) plan allows employees the ability to boost their savings for retirement. Many participants in other qualified plans are unable to deduct IRA contributions. With a 401(k), they have an absolute tax-advantaged retirement savings option. The other major advantages over an IRA are that the annual contribution limit is higher, there are potential beneficial tax treatments for distributions, participants can borrow from their accounts, and the employer may make a matching contribution.

Summary of 401(k) Plan Features

- Maximum flexibility
- No required contributions
- Maximum allowable employee contribution is $7979 in 1990 (indexed for inflation); employers can make matching contributions

- Should be considered by most companies—employees benefit even if the employer makes no contribution

Defined Benefit Plan

A defined benefit plan provides a set monthly payment to participants either for life or a set term.

If the client's goal is to benefit mainly older, highly-compensated employees with substantially longer terms of service then the rest of the work force, a defined benefit plan would be the best.

Defined benefit plans differ from defined contribution plans in many ways. Instead of separate accounts being maintained for every participant, a pool of assets is dedicated to providing stated benefits to all participants. As participants become eligible for distributions, payments are made from this fund. The benefit is generally defined as an average of annual preretirement compensation, often based on either the participant's last five years with the company or the highest consecutive five years of compensation.

The maximum annual benefit as of a participant's social security retirement age cannot exceed the lesser of $102,582 in 1990 (indexed for inflation) or 100% of the average of the three consecutive highest years' compensation.

At the other extreme, a *de minimis* rule allows employers to provide up to a $10,000 annual retirement benefit to any employee, regardless of current age or compensation. If there is a spouse or family member who works part time, this could be a valuable option.

The employer has considerable latitude in setting up a defined benefit plan; however, once the plan is established there is not much you can do to change it. The employer is required to make a sufficient annual contribution to fund the projected benefits regardless of what kind of year the employer has. Quarterly deposits are now required, just like estimated tax payments.

Though administrative costs may be high and flexibility low when compared with many defined contribution plans, this plan is a valuable option if the employer's goal is to benefit older, higher-paid employees.

Characteristics of Defined Benefit Plans

- Not extremely flexible once created
- Relatively high administrative costs
- Employer is required to make an actuarially determined contribution
- Maximum and minimum contributions vary according to benefit promise and investment results
- Usually more beneficial for older or highly compensated employees

Specific Requirements of Defined Contribution and Defined Benefit Plans

A qualified plan must satisfy mathematical nondiscrimination rules as well as definitional requirements imposed by Code Section 401(a). In contrast, a pension plan is a definite written program and arrangement that is communicated to employees and which is established and maintained by an employer to provide for the livelihood of the employees or their beneficiaries after retirement of such employees through the payment of benefits, determined without regard to profits.

The Employee Retirement Income Security Act of 1974 (ERISA) requires that a qualified retirement type plan be in writing and that the plan's assets be held in trust by one or more trustees. Each trustee must be named in the trust or plan instrument or appointed by a named fiduciary.

The plan and the trust are often incorporated in a single document, with the trust provisions contained in a separate article or articles. The plan provisions, whether or not they are contained in a separate document from the trust, deal with such matters as participation, vesting, benefit accrual, and retirement eligibility, among others.

The trust provisions govern such matters as the trustee's standard of fiduciary responsibility, powers, and investment duties.

The trust documents also generally contain the anti-alienation rule of Code Section 401(a)(B). A trustee shall not be a qualified trust unless the plan of which it is a part prohibits the assignment or alienation of plan benefits. This helps ensure that the plan benefits will be available for distribution to participants and beneficiaries upon retirement. The Retirement Equity Act of 1984 provides a limited exception to the general anti-alienation rule for certain qualified domestic relations orders.

A qualified trust is a trust created or organized in the United States. This rule does not prohibit a U.S. trust from holding foreign assets, with certain exceptions. The trustee must hold the plan assets in a manner that renders them subject to the jurisdiction of the U.S. district courts.

Plan Must Be Established by the Employer

A qualified plan must be established and maintained by the employer. Employee and employer contributions are allowed. A qualified plan can also consist entirely of employee contributions, so long as it is established by an employer. An affiliated group of employers may establish a common plan and, in the case of a profit-sharing plan, profitable members of the group can make certain "make-up" contributions on behalf of an employer who failed to make a profit for the plan year.

The employer must act affirmatively to adopt the plan. For corporations, this generally means that the adoption of the plan must comply with the relevant state requirements for similar corporate acts. The plan should be presented to the board of directors at the annual or special meeting held before the proposed effective date. The plan can then be adopted by a board resolution. Once the plan is formally adopted, the board may delegate day-to-day administrative authority, including securing a favorable determination letter from the IRS, to the plan's attorney or actuary or to a subcommittee of the full board.

Plan Must Be Communicated to Employees

The existence of the plan and its basic terms must be communicated to employees. This communication is to be "written in a manner calculated to be understood by the average plan participant and . . . sufficiently accurate and comprehensive to reasonably apprise such participants and beneficiaries of their rights and obligations under the plan."[*]

The statute requires a written notice in addition to a summary plan description (SPD). The employer can satisfy both requirements by providing employees with an appropriately drafted SPD as notification of the plan terms.

Summary

Pension plans can be either defined contribution or defined benefit programs. Various plans can be designed that fit under either of these two definitions.

In order to decide which plan (or combination of plans) best suits your requirements, you should analyze your business from the point of view of who your employees are, your annual profitability and the stability thereof, and your own personal characteristics and requirements. Each of the plans has definite rules, and some of the plans require that you commit to an annual amount that must be paid to the plan. Some of the plans have greater flexibility than others, and some plans provide a degree of latitude in providing greater benefits to owners.

There are a number of resources that can be drawn upon to help you to analyze your options as well as provide ongoing administration for your programs. Your accountant or attorney is a good place to start.

Suggested Reading

[*] Source: Employee Retirement Income Security Act of 1974 (ERISA).

37 | Short-Term and Long-Term Personal Financial Planning

BARRY A. LITZER

The financial world is foreign to most people. It is the lack of familiarity with financial concepts that inhibits making appropriate decisions. However, with a little reading, figuring, and planning, you can make the right choices for yourself and your family.

The Need for Financial Planning

Not too many years ago financial planning was much simpler. You put money into a savings account, bought some insurance, and hoped for the best. Then came a series of changes that left the financial system in the United States forever altered. Interest rates, which used to move half a percentage point at a time, at most, began to move sharply up and down. Inflation hit double digits, then plummeted. The government continued to change the rules by enacting four major tax bills over a five-year period. These factors, combined with the partial deregulation of banks and other financial institutions, brought hundreds of new investment possibilities to the average person. People began to realize that the decisions they made about budgeting, credit, taxes, investments, insurance, and retirement planning could affect the quality of their lives—today and in the future.

Common Concerns

Professional people also have issues confronting them which can be addressed only with an organized approach. Among the primary concerns are the following:

- Expectations for relatively high life style
- Income does not significantly exceed expenditures
- Investments may not keep up with inflation
- Retirement plan payments may be insufficient to meet needs at retirement
- Taxes
- General uneasiness due to the lack of an organized and systematic approach to family financial management

Developing an overall strategy from an informed perspective is the only practical way to address these concerns.

A good financial plan should consist of a few basic but very important elements:

- Goal setting—short and long term
- Budgeting
- Establishing and monitoring your net worth
- Realistic projections of income from salary, business profits, and investments
- Asset allocation—portfolio diversification
- Tax planning
- Estate planning
- Retirement planning

Goal Setting

It is essential to set realistic goals for your investments. This will help you to make appropriate investment decisions, allow you to establish investment parameters, and enable you to maintain the proper diversification in your portfolio. Your personal financial goals might include some or all of the following:

- Purchase of a home
- Savings
- Funding children's education
- Retirement
- Capital reserve for starting or expanding business
- Emergency funds
- Adequate insurance protection
- Reducing taxes
- Building investment portfolio
- Annual income and total return expectations from your investment portfolio
- Travel/vacations
- Other major expenditures (second home, R.V., boat, etc.)

Your expectations must also be realistic. For example, you cannot expect an income-oriented investment to yield 20% annually if interest rates overall are 10% to 12% without taking on an undue or inappropriate degree of risk.

Your portfolio should be reviewed regularly (i.e., quarterly, semi-annually, or annually) so that adjustments can be made as necessary. Any investment professional should be willing to provide you with regular profit and loss reports and income statements.

The main objective is to attain the highest possible total return (income + capital appreciation) over a long period of time, while maintaining the proper risk/reward ratio in your portfolio. At a 10% average annual yield, your portfolio will double in 7.2 years; at 15%, in 4.8 years.

Keep in mind that goals can be changed and/or adjusted. They should be flexible enough to reflect changes in your income level and availability of investment capital. Further, they should allow for new investment opportunities.

Investment Allocation

Your portfolio should consist of various investment instruments, balanced according to your personal investment profile. No single investment is appropriate in all circumstances. Rather, it is the combination of your investment holdings working together that will enable you to achieve your goals. A proper investment allocation strategy will help you construct a diversified portfolio tailored to your personal situation.

Investment Attitudes

What type of investor do you consider yourself to be? (See Fig. 37.1 below.)

Investments with little risk of principal fluctuation typically produce relatively low returns in the form of income. Investments seeking higher returns through capital appreciation normally experience fluctuations in principal and enjoy a lesser degree of liquidity. Figure 37.2 will help you to choose the investment return characteristics for which you are best suited. For example, if you are a relatively aggressive investor—say, an "8"—20% of your investments might be income producing whereas the balance might be allocated principally for their growth potential.

Your Investment Profile

To develop an appropriate investment strategy, you need to first assess your investment profile. Several essential factors should be considered, including your risk tolerance, age, portfolio size, level of income, and liquidity needs. Your investment decisions should be consistent with your personal goals and investment attitudes.

Second, your investment decisions should reflect the current economic outlook and opportunities available in the financial marketplace as well as provide for present portfolio holdings. Taken together with your invest-

Conservative				Moderate			Aggressive		
1	2	3	4	5	6	7	8	9	10

Figure 37.1. Investor type

Income

100%	90%	80%	70%		50%		30%	20%	10%	0%
1	2	3	4	5	6	7	8	9	10

0%   10%   20%   30%   50%   70%   80%   90% 100%
Growth

Figure 37.2. Investment return characteristics

ment profile, these factors culminate in an appropriate investment allocation being developed for your portfolio.

Once an appropriate allocation of your holdings is derived, the next step is to examine the various types of investments available and determine whether their characteristics are suitable for your situation.

Investment Characteristics

Investments can be generally categorized as offering the following characteristics:

Liquidity. Liquid investments provide you with access to your funds for short-term or unexpected needs, afford principal protection, but offer relatively low returns.

Safety of principal. Such investments offer reasonable returns of current income with little risk of principal fluctuation. They are the investments that offer a secure foundation in a portfolio.

Purchasing power protection. These vehicles afford protection against inflation eroding the value of your money. These investments generally are based upon real assets rather than financial assets.

Capital appreciation. These investments provide potential growth of capital with reasonable safety of principal. They are the principal element in building your overall wealth for the future.

Aggressive capital appreciation. For investors willing to accept an above-average level of risk, these investments offer potentially higher returns. These investments are often characterized by significant principal fluctuations and are therefore better suited for longer-term diversified investment portfolios.

Currency fluctuation protection. These investments have historically provided investors a hedge against adverse currency fluctuations in the international economic climate. They can provide protection against unstable and unpredictable political and economic environments.

Figure 37.3 illustrates how an investment allocation may appear for a

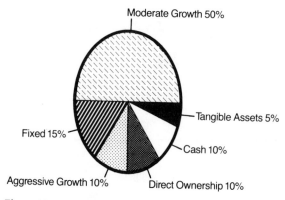

Figure 37.3. Recommended investment allocation

person who is more interested in growth of capital with moderate risk than in current investment income, as indicated by Level Six in Figure 37.1.

Investment Categories

Cash or Cash Equivalents

Money market funds

Tax-free money market funds

Short-term certificates of deposit

Short-term municipal obligations

Intermediate government funds

Fixed-Income Investments

Municipal bonds

Fixed rate annuity/fixed rate life insurance

Government agency obligations

Corporate convertible bonds

Government mortgage obligations

Moderate Growth Investments

Variable rate annuity-variable rate life insurance

Blue chip common stock

Common stock with covered option strategies

Common stock—broad-based issues

Aggressive Growth Investments

   Option growth mutual funds

   Managed commodities accounts

   Aggressive growth mutual funds

   Global growth mutual funds

Direct Ownership Investments

   Energy-producing income programs

   Leveraged real estate programs

   Net lease programs

Tangible Assets

   Gold and silver coins

   Precious metal and mining company stocks

   Timber company stocks

Changes in your personal situation can trigger the need to reposition assets. For example, a change in your income, tax status, or family responsibilities should alert you to the need to reexamine your investment portfolio and financial goals.

External factors, including changes in economic conditions, tax laws, and new investment opportunities, may affect how well your current portfolio is meeting your needs, even if your goals and personal situation have not changed.

Estate Planning

Estate planning is an important part of financial planning which is often misunderstood. In simple terms, it may be defined as lifetime planning for the passage of assets in the event of your death in accordance with the estate owner's wishes and at the least possible tax cost. A properly structured estate plan allows you to choose your beneficiaries, provide for the management of your assets, and eliminate or reduce estate taxes. Without careful planning, your estate may pass to unintended beneficiaries or be reduced in value by unnecessary taxes or unsound investments.

Estate planning also addresses such questions as who should own property, what property to own, and how it should be owned—jointly or separately.

Further points to consider are whether trusts are needed for management or tax savings and whether lifetime gifts should be made.

Passage of Assets

Should you draw up a will? Experience has proved the wisdom of those who executed a properly planned will. By doing so, they ensured that their property would go where they wished and that those who would be faced with the settlement of the estate could do the job as efficiently as possible. If you do not draft a will your probate property will be distributed according to laws of the state in which you resided at the time of your death. This may result in unnecessary federal and state death taxes. A will may not control the distribution of all of your assets. Some assets pass outside the control of the will. The will does not control those assets that pass because of their nature of ownership or by contract. Property that passes under a will is called *probate property* because it is subject to the supervision of the probate court or probate fees (see Table 37.1).

Nonprobate assets include:

1. Assets owned jointly with the right of survivorship which will pass to the surviving joint owner. (An example might be a married couple's home, except in community property states).
2. Assets held in trust which will pass in accordance with the trust agreement.
3. Life insurance proceeds which will be paid to beneficiaries. (This includes your group life insurance.)
4. Pension, profit sharing, deferred compensation, or other corporate plans as well as individual retirement or Keogh accounts, which will be paid to the beneficiaries you designate on the beneficiary form.

All other property is categorized as probate property, which will be distributed according to the terms of your will and under the supervision of the probate court. Such assets include personal property, real estate, and assets for which you have named your estate as beneficiary.

Table 37.1 The Cost of Probate

Assets	Minimum fees
$ 200,000	$ 10,300
300,000	14,300
400,000	18,300
500,000	22,300
750,000	32,300
1,000,000	42,300
2,000,000	62,300
3,000,000	82,300
5,000,000	122,300

California's probate fees—set by law—are about average among states. These fees to settle an estate in court don't include special fees for the sale of assets, tax preparation, and litigation.

Trusts are frequently used in conjunction with wills. A trust is created when the owner of property transfers an asset to a trustee to manage on behalf of specified beneficiaries, subject to directions contained in the trust agreement as well as to guidelines established by state law. Trusts can provide the benefits of professional management, tax savings, flexibility, and privacy. A variety of trusts can be created to implement your specific objectives. Trusts may be revocable or irrevocable, short term or long term, effective during your lifetime or dormant until your death, funded or unfunded. More Americans are putting their assets in revocable living trusts. In such a plan, titles to real estate, securities, and other assets are placed in a trust while the owners are still alive. The trust document outlines instructions for managing the assets and distributing them after the individual's death. The people who create the trust can act as their own trustees, so there are no management fees or loss of control. They can change the trust at any time.

The advantages of living trusts over wills are considerable. Under a will an estate must be settled in probate court. Lawyer's fees and court costs often are substantial; there may be exasperating delays, and the proceedings are a matter of public record. In contrast, a living trust is settled without a court proceeding; a successor trustee simply distributes assets according to the trust's instructions, with an accountant, notary public, or lawyer certifying any transfer of titles. The process is much quicker, cheaper, and more private than settling a will, and it may save on estate taxes.

Trusts can be contested, but not as easily as contesting a will. When an estate goes to probate in some states, the court freezes its assets for four months and invites anyone to come forward and contest the will. Someone contesting the will does not even need to hire a lawyer. However, to contest a trust, a disgruntled heir needs to hire a lawyer and file a civil suit. The assets of a living trust are not frozen, however, and the trustee can distribute them to the beneficiaries immediately. The disgruntled heir then would have to sue each beneficiary.

Many other kinds of trusts are used for estate planning, but the revocable living trust is growing in popularity. An irrevocable living trust offers the same advantages of avoiding probate and perhaps saving on estate taxes, but causes problems because it cannot be changed. A testamentary trust, created after death, must go through probate.

Estate and Gift Taxes

Simply stated, an estate tax is a tax upon the value of all property owned by a decedent which is transferred or transmitted to the decedent's heirs or beneficiaries upon the decedent's death. On the other hand, an inheritance tax is a tax on the value of property received by an heir or beneficiary on account of the decedent's death.

The federal government imposes a gift tax on lifetime gifts and an estate tax on transfers at death. The estate tax is based on the market value of your property, cash accounts, securities, partnership interests, real estate, personal and group life insurance, individual retirement accounts, pension and profit sharing plans, deferred compensation, and stock options. Since the federal estate tax rates start at 37% and increase with the size of your estate, the estate planning process should emphasize reducing or eliminating these taxes. This may be accomplished by taking maximum advantage of deductions and credits that include:

1. the "unified credit," which exempts a specified amount of your estate from tax ($600,000 as of January 1, 1987);
2. the "unlimited marital deduction," which permits married couples to postpone the tax until the survivor's death; and
3. deductions for funeral expenses and other costs associated with administering the estate (eg, attorney fees and court costs).

For the married person who wants the spouse to inherit some or all of the estate, the marital deduction is the easiest way to eliminate federal estate taxes. In order to qualify property in your estate for this deduction, it must benefit your spouse in one of two ways: either the assets must pass directly to the spouse or they must be held in trust that benefits the spouse's estate exclusively. If one of these requirements is met, you may leave your spouse as much property as you desire without incurring federal estate taxation upon your death. However, unnecessary taxation may result upon the death of the surviving spouse if you and your spouse's estate exceeds $600,000.

Lifetime Gifts

Next to the marital deduction and unified credit, gift giving is probably the most common form of reducing estate taxes. Lifetime gifts are subject to a federal gift tax, which is imposed at the same rate as the estate tax. However, you are entitled to give up to $10,000 ($20,000 if you are married) annually to each of as many persons as you like without paying gift tax or having to file a gift tax return. For example, if you are married and have two children and two grandchildren, you and your spouse together can give $20,000 annually to each of the four young family members for a total of $80,000 annually. Gifts that exceed the annual exclusion will, however, reduce the amount that can be transferred tax free at your death, because they will use up the credit that would otherwise be available to your estate. In addition, tuition directly paid to a school for another person is not a taxable gift, nor is the payment of medical expenses paid directly to the provider.

Executors and Trustees

The need for a professional executor and/or trustee will depend in large part upon the complexity of your personal and financial circumstances.

However, any executor that you select should have the professional expertise to manage the portion of your estate left in trust. If you appoint your
spouse as executor and/or cotrustee you may also appoint a professional
coexecutor and/or cotrustee to assist your spouse.

Summary

There are many more aspects to financial planning, but they all cannot be
covered in one chapter. However, many good financial professionals are
available to help you develop and implement a financial plan.

Choose a financial professional carefully. Experience and expertise are
very important. However it is important to choose a professional with
whom you can be comfortable. It is not necessary to hire a financial planner
who will charge you a fee just to develop a financial plan. Instead, most
financial professionals should be willing to work with you to develop,
implement, and administer a financial plan on an ongoing basis as part of a
working relationship.

A proper investment strategy is a road map to your long-term financial
future.

Suggested Reading

Brosterman, Robert, and Brosterman, Thomas, *The Complete Estate Planning Guide.*
  Chula Vista, CA: Mentor, 1990.

Clifford, Denis, *Plan Your Estate.* Berkeley, CA: Nolo Press.

Dolan, Ken, and Dolan, Daria, *Smart Money.* New York: Berkeley Publishing Group,
  1990.

38 | Adding a Partner or Physician Associate

LAWRENCE LEITER, MD, MBA

Adding a partner or physician associate to one's practice has both advantages and disadvantages. If approached in an organized manner, the process of interviewing and hiring an associate can be a rewarding one. However, the process also has its frustrations. This chapter will present some basic strategies for a successful search.

Determine Need and Locate Candidates

The first step in adding a partner is to determine need. Need can be based on a variety of factors: increased volume of patients seen, a projected increase of patient volume, or the imminent loss of a present associate. The managing partner (or sole proprietor) should make the decision to add a partner very carefully, because to hire a qualified person and then be forced to lay off this physician because of a lack of business would be disastrous. In assessing the need for a partner, you should outline on paper the projected volume of increase for your practice. If you are certain that the need exists, the next step will be to locate your applicants.

Advertising for a Partner

There are four ways to find potential partners or employees. The first way is to place an advertisement in a journal. A commonly used outlet is the *Journal of the American Medical Association*. In most areas, the local county medical association journal is an excellent choice. One common misconception about placing ads is that they will immediately bear fruit; it can sometimes take as long as a year before an ad is answered by an appropriate candidate.

It is important to compose your ad in the most desirable way possible. Do some preliminary research—read through the advertising section of your target journals to get an idea of how others present their positions to be filled. Try to frame your ad in a comparable way. You may want to respond to other ads to inquire about salary and working terms, so that you can compare those with what you are offering. Table 38.1 gives a list of items to include in your ad; Table 38.2 is a sample advertisement.

Table 38.1 Physician/P.A. Advertising

Things to Include in an Advertisement:
1. General description of location
2. General description of practice
3. Urgency of opening
4. Salary
5. Requires board certification or eligibility
6. Specialty needed
7. Benefits
8. Opportunity for partnership after one year

Headhunters May Be Helpful

Headhunters can be a second source for partner candidates. Some practices report good results from using a headhunter, while others have experienced disappointments. It may be useful to consult other medical groups for references so that you can select a good headhunter. Remember that headhunters will coach their applicants to make them as presentable as possible. Despite a headhunter's assurances that he or she has selected only candidates who meet your needs, this may not always be the case. Sometimes the applicant only *appears* to meet your needs, and you may need to do additional background checks to corroborate information furnished by the headhunter.

Residency Training

Certainly, if one can penetrate a residency program, this can be a worthwhile third source of potential candidates. Generally, though, people who are hired from a residency training program have come from referral directly or indirectly related to current associates. Residency programs are frequently controlled by headhunters or other physicians who work in the residency for the purpose of filling positions in their offices.

The Old Standby: Word of Mouth

The fourth and final source of potential applicants is often through word of mouth. Let your associates and colleagues know that you are looking for a

Table 38.2 Sample Advertisement

Board Certified or eligible family practitioner and pediatrician needed for rapidly growing multispecialty group of 15 physicians in the Southern California area. Excellent starting salary and benefits. Opportunity for partnership after one year. (state phone number).

partner. Mention your search at association gatherings, even social gatherings. Sometimes the best candidates come through referrals by friends or associates.

The Telephone Interview

There are many phases to the process of hiring a partner. At each step of the way, you will be filtering through candidates, eliminating some and going further with others. The telephone interview is the first step in this process. Keep in mind that in addition to the actual accomplishments and qualifications of the candidate, you should like the person. There is no replacement for your positive response to a person.

Talking to the applicant over the telephone can give you some sense of his or her expectations of the job. You may decide to eliminate some applicants at this stage. For those who sound satisfactory, send them a copy of your partnership contract and request that they, in turn, send their curricula vitae (CVs) to you.

Researching the CV

It is extremely important to review the CV of each applicant carefully. Some partnerships go so far as to require that applicants obtain letters vouching for their character and abilities. Whether you choose this method or another, the object is to verify your applicant's verbal and written representations. Some additional ways to verify the CV include calling the Board of Medical Quality Assurance, the local medical association, and people with whom the applicant has worked.

Gaps in an applicant's CV might indicate periods of time that the person does not wish to reveal. Investigate these, if you can, by questioning either the applicant or his or her references. Keep an open mind on the subject of training and degrees. An internship at a prestigious institution does not necessarily guarantee a superior physician. Some graduates of foreign medical schools can work out well, and there are no generalizations that hold true about graduates of U.S. schools always working well.

After you have reviewed the applicant's CV, the next step is to arrange the personal interview.

The Personal Interview

The purpose of the personal interview is to meet with your applicant and to discuss questions the applicant may have regarding your partnership contract and any questions you have regarding his or her CV.

Some practices have existing formulas for paying associate physicians. These formulas often include health insurance and other benefits in addition to a fair salary. If you have not hired a partner previously, you should consult an attorney to draw up the contract.

Make sure that every aspect of your contract is clear. It is crucial that your candidate understands his or her responsibilities and what you expect of him or her. In addition, you need to know what your prospective associate expects of you—especially in the areas of working hours and salary; misunderstandings at this stage of the partnership can portend major problems to come. The objective is to find an applicant who is happy with the arrangement you are offering, so that you (not to mention your patients) do not have to go through the aggravation of switching from one physician to another.

Most applicants will have questions concerning the proposed contract. This is not unusual; indeed, it should be encouraged so that you have the opportunity to clarify any questions. However, there are some warning flags that can signal potential problems. When the applicant has many, many questions and/or wants to make a lot of changes to the contract, this can predict problems.

Too much concern about the benefits offered, about the practice's reputation in the community, about the issue of life insurance, and so on, can also signal problems. Some potential employers may feel that these questions demonstrate the candidate's basic distrust, which will make it difficult to work with him or her. Some employers believe that the fewer the questions, the easier it will be to work with the person. This may or may not be your belief. However, if coming to terms is too much work, the question to ask yourself is, Do I want this person as a partner? If the encounter already seems difficult, perhaps this is not a person with whom you would be comfortable working.

As with hiring any employee, you should note certain details when you meet with applicants. Did the applicant dress in a way that you feel is appropriate? Dressing well does not mean that the physician will always dress appropriately when seeing patients, but it does connote a concern and respect for making a good appearance during this business encounter.

Assuming the personal interview goes well, the next meeting will be with your existing partners, yourself, and the applicant. The person responsible for hiring may feel that he or she has all the answers. This is an attitude to be avoided if you want the hiring of a new associate to go smoothly. It is important to see whether the other partners have something valuable to contribute. In addition, excluding the other partners from the hiring decision can sabotage the new person's adjustment to the practice.

Other Considerations

The third meeting can be considered a social meeting. The candidate and his or her spouse (or significant other) are invited out to dinner with the hiring partner and spouse.

Some authorities on techniques for hiring partners do not place emphasis on the candidate's mate. However, a candidate's spouse can be extremely important. Emotional issues in relationships will often have an effect on a person's job performance. If a spouse visits the office too much, asks meddlesome or overly personal questions about the practice, or is overly involved in the spouse's career, you are essentially including that person in your office partnership. This can place undue stress on your future working relationship. Whether you are dealing with a male or female applicant, the spouse's career should at least be discussed. With two-career couples, conflict can arise when one gets a job offer in another city or state. As the hiring partner, you should be concerned about the stability of your candidate's mate and should take such possibilities into account when evaluating your candidate.

When interviewing physician candidates of a race or religion different from yours, openness is essential. Talking openly about the candidate's race and religious beliefs contributes to understanding and mutual trust.

Generally, it is best if your prospective partner lives in or intends to move to your community. If the physician lives more than 15 to 20 minutes' drive from the office, you may have problems covering office hours during periods of high volume or absence attributable to illness and other factors.

Some management groups recommend that the prospective physician make a complete evaluation of the hiring physician and the partnership. Although this may be helpful to your candidate in making a decision about an offer, it can also create problems. Depending on who they talk to, you may or may not appear in a favorable light.

If the prospective partner wants to bring in a consultant to evaluate your business, you may have a problem. Some physicians may not be concerned about such a request; however, the consultant may not be competent. In order to assure the applicant that they are earning their money, consultants sometimes find fault with elements in a practice which are not critical and may tell the applicant to modify the partnership contract. This can cause other problems arising from rivalries with existing partners.

Hire for One Year

Assuming that your candidate checks out well, is acceptable to your associates, and is a person with whom you believe you can work well, you may want to hire him or her for an initial one-year period. After one year's time you can determine whether this person is eligible for partnership. A one-year trial period is usually a good idea because any problems will almost certainly have surfaced within that time. How those problems are confronted and solved by your new associate, yourself, and your other partners will be invaluable considerations in making the decision of whether to extend a partnership offer.

Business partnerships have often been compared with marriages. Using that analogy, keep in mind that it is not so much the problems as the handling of the problems that should determine whether you stay in the relationship. Has there been an uncomfortable level of stress when dealing with your new associate? If you think you would be better off without the relationship, perhaps you should not offer a full partnership contract.

As with any venture, the more information you have about the process of hiring a partner, the better. Begin your search with a clear idea of your practice's needs and advance to filling those needs with the best possible candidate.

39 | Practice Mergers and Forming a Medical Group

ROBERT A. STEINBERG, ESQ.

This article addresses some of the legal and practical considerations that arise when physicians with existing practices (hereinafter called *individual practices*) combine their individual practices into a single integrated medical group. This chapter does not address the establishment of a new practice by physicians, or the expansion of an existing practice by the addition of one or more partners or associates. Instead, this chapter will focus on the reasons for forming a medical group and the reasons not to form a medical group, the mechanics of forming a medical group, and some of the operational issues physicians must confront when melding their practices.

Reasons to Form a Medical Group

There are two basic types of group medical practices: single-specialty and multispecialty groups. Many of the reasons for forming a medical group are common to both these types, but there are certain differences.

The primary reason to form a medical group, regardless of type, is simply economics: the sharing of costs and personnel. The economics of group practice, however, manifests itself in other ways as well. For example, although two obstetricians may benefit by joining together to eliminate duplicative office space, equipment, and personnel, additional profit may be derived by a group practice of physicians with complementary practices. These complementary practices afford the opportunity for cross-referrals, increasing the aggregate available patient base per physician.

The ability to cross-refer patients is obviously greatest with the larger multispecialty medical groups. Individual physicians within these groups form a network of primary care and specialty care physicians who can provide virtually all of the medical care needs of a patient. Such groups constitute, in essence, the medical equivalent of "one-stop shopping." Such groups, because of their economic clout, have significant leverage in their relationships with third parties, including insurance carriers, hospitals, and suppliers of medical equipment and other supplies. Such economic clout is a principal reason and benefit of forming a large multispecialty group.

Many of the foregoing benefits also apply to single-specialty groups. Here, the opportunity for cross-referral is at least as great. Moreover, there are the additional benefits of scheduling flexibility to accommodate an individual physician's personal life-style. If a physician knows that another member of the group is available to handle a patient's needs, he or she will be less likely to feel uncomfortable in taking time away from the practice for personal needs.

An additional benefit of forming a medical group may arise if various legislative proposals that would prohibit most patient referrals of Medicare patients are ultimately implemented. Most forms of such legislation would exempt referrals within an integrated medical group from the general prohibition against patient referrals. Consequently, if a particular referral network of unaffiliated physicians desires to maintain its ability to cross-refer after the enactment of such proposed legislation, it could continue to do so simply by forming an integrated medical group.

Another benefit of going into group practice is the greater time availability resulting from each participating physician's proportionately smaller involvement in managerial and administrative matters. To the extent that physicians are no longer responsible for running their entire practice, they presumably have additional time available for their other professional and personal needs.

There are certain disadvantages of group practice, however. Perhaps principal among these is the loss of autonomy that an individual practitioner previously enjoyed. The physician no longer has complete control over his or her practice. Instead, the physician must answer to his or her partner or partners. For this reason, a major fundamental issue arises when considering the formation of a medical group: compatibility with one's partners. Without such compatibility and mutual trust, the new medical group is in all likelihood doomed to failure.

A second significant disadvantage of group practice is the loss of flexibility with respect to certain business aspects of the practice. For example, administrative commitments, compensation arrangements with partners, pension plans, and certain other commitments (financial or otherwise) are circumscribed by the needs of the group as a whole rather than the individual desires of the group's members.

In sum, when determining whether to form a medical group, and with whom, it must at all times be recalled that the practice of medicine also constitutes a profit-making activity. In conducting the business of medicine, one should choose one's partners wisely and with full awareness of both the benefits and detriments group practice will provide.

How to Form a Group Practice

Once it has been decided to combine individual practices into a group practice, the actual mechanics of formation must be considered. Although fundamentally this decision primarily belongs in the province of lawyers and accountants, the physicians should be aware of the business implications of the decision. Moreover, at a minimum, the physician should be able to converse in the vocabulary of his or her other professional advisors so that he or she understands the implications of the decision. This section will therefore address the types of legal entities that may serve as vehicles for group medical practice; it will then discuss the methods of accomplishing the combination of individual practices into a single group practice, and it will consider the relevant tax issues that arise from both the choice of entity and the method of combination.

Types of Legal Entities

There are two primary legal entities that serve as vehicles for group medical practice: corporations and general partnerships (hereinafter called simply *partnerships*). These two are the only entities recognized by most state laws as appropriate for the conduct of a profession. Moreover, there are combinations of these two entities—and variations on each entity—which may also afford suitable vehicles for the group practice.

There are two primary differences between a partnership and a corporation. First, a partnership is a so-called pass-through entity—that is, all of its tax attributes are shared directly pro rata by the partners. That is not the case with a corporation, which is a taxable entity separate from its shareholders. Because both the corporation and its shareholders are subject to taxation, the tax burden of corporate conduct of a group practice is somewhat greater than the tax burden imposed on a partnership. A partnership form of group practice exposes the individual partners to the general liabilities of the partnership, whereas a corporation is a limited liability entity and its shareholders are generally shielded from personal liability for corporation debts (other than professional malpractice liabilities).

These differences in practice are sometimes muddied. For example, a group medical practice may be a partnership of professional corporations, in which case the physician shareholders of each professional corporation partner may not be personally subject to the liabilities of the partnership in many instances. Moreover, most such partnership liabilities can be insured against, thus reducing the risk to the individual partners, whether or not they are independently incorporated.

On the other hand, a corporate group practice may achieve the primary benefit of a partnership (namely, a single level of taxation on corporate profits) by electing under applicable tax law to be an "S corporation." An S corporation has elected under the Internal Revenue Code and relevant state law to be subject to tax in the same general manner as a partnership. Thus the S corporation itself generally is not subject to federal income taxation at all, and the shareholders will be taxed on their pro rata share of each item of the S corporation's income, gain, loss, and deductions. (Some states do not recognize S corporations as a pass-through tax entity at all, however, and other states, such as California, will impose a corporate-level tax on them which is generally lower than the basic corporate tax rates.)

Even if the shareholders decline to elect S corporation status, or the corporation cannot qualify to be an S corporation, a single level of taxation may nonetheless be achieved simply by paying out what otherwise would be corporate profits as deductible bonuses or other compensation to the physician-shareholders. There are certain limitations on a corporation's ability to "zero out" its profits in this manner, but if the aggregate compensation payable to each physician is "reasonable," then the result achieved can be virtually identical to that of a partnership.

Methods of Forming a Medical Group

If it is determined to conduct the group medical practice as a partnership, then the physician members simply need to enter into a partnership agreement to form the group practice. It will be of critical importance for the physicians to anticipate concerns that may arise during the life of the medical group and to address those concerns in their partnership agreement. Obvious issues of importance are the method of compensation, the method of and criteria for bringing in new partners, how profits are to be allocated, the size of the capital contributions of each partner, whether partners must be individuals or may be permitted to be professional corporations, how control of the partnership is to be allocated among the partners, and creation of a dispute resolution mechanism among the partners if they are unable to agree with respect to any subsequently arising issue.

Partners may desire to delegate management control to a management or executive committee. If so, careful thought must be given to the nature of the powers to be delegated to such a committee and its size and makeup. For example, such a committee might operate in the same manner as the board of directors or officers of a corporation might operate. That is, the management committee might be empowered to make and/or implement policy for the group. How large or small to make the committee would in large part be a function of the size of the group itself. If there are too few members of the committee empowered with too great authority, then the committee may not be adequately representative of the desires of the members of the group. Conversely, too large a management committee could defeat the reasons for its formation, in that authority will not be adequately centralized for making appropriate management decisions that need not concern the individual partners. Other issues of importance with respect to the management committee are the term of office of committee members, the vote necessary for both electing and removing members of the committee, criteria for selection, criteria for removal, and clear enumeration of the committee's authority. To a very large extent, the resolution of these issues will reflect the degree of trust and desire for autonomy of the individual members of the group.

Another important issue to resolve is who may be a member of the partnership. There may be differences of opinion as to the future growth of the partnership, both in terms of size and the qualifications of future partners. Some physicians may want to aggressively recruit other physicians and rapidly expand the partnership, whereas others may want to maintain a smaller organization. Some physicians may desire to establish qualifications for members of the group so that only a limited number of a selected class of physicians may be included. Such limitations may be desired because (a) the medical group may wish to restrict its practice to a specific geographical area or (b) it may wish to limit the scope of its practice to one or more specialties. These kinds of issues *can* be dealt with after the group's formation. It is probably better, however, to discuss these issues in advance so that the issues can be dispassionately resolved.

Many of the foregoing issues are also relevant to the formation of a corporate group practice. These issues could be resolved through a shareholder agreement among the shareholders or through provisions in the instruments of corporate governance (namely, the corporation's articles or certificate of incorporation and/or its bylaws). Indeed, in many states, such as California, many of the issues involving corporate control (such as shareholder or director qualifications) must be addressed in the corporation's governing instruments in order to have legal effect.

The manner in which the corporate group practice is formed is somewhat more complex than the formation of a partnership. The reason is that corporation law, unlike partnership law, is primarily set forth in statutes, which can be modified only in very specific cases. The two primary methods of combining practices into a single corporation are (a) combining the separate practices into one of the existing corporations (the combination method) and (b) forming an entirely new corporation into which the assets of the individual practices can be contributed in exchange for shares of the new corporation (the corporate formation method). Moreover, there are combinations and variants of those methods that may be appropriate in particular instances. Although these methods are superficially similar, there are significant corporate law and tax law differences that mandate that the choice of corporate group practice formation be examined closely.

Before proceeding to such examination, however, it is pertinent to note that the professional corporation laws of many states require that the shareholders of the professional corporation be individuals. Corporate shareholders in those states are prohibited. Thus under either the combination method or the corporate formation method, the end result must be the elimination of the physicians' individual professional corporations and the replacement of those corporations by one single group corporation that is collectively owned by the individual physicians themselves.

Combinations of the individual practices under the combination method can be accomplished in several ways under relevant corporate and tax law. One way is the direct merger under state law of separate professional corporations into one of the existing individual corporations (the surviving corporation) or into a newly formed corporation (the merger variant). This merger will be tax free (except as indicated below) but has the drawback that the new or surviving corporation by operation of law will be assuming all of the existing and contingent liabilities of each individual corporation. Physicians who wish to combine their practices may understandably not desire to assume each others' preexisting liabilities. For this reason, a simple merger of corporations may be unacceptable in certain circumstances.

A second variant of the combination method is what is styled by the tax law as a "C" reorganization (the C reorganization variant, named after the subsection of the Internal Revenue Code, Section 368(a)(1)(C), in which this method is described). Essentially, this method involves the contribution of substantially all of the assets of the existing corporations into the new corporation (or the surviving corporation) in exchange for the stock of that corporation. In order to be effective, however, the shareholders of the former individual corporations must in the aggregate own not less than 80% of the stock of the new corporation immediately after the transaction. Moreover, the existing individual corporations must be liquidated immediately after the transaction as part of the reorganization. This requirement is imposed by the relevant tax law but is also consistent with the professional corporation law of most states that require that the shareholders of a professional corporation be individuals.

The C reorganization variant may be preferred over the simple merger variant because the preexisting liabilities of the individual corporations remain with such corporations (assuming certain procedural technicalities are complied with, namely, the state's "bulk transfer" law). When the individual corporations are liquidated pursuant to the plan of reorganization, these liabilities will have to be paid off or otherwise provided for by the individual shareholders. Thus if the procedural requirements of state law are complied with, the new corporation should start afresh without the baggage of the preexisting liabilities of the former individual corporations.

The second method of combining individual practices, the corporate formation method, is most suitable in the circumstance where some of the separate practices are conducted by individuals rather than their corporations. The corporate formation method is like the C reorganization variant of the combination method, except that the assets are being contributed by individuals to a new corporation in exchange for stock in that new corporation. Like the C reorganization variant, the corporate formation method is also tax free, assuming that the former individual practitioners in the aggregate own at least 80% of the stock of the new corporation immediately following the transaction.

Each of the foregoing methods in most cases will not result in income taxation to physicians. If the new corporation, however, will be assuming liabilities of the old corporations (for example, bank loans, financing equipment leases, accounts payable, and similar liabilities), the amount of which exceeds the tax basis of the assets being acquired by the new corporation, then, to the extent of such excess, the old corporations and/or individuals who contributed such assets subject to such liabilities in exchange for stock in the new corporation will be subject to federal and state income taxation.

If the group practice is to be conducted as a corporation, it may be prudent for the corporation to elect to be a so-called close corporation under relevant state law. In many states, this election enables the shareholders to deal with one another as if they were true partners, while nonetheless conducting their business in a corporate form. The principal practical benefit of such an election is that the shareholders agreement in essence becomes a governing instrument of the corporation. In other words, profit allocations and control provisions contained in the shareholders' agreement, for example, will have the same efficacy as if they were set forth in the articles of incorporation and bylaws of the corporation. This circumstance permits the individual shareholders a wide degree of flexibility because they can make whatever changes they desire to their mutual arrangements without going through the administrative inconvenience of filing amended articles of incorporation. Physicians forming a group practice should consult with their professional advisors regarding the desirability of electing to be a close corporation.

Operational Issues

A number of business and operational issues must be addressed once it has been decided to form a group practice. The following section will address some of these issues.

Physical Plant

Prospective individual members of the nascent medical group will frequently be conducting their respective practices in more than one location prior to the group's formation. Initially it will be important to identify all of the existing obligations of the physicians in this regard and to ensure that such obligations can be met or terminated on a satisfactory basis. Then, even more importantly, it will be necessary to decide where the group's practice ought to be conducted. Such a decision will depend in large part upon the purposes for which the group is being formed. For example, if the individual physicians want the group to add new members and to grow over time, then they may need to take new space for the group which will contain room for such expansion. If, on the other hand, the group is being formed by only a few physicians, none of whom harbors any ambition to expand the size of the group significantly, then the existing offices of one or more members of the group may well be sufficient for anticipated needs. Such will especially be the case if the physicians are currently operating out of a single suite or on a single floor of the same building.

Physician Compensation Arrangements

This issue may well be the most difficult to address. As indicated earlier in this chapter, it is an issue that will need to be addressed in the partnership or shareholder agreement among the parties.

Retirement Plans

As part of physician compensation, it will be necessary to consider how best to combine existing retirement plans. Physician owners may be of different ages and have different interests in planning for retirement. Moreover, existing plans of some of the physicians may be incompatible in certain respects with the retirement plans of other physicians. In any event, once physicians determine to form a group practice, they will no longer be permitted to carry on their individual plans under relevant pension law and they will be required to agree upon some legally permissible method of amalgamating their plans.

Employees

Given that one of the principal purposes of forming a group practice is to achieve economies of scale and eliminate duplication of costs, it will, of course, be necessary to determine which employees of which individual practices will be retained and which will be let go. For example, a group practice rarely will need more than one receptionist and may not need more than a few nurses and technicians. In view of preexisting loyalties to employees, this issue may be a sensitive one for physicians. Nonetheless, unless the physicians take a realistic view toward their personnel needs, one of the primary benefits of group practice will be lost.

Insurance

In many cases, professional liability insurance carriers will not insure the new group practice entity unless all of the individual members of the group practice are covered by that same carrier. Thus one or more of the physician members of a group practice may have to switch carriers. Because physicians generally have claims-made coverage, it will be important to ensure that any such switch does not result in a "coverage gap." The physician switching carriers might have to maintain tail coverage regarding any unasserted claims. Alternatively, it is possible that the insurance carrier retained by the group might provide nose coverage, which will cover unasserted but preexisting claims.

Fee Schedules and Third-Party Payor Contracts

Individual members of the group may have utilized very different fee schedules when they were practicing independently. Generally, it will be necessary to consolidate such fee schedules. In addition, individual members of the group may have had different experiences with third-party payor arrangements. Some of the members may be involved in one or more independent practice associations (IPAs), and members may have individual contracts with various third-party payors, including HMOs and PPOs. In many cases the members will conclude that it would be best to transfer such agreements to the group itself, which will generally require the approval of the third-party payors. Alternatively, if the group decides that it is acceptable to allow members to maintain individual contracts with IPAs or third-party payors, the group should consider developing standards and protocols regarding such individual agreements, because such agreements, whether applicable on an individual or group basis, will have a financial impact on the group.

It is generally conceded that the health-care industry will continue to see accelerating growth in health-services contracting. One of the primary advantages of a group practice is that it gives the individual physicians increased opportunities and leverage in the contracting arena.

Medical Record Consolidation

Each individual practice that is consolidated into a group practice will have its own set of medical records. It will be very important for the physicians to decide how such records will be consolidated. In the long run, such medical records should generally be fully integrated, but in many cases the individual physicians may want to maintain segregated records for a limited period of time until they feel assured that the new medical group is viable.

Professional Advisers and Billing Services

As discussed earlier, many of the benefits of consolidating individual practices into a medical group are derived from the efficiencies of consolidating space and personnel. In addition, it is necessary to consider the consolidation of various services used by the individual physicians. First, it is essential that the physicians agree on the use of a single billing service; in fact, the increased volume of a group practice may enable the new group to negotiate a better rate than that available to any of the individual physicians. The physicians should also seek agreement on the use of professional advisers, including attorneys and accountants, for the new entity. (In this regard, it is often advantageous to have the same advisers for the individual physicians as the entity.)

Noncompetition Agreements

In working together in a group, the individual physicians will, in many cases, be sharing important information and opportunities with one another. If one of the physician members should subsequently leave, he or she could use such information to the significant competitive disadvantage of the medical group. Therefore many medical groups consider the adoption of noncompetition provisions precluding departing physicians from competing with the group during some reasonable period of time following departure. In many states such noncompetition provisions are enforceable only in certain circumstances.

Conclusion

Definite benefits are associated with group practice, but there are also certain drawbacks. Whether individual physicians should combine their practices, and how such combination is best accomplished, must be carefully considered in view of the many factors described in this chapter.

40 | Coping with Stress and Burnout

BARBARA L. INGRAM, PHD, AND
RICHARD S. CHUNG, MD

Wanted: highly skilled professional who can (1) remain sensitive, alert and all-knowing, even during long work days serving cranky or demanding clientele, (2) answer calls day and night from the ill and the distraught, and (3) juggle a growing load of paperwork unrelated to previous training. Also must be part accountant, part defense attorney, and part Prince Charming. Family sacrifices frequently a must and vacations sometimes few and far between. Prefer someone with lots of stamina, unending supply of compassion, and immunity to burnout. (Anne Scheck, 1989)

Stress has always been an inevitable consequence of the responsibilities, challenges, and long working hours of learning and practicing modern medicine. Today's physicians, however, are experiencing new demands and stresses, for which their medical training has not prepared them, as they cope with the bewildering array of "alphabet medicine" (PPOs, IPAs, HMOs, DRGs, etc.) and the increasing scrutiny from third-party payors and government agencies. The respect and reverence awarded to physicians in the past have been largely supplanted by attitudes of challenge, skepticism, and blame. "Defensive medicine" results from the fear of malpractice suits; even though high insurance premiums may protect against financial disaster, the emotional consequences of being sued can affect the physician's well-being for several years. One recent survey by Shortt even reports that fear of violence from patients can be added to the list of doctors' concerns.

A physician's stress level is affected by the social transformation of the U.S. health-care system in the last 20 years, through which concern with profit has displaced the traditional value of providing care. Only a minority of physicians work as independent practitioners. Over 50% work in group practice, most commonly a health maintenance organization (HMO), and are thus transformed from professionals into employees. The financial consequences of clinical decisions are scrutinized by people who are more concerned about profit and cost effectiveness than about quality of patient care. Stress comes not only from the loss of control over professional decisions but also, more painfully, from the erosion of ideals by the compromises of daily work life.

The following discussion proposes a method of identifying and dealing with stress and burnout, which threaten professional performance, emotional and physical well-being, and the mental health of the doctor's spouse and children. The high incidence among physicians of substance abuse, emotional disorders, suicide, and marital and family problems documents their need for better stress management tools.

Figure 40.1 presents a four-phase model of stress management, which incorporates education and prevention as well as the resolution of stress-related problems before they develop into professional impairment.

Understanding Stress and Burnout

Stress is a normal part of life and certainly an inevitable part of any career in medicine. Although this word generally has the negative connotation of hardship or adversity, its more accurate meaning is *strain on personal endurance*. Moderate levels of well-managed stress can motivate, stimulate, and provide challenge for creativity and heightened performance. Too

Figure 40.1. Model for coping with stress and burnout.

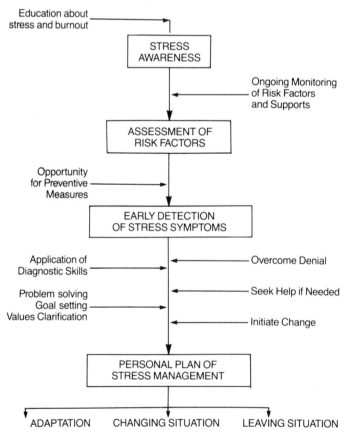

little stress—meaning the absence of any demand to cope—can be associated with boredom and lethargy. In contrast, stress that builds up beyond the individual's threshold of endurance will result in distressing physical and emotional symptoms and the potential for impairment in professional and interpersonal functioning.

Components of Stress

To reduce ambiguity and confusion, it is useful to study stress as a process that consists of four components of interaction.

Stressor: any stimulus that presents a demand to cope or respond. Stressors can be external (eg, loss of employment) as well as internal (eg, shame over imagined public ridicule). Life changes, whether positive or negative, function as stressors, and the accumulated stress-producing effect of unremarkable daily hassles can sometimes surpass that of dramatic disasters. In fact, with the exception of clearly traumatic stressors such as rape or airline disasters, clinically significant stress usually involves multiple strains whose impact is cumulative. The current psychiatric diagnostic system attempts to objectively quantify the severity of stressors. Consideration of cultural differences and learning history, however, is necessary to predict the actual severity level experienced by a specific individual.

Appraisal: cognitive labeling or interpretation of the stressor—for instance, the meaning attributed, the conclusion drawn, or the expectation violated. This cognitive appraisal determines whether the autonomic arousal elicited by the stressor will be experienced as distress or as a more positive emotion. For example, a physician berated by a dying patient may feel angry, depressed, and unappreciated; in contrast, the physician might actually feel pleased if he or she appraises the hostile reaction as a healthy sign that the patient is finally progressing past the stage of denial.

Response: physiological, behavioral, and psychological reactions. Selye used the term *general adaptation syndrome* to describe the organism's physical mobilization in the face of stress, sometimes referred to as the *fight or flight reaction.* Behaviors that attempt to effect change in the stressful situation are examples of adaptive channeling of fight impulses; defense mechanisms are internal, often unconscious, flight responses that involve varying degrees of distortion of reality in the service of reducing emotional discomfort. Three physicians working for a well-known HMO give examples of different responses to the pressure to increase their patient load by reducing the time spent with each patient. Dr. A organized her fellow physicians into a cohesive group and retained an attorney, a strategy that ultimately led to a modification in the policy. Dr. B complied with the policy and even praised it as ultimately more profitable, yet began to develop gastrointestinal symptoms. Dr. C. decided to leave the corporation and find a small, congenial group practice where he would have more autonomy and job satisfaction.

Consequence: the impact of stress is on one's physical and psychological functioning as well as the outcome of one's coping and defensive responses on the environment. Successful consequences include adaptation to demands, increased personal resilience, and effective environmental change, such as changing jobs or reducing workload. Conversely, unsuccessful outcomes can include professional and personal impairment, job burnout, and varied symptoms of stress reactions, including pain, illness or injury, and psychiatric disorders. One unfortunate consequence of excessive stress is that it impairs one's capacity to cope with whatever new stressors arise. A problem that might have been easily resolved under normal circumstances may be experienced as overwhelming. Furthermore, inadequate efforts to resolve that problem may in fact create new difficulties (stressors), which further tax the overloaded coping capacity. Hence a downward vicious cycle is a common consequence of excessive stress.

Burnout

Burnout is a consequence of job stress that arises from the chronic emotional strain of dealing extensively with people who need help. Caregivers are especially vulnerable to developing this syndrome when the dependency of the patient extends over a long period of time and the efforts of the provider appear to have little effect. A lack of autonomy and control also contributes to burnout. People are at greater risk when they feel powerless and trapped, either because of their unassertive personal style or because of the rigidity and irrationality of institutional regulations.

The various symptoms of burnout can be grouped into three categories.

Emotional exhaustion: Professional functioning can be impaired by chronic fatigue, low energy, irritability, and difficulties with concentration, short-term memory, and decision-making. The subjective experience is described as "trapped," "weighed down," or "drowning." The sufferer dreads facing a new day of work, longs to escape, and feels overwhelmed by insurmountable obstacles.

Depersonalization: A certain degree of *detached concern*—blending compassion with objectivity—is an adaptive deterrent to burnout. When detachment develops into dehumanizing, callous insensitivity, then the diagnosis of burnout is justified. Those physicians who are initially the most idealistic and enthusiastic and who cannot develop healthy ways of maintaining some emotional distance are at greatest risk for this disillusionment and cynicism.

Reduced personal accomplishment: Impaired functioning in professional duties is often accompanied by feelings of guilt and inadequacy, further contributing to a downward vicious spiral. It is common for the burned-out physician initially to elicit concern from friends, peers, and family, only to alienate them later by his or her attitudes and behavior.

Assessment of Risk Factors

An understanding of stress and burnout should be part of an ongoing monitoring of the risk factors in one's life. Three major categories of variables interact to determine one's susceptibility to stress: personal vulnerability (or resilience), the cumulative level of environmental stress, and the quality of available social support. Each of these factors is summarized below. Table 40.1 provides a simplified self-assessment inventory, highlighting the more important topics, in order to encourage an honest self-appraisal of one's coping resources and liabilities. It is hoped that the commitment to a periodic checkup will contribute to the initiation of timely preventive interventions.

Personal Vulnerability

Biological Factors. Although certain biological givens influence the stress reaction process (eg, physiological reactivity, predisposition to certain illnesses), life-style and behavior have a major effect on biological vulnerability or resilience. Maintenance of good health serves as a buffer against the effects of stress, whereas poor health reduces coping resources and creates additional stressors. Excessive use of alcohol and medications undermines more adaptive approaches to stress management and adds the problems of addiction and family dysfunction to the burden of stressors. Recreational activities and self-care (sleep, nutrition, and exercise) are important coping resources in reducing stress. One irony of medical training is that the heavy work schedule, including excessive on-call hours, deprives the new physician of using these proven methods of stress management during the period of professional development when stress is greatest.

Personality Traits. Another irony of training is that the very personality traits that contribute to selection for and success in medical school are also risk factors, when amplified, for depression and other stress-related reactions. Examples of these traits can be clustered into two broad interrelated categories, both of which contribute to the quantity of life stress as well as to difficulties in applying stress management strategies.

Obsessive-compulsive style: Studies of the personality traits of medical students describe them in terms of obsessionality, compulsiveness, lack of pleasure-seeking, conscientiousness, feelings of indispensability, devotion to duty, and high need for order and control.

Control over emotions: Intellectualizing and obsessive-compulsive defense mechanisms serve to protect the medical student from experiencing unpleasant emotions such as inadequacy, anger, or fear. The medical school environment reinforces these tendencies toward emotional constriction.

Table 40.1 Self-Assessment of Risk Factors

Instructions: Decide whether item increases risk of stress problem, reduces risk (buffer), or is neutral	Risk Factor	Neutral	Buffer/ Support
Current state of health			
Amount and quality of sleep			
Nutrition			
Exercise and level of fitness			
Recreational breaks from work			
Use of alcohol/medication for relaxation			
Compulsive, "workaholic" traits			
Personal security/self-esteem			
Acceptance of "weak" feelings			
Facade of invulnerability			
Detached concern vs. overinvolvement			
Tendency toward perfectionism			
Ability to seek help and nurturance			
Current work load: available time			
Performance expectations: level of competence			
Work relations (adversarial vs. cooperative)			
Availability of supportive mentor			
Proportion of chronic/terminal patients in practice			
Amount of personal control over decisions and work activities			
Presence of prejudice or unfair treatment at work			
Quality of marital relationship (amount of support, conflict)			
Amount of responsibility/help for children/home			
Availability of confidante			
Formal or informal support group			

Medical students and house officers, when compared with peers in other professions, are found to be less impulsive and playful and less able to access and express their natural feelings of rage and dependency or to comfortably seek nurturance from others.

Attitudes and Expectations. The ability to view conflict as a challenge rather than a threat and to see opportunity instead of disaster in a crisis are examples of how the intensity of stress can be lowered by an adaptive appraisal process. Physicians who perceive that they have personal control in a situation have lower stress than those who attribute more control to external factors. Inevitably, all physicians are faced with situations over which they have no control. For instance, patients die, regardless of one's best efforts. In such situations the tendency to angrily assign blame, either to oneself or to others, will increase one's stress level; attitudes that are more objective and philosophical will not. Those physicians who cope well when they do have control may be more at risk in situations where they must accept the existential fact of their powerlessness.

Expectations that physicians set for themselves tend to be unrealistic and excessively demanding. The desire to help others and a tendency to perfectionism lead many physicians to what Sandroff called the "M.D.-eity syndrome." This expectation of being able to cure their patients clashes with the reality of death and chronic illness in their practices, leading to self-doubt and recriminations or emotional distancing and anger. Physicians who work with the terminally ill need to define goals for success in terms of caring rather than of curing. Otherwise, they will easily become submerged in a sense of futility and hopelessness.

Level of Environmental Stress

Respondents to a survey by Alexander et al. on sources of stress in physicians perceived their major stress as role overload, noting that their job demands exceeded the resources available. The assumption that there are character-building benefits of extreme stress during medical training is slow to yield to the substantial research evidence of its harmful effects on the medical student, on his or her family, and on the quality of patient care. This stress is exacerbated by the lack of supportive relationships; competitive and adversarial interactions are more common than mentorship and collaborative teamwork.

Medical practice, though less stressful than residency, provides a continuing overload of demands in one's responsibilities for patient care, office management, and continuing education. One of the occupational hazards of practicing medicine is the ready availability of self-destructive remedies for stress. As Burrows stated, it is "too easy for doctors under stress to quietly and surreptitiously start eating their mail from drug companies, instead of reading it." One factor that is related to burnout is the lack of control the physician actually has over the outcome of his or her efforts, whether as an employee of a corporate entity or a caretaker of chronically ill and frequently uncooperative patients.

Physicians who work predominantly with the terminally ill experience additional sources of stress. For example, they suffer emotionally from uncertainty, helplessness, and loss; serve as targets of anger, resentment, and dependency; and experience more urgent pressures to keep current and invest in continuing medical education. In addition, doctors treating AIDS patients quickly develop an overloaded practice as soon as other physicians and AIDS patients learn of their expertise in this area.

Female physicians, as a minority group, are likely to experience greater levels of stress than do their male counterparts; they report negative treatment and prejudiced attitudes and are disadvantaged by the relative lack of female role models. Stress is further compounded by their own sex role socialization and internalization of societal norms about the proper relationship between women's professional and family lives. Thus women experience greater role conflicts when their work schedules interfere with family life and tend to assume full responsibility for home and children, even though their professional commitments are equal to or greater than those of their husbands.

Quality of Social Support

The risk factors in the environment are determined by the types and intensities of the stressors as well as by the quality of social support available to buffer the physician from these stressors.

Ideally, a medical student will draw support from his or her marriage. It is more likely, however, that the stress of medical school will destructively affect family life and that conflicts originating at home will be additional sources of stress. Furthermore, the transitions in the career of the physician, from medical school to internship to residency and finally to practice, are times of additional strain for marriages. Not surprisingly, physicians who rate themselves high in family support report lower levels of professional stress. Although female physicians receive less support from their spouses than do male physicians, male physicians can no longer expect that their wives' needs will be subordinated to their careers, as was common 20 years ago.

Peer support, like cohesive family life, is a potent buffer against stress. The existence of a confidante—someone with whom one can share, without reservations, all of one's problems and emotions—is associated with greater resilience against depression. Social support systems are protective against burnout or job-related tedium and are even found to protect against the negative effects that life stress has on health. Notwithstanding, physicians are notoriously resistant to sharing problems with peers and to admitting any need or weakness. Medical training, by fostering competitive relationships, can undermine the development of peer support. If, in spite of these pressures, the medical student or resident succeeds in building a supportive network, it is often destroyed through the geographical relocations of their postresidency career choices.

Early Detection of Stress Symptoms

Emotional Awareness

A recognition of one's own emotional state is the most obvious route to detecting the level of stress and burnout in one's life. Moodiness, irritability, anger disproportionate to the cause, depression, worry, tension, frustration, and garden-variety unhappiness would inform most people that something needs attention in their lives. Unfortunately, as noted earlier, doctors are experts in avoiding and denying their own emotional states. When unpleasant feelings intrude, they can be staved off with greater immersion in work, the very solution that often caused the problem in the first place. Fortunately, there are ways in which stress is revealed that do not require emotional awareness: bodily reactions, behaviors, and cognitive functioning.

Body Awareness

Physicians are well-trained in recognizing the early physical signs of stress, which, if unattended, can develop into conditions such as ulcers, colitis, or hypertension. Complaints of tension headaches, neck and shoulder pain, tachycardia, or chronic fatigue, should be the cue to planning stress management intervention. Other, more subtle, signs of stress can be read by paying attention to body language. Nervous foot tapping may mean impatience or irritability; nail biting, teeth grinding, or clenched jaws suggest anxiety and worry; restlessness or tightly folded arms may signal boredom and anger.

Behavioral Awareness

Signs of excessive stress can also be revealed in one's actions and behaviors. Examples of stress-related behaviors include frequent absences and lateness; impulsivity; conflict with coworkers, family or friends; inability to stay with any one task; and social withdrawal. An objective record of one's consumption of alcohol and medications can offer evidence that substance abuse is compounding the problems created by job-related stress. Signs of anxiety or depression, such as disturbances in sleeping, eating, or sexual activity, can be clues that stress is exceeding endurance.

Soliciting feedback from others about our behavior should be part of an objective assessment of stress. If we manage not to respond defensively, spouses, friends, and coworkers can report their impressions of changes in our functioning—for instance, increased impatience and sensitivity, lowered frustration tolerance, and a decline in the quality of our job performance.

Cognitive Awareness

The presence of excessive stress can also be recognized in our cognitive functioning. Forgetfulness, difficulty concentrating and paying attention, preoccupations and rumination, and impairment in decision-making are definite signals of stress. Daydreaming can inform us of our wish to escape. The way we "talk" to ourselves can reveal stress-inducing messages. For instance, frequent use of self-critical and self-blaming messages can increase our own depression, whereas frequent criticism of others increases impatience and irritability.

A Personal Plan of Stress Management

The challenge for the physician is to be able to bring professional diagnostic skills to his or her own life. The first, and perhaps most important, step in a stress management program is to overcome the tendency toward denial of personal difficulties. The most common cause of physician suicide, which occurs at a rate higher than in the general population, is the failure to recognize depression. Physicians are known to be "notoriously reluctant to seek help," according to Shortt. In addition to a defensive need to deny weakness and dependency, there are realistic fears of the threat to one's professional reputation and livelihood associated with openly acknowledging that stress has impaired one's functioning.

Applying Problem-Solving Skills

It is not unusual for people who have demonstrated superior problem-solving skills in academic and occupational settings to have great difficulty applying them to their own emotion-charged problems. For this reason it is often helpful to seek assistance from a more objective outsider. Problem-solving skills, as a part of stress management, entail the following:

Defining the problem as clearly as possible, usually in concrete terms: who, what, when, where, how often, and why? The generic problem definition, excessive stress, may lead to palliative measures, but may not be useful in eliminating the source of the problem. To pinpoint the aspects of work that create stress and dissatisfaction, it may be helpful to use a daily log, entering observations under column headings that reflect the four components of stress: *stressor, appraisal, response,* and *consequence.*

Defining goals for the particular problem you have identified. *Goal* refers to the desired outcome, not the method of achieving it. "Spend more time with my children," "reduce amount of hostile and competitive interactions with my colleagues," and "develop more satisfaction in my contacts with patients" are examples.

Brainstorm solutions to reach your goal, aiming for quantity and creativity, avoiding premature censorship of the proposed solution.

Choose a solution after assessing the quality of alternatives. Consider who can help you and what obstacles need to be worked through.

Implement the chosen solution and evaluate its effectiveness.

Goal-Setting and Values Clarification

As you review the range of stressful situations in your life, it is useful to put aside prior assumptions and ask yourself these three questions: (1) Can I change the situation? (2) Can I change myself to improve my adaptation to the situation? and (3) Can I leave the situation and find satisfaction elsewhere? The ultimate choice of strategy requires reality testing, clarification of values, and a cost-benefit analysis. One does not need to be an alcoholic or addict to benefit from the prayer of "12-step" programs such as Alcoholics Anonymous:

> Grant me the serenity to accept the things I cannot change
> The courage to change the things I can
> And the wisdom to know the difference.

Solutions will fall roughly into three categories: *adapt* to the situation and learn to find additional satisfactions outside of work; actively pursue a course intended to *change* some aspect of the situation; or *leave*. Because it takes time and planning to change or leave a situation, strategies for adapting better and reducing one's own stress reactions are necessarily a part of every intervention plan.

Strategies for Stress Management

Self-care. Physicians find it easy to prescribe the basics of maintaining good health—nutrition, exercise, adequate rest—to patients and very difficult to practice what they preach. The frequently given admonition to reduce intake of alcohol, caffeine, fat, and cholesterol should be given to oneself. The relation of regular aerobic exercise to reduction of occupational stress is now so widely recognized that many companies are including aerobic classes in their facilities as part of their employee health programs. Certain more aggressive physical activities, such as racketball or use of punching bags, provide healthy outlets for stress-related anger. The suggestion to pamper yourself and find self-nurturing alternatives to drugs and alcohol is part of a self-care strategy.

Relaxation training. More formal techniques to induce relaxation are recommended for people who cannot achieve the "relaxation response" through their own preferred pursuit of exercise and pleasurable activities. Regular use of relaxation exercises, yoga, or meditation actually alters physiological reactivity and provides a welcome respite from daily pressures. A relaxation state can be induced in only 10 to 20 minutes with the following instructions:

> Sitting quietly in a comfortable position with your eyes closed, begin by relaxing the muscles in your toes and gradually move up to your face. Breathing through your nose, concentrate on your breathing. As you breath out, say the word "ONE."

People who say they do not have time to relax should be aware that just three deep breaths exhaled slowly can provide on-the-spot relaxation.

Cultivation of nonwork interests. Prevention of burnout requires the physician to have varied interests outside of work, maintaining friendships and enjoying scheduled vacations. It is important to learn to limit work activities to a reasonable number of hours per week and to keep work from spilling into nonwork hours. Behavior therapists set as a clinical goal the ability to "goof off" comfortably. Successful stress management may simply require development of the ability to postpone thinking about work-related problems outside of work and to absorb oneself in other activities that provide meaning and pleasure. Often people who have been living with stress for a long time have forgotten the leisure activities that used to give them enjoyment and need their memories jogged with structured checklists or trips to a public library.

Sometimes the best available option is to live with a stressful professional situation and find your sources of satisfaction in other areas of life. Physicians, who expect their work to be a major source of fulfillment, may initially find this solution unacceptable. When a rational cost-benefit analysis yields no better alternative, then the cognitive restructuring strategies discussed below may help physicians to accept that just because medicine does not live up to their adolescent hopes and dreams does not mean that they are failures or that they cannot find greater satisfaction in other parts of their lives.

Time management skills. All of the above strategies assume that the busy physician has the ability to set priorities on various activities, to schedule time to achieve goals, and then to adhere to self-imposed commitments. Those who feel as if their life controls them may need to include the development of time management skills in their overall plan of stress management. The following suggestions may help overcome common pitfalls.

1. In estimating the amount of time needed for each activity, refer to a record of the actual time it has taken you in the past, and then add a "fudge factor."
2. Categorize your activities by three criteria: (1) what is under your control, (2) what is under someone else's control, and (3) what activities are most important. Then, when scheduling blocks of time for activities, start with the most important activity that is not under your control.
3. Learn to set limits on new activities, saying "no" instead of accepting new commitments. (This may require new skills in assertiveness, discussed later in this chapter.)
4. As much as possible, delegate routine tasks and allow the other members of your team to take more responsibility.
5. Structure your work day so that you warm up slowly, and allow a "decompression" period at the end of the day.
6. Modify perfectionistic standards that are costly in terms of time.
7. In developing a written schedule, be sure to leave at least two blocks of time per day that are for your use only.

A systematic examination of one's use of time will usually result in the decision to cut back on one's workload, or at least selected aspects of it. Because burnout is associated with the intensity of the care-giving relationship, a recommended treatment is reducing the amount of continuous direct contact with patients.

Alteration of attitudes and expectations. When the obvious solution is to set limits and cut back on the commitments in our lives and we refuse to do so, the problem may lie in perfectionistic expectations that need to be modified. An important coping strategy for someone in the throes of burnout is to examine and alter the myths, ideals, and expectations that have been unsupported in daily practice. The physician needs to lower his or her expectations, attain detachment without becoming cynical, and set realistic and personally meaningful goals.

In keeping the log of stressful events described on p. 486 (Defining the problem), it is helpful to use the Appraisal column to enter cognitive processes that intervene between the stressful event and the emotional response: the self-talk, the value judgments, the irrational beliefs, and the "shoulds" and "musts." A variety of strategies fall under the rubric of cognitive restructuring:

1. Logically disputing the irrationality of beliefs such as, "If I'm not perfect, I'm no good," or "I need to be liked and appreciated by everyone to be a worthwhile human being."
2. Internally screaming "STOP" or even using mildly aversive physical sensations, such as a rubber band snapped against your skin, when persecuted by an internal message such as "You idiot, can't you do anything right?"
3. Substituting adaptive alternatives for those self-statements that seem to increase one's stress level. For instance, "That jerk, he deserves to be shot," is more likely to produce dysfunctional anger that leads to inappropriate outbursts and interpersonal conflicts than, "He doesn't do it as well as I do, but he's not really harming anyone, and I can't expect everyone to live up to my standards all the time."
4. Recognizing the arbitrary and moralistic tone of all "should" statements, and deliberately shifting to more tolerant and relativistic positions. Using wordings such as "It would be better," or "I would prefer it," or "Most people I respect would . . ." will reduce the sense of outrage, feelings of worthlessness, and attitudes of superiority that add stress to one's working relationships.
5. Challenge some beliefs as if they were tentative hypotheses requiring empirical validation, rather than absolute truths. The stress-producing conclusion, "No one around here ever shows any appreciation," is easily disconfirmed by objectively recalling the exceptions to that generalization.

Mobilization of social support. As part of the problem-solving process, difficulties in family and interpersonal relationships may have been identified as sources of stress. It is not uncommon for an individual to experience dissatisfaction in the work sphere when in fact the major root of unhappiness and tension is found in the marital relationship. Hence a stress management program may evolve into efforts to resolve marital conflicts and strengthen the cohesiveness of the family. In the work setting, development of supportive team approaches to patient care, especially when working with dying and chronic patients, can reduce the risk of burnout and eliminate stressors that come from assuming an authoritarian, aloof role in staff relations.

Developing peer support and cultivating those relationships where one can admit problems and openly communicate about feelings are effective strategies in dealing with stress and burnout. Turning to friends and former teachers for support and help may first require some of the cognitive restructuring described above in order to overcome beliefs such as, "I should be able to handle everything on my own." The use of counseling for stress, marital problems, or assistance with problem-solving does not need to be saved as a last resort. The days of therapy meaning years on an analyst's couch are past, and many varieties of brief therapy and counseling can help resolve difficulties in a matter of a few visits. The group support available in AA and other 12-step programs can infuse the lonely struggle against addictions with hope and encouragement.

Development of interpersonal skills. Deficiencies in interpersonal skills may interfere with the ability to maintain supportive relationships and have a direct causal role in the creation of stress. Thus a systematic analysis of stress-related problems often leads to the recognition that improved interpersonal skills would either eliminate causes of stress or help provide solutions. Books, courses, and counseling are all routes to developing skills in the following areas:

Communication: includes active listening skills; skills of self-disclosure and honesty; methods for reducing defensiveness in self and others; awareness of nonverbal messages.

Assertion: clarification of individual "assertive rights"—for instance, the right to your own feelings and opinions, to change your mind, to make mistakes, and to avoid what you do not want; recognition of nonassertive, assertive, and aggressive behaviors; development of skills in assertion—for example, asking for what you want and saying "no."

Conflict resolution: negotiation skills, including the ability to build a point of agreement between adversaries, and identify common goals ("win-win" solutions); skills in the use of positive and cooperative language.

Career change. Sometimes the best solution for stress and burnout is to leave the current situation: to find another position, change one's specialization or type of practice, or even give up the practice of medicine completely. Before misery drives you to an impulsive decision to pack up and quit, it is recommended that you first pursue a systematic exploration of your values, interests, needs, and life goals, perhaps following some of the structured exercises in books in the field of career planning or attending intensive seminars or counseling institutes in the area of adult career transitions.

The term *career* no longer refers exclusively to work; it incorporates the entire life-style, including leisure, peer affiliates, and family. A systematic life-planning process will include a review of significant life events, identification of the specific skills you enjoy using, and clarification of the environmental and interpersonal factors that will increase your satisfaction.

Although the changes selected will ultimately reduce stress, any life change, even a desired one, is inherently stressful, placing huge demands for coping and adjustment, Awareness of this fact means accepting that the rewards for change are not immediate. In fact, sometimes it is advisable to postpone the riskier choices until stress-induced dysfunctions have been alleviated.

Helping Others

This chapter has offered ideas for the individual physician to cope with stress. Nonetheless, the prevalence of stress reactions within the medical profession indicates the need for broader solutions on an organizational level, involving medical professionals who are willing to translate their concerns for over-stressed colleagues into action.

In Medical School, Internships, and Residency Programs

Replace stress-inducing training practices with more supportive measures and offer programs of early remediation for stress-related problems. For instance, some recommended strategies include reduced workload, part-time residencies, peer support groups, supportive mentorship, finding ways to strengthen marriages instead of subjecting them to strain and neglect, and didactic instruction in stress management.

In Medical Organizations

Create policies that reduce risk of burnout, enter the value of physician satisfaction into the cost-effectiveness equation, develop nonpunitive and fair models for rehabilitating impaired physicians, and lobby for public policy that reduces the stress of the malpractice crisis.

The ideas for stress management in this chapter can be applied to helping friends and colleagues on an informal basis. For instance, when we detect the symptoms of stress in our fellow physicians, instead of colluding in denial, we can give constructive feedback and offer our services as confidantes and problem-solving consultants. Each of us has the power to be a support or a stressor in another physician's life, and the choice we make can influence the stress level in the entire profession.

Suggested Reading

Albeti, R. E., and Emmons, M. L., *Your Perfect Right.* San Louis Obispo: Impact, 1974.

Alexander, D., Monk, J. S., and Jonas, A. P., "Occupational Stress, Personal Strain, and Coping among Residents and Faculty Members." *Journal of Medical Education* 60(11, 1985):830–839.

American Psychiatric Association, *Diagnostic and Statistical Manual of Mental Disorders* (3rd ed.). Washington, DC: APA, 1987.

Battle, C. U., "The Iatrogenic Disease Called Burnout." *Journal of the American Medical Women Association* 36(12, 1981), 357–359.

Benson, H., *The Relaxation Response.* New York: William Morrow, 1975.

Bolles, R. N., *What Color is Your Parachute?* Berkeley, CA: Ten Speed Press, 1989.

Burrows, T. M. O., "Stress and the Medical Profession: Doctors Are People, Too." *Journal of Holistic Medicine* 4(1, 1982):68–79.

Coombs, R. H., and Fawzy, F. I., "The Impaired-Physician Syndrome: A Developmental Perspective." In C. D. Scott and J. Hawk (Eds.), *Heal Thyself* (pp. 44–55). New York: Brunner/Mazel, 1986.

Gibbs, N., "Sick and Tired." *Time* (July 31, 1989):48–53.

Jackson, S. E., "Organizational Practices for Preventing Burnout." In A. S. Sethi and R. S. Shuler (Eds.), *Handbook for Organizational Stress Coping Strategies* (pp. 89–111). Cambridge, MA: Ballinger Publishing Company, 1984.

Kelner, M., and Rosenthal, C. "Postgraduate Medical Training, Stress, and Marriage." *Canadian Journal of Psychiatry* 31(1, 1986):22–24.

Lakein, A., *How to Get Control of Your Time and Your Life.* New York: New American Library, 1973.

Lange, A., and Jakubowski, P., *Responsible Assertive Behavior.* Champaign, IL: Research Press, 1976.

Lazarus, R., and Folkman, S., "Stress as a Rubric." In A. Eichler, M. M. Silverman, and D. M. Pratt (Eds.), *How to Define and Research Stress* (pp. 49–53). Washington, DC: American Psychiatric Press, 1986.

LeBourdais, E., "Hopelessness and Helplessness: Treating the Doctors Who Treat AIDS Patients." *Canadian Medical Association Journal* 140(Feb. 15, 1989):440–443.

Levin, R., "Beyond 'the Men of Steel': The Origins and Significance of House Staff Training Stress." *General Hospital Psychiatry* 10(2, 1988):114–121.

Loughary, J. W., and Ripley, T. M., *Career and Life Planning Guide.* Chicago: Follett Publishing Company, 1976.

Martin, C. A., and Julian, R. A., "Causes of Stress and Burnout in Physicians Caring for the Chronically and Terminally Ill." *Hospice Journal* 3(2–3, 1987):121–146.

Maslach, C., *Burnout—The Cost of Caring.* Englewood Cliffs, NJ: Prentice-Hall, 1982.

May, H. J., and Revicki, D. A., "Professional Stress among Family Physicians." *Journal of Family Practice* 20(1985):165–171.

McCue, J. D., "The Distress of Internship: Causes and Prevention." *New England Journal of Medicine* 312(7, 1985):449–452.

Nadelson, C. C., and Notman, M. T., "What is Different for Women Physicians?" In S. C. Scheiber and B. B. Doyle (Eds.), *The Impaired Physician* (pp. 11–25). New York: Plenum Medical Book Company, 1983.

Nunnally, E., and May, C., *Communication Basics for Human Service Professionals.* Newbury Park, CA: Sage Publications, 1989.

Pelletier, K. R., *Healthy People in Unhealthy Places: Stress and Fitness at Work.* New York: Delacorte Press, 1984.

Pines, A. M., Aronson, E., and Kafrey, D., *Burnout: From Tedium to Personal Growth.* New York: The Free Press, 1981.

Roeske, N. C. A., "Risk Factors: Predictable Hazards of a Health-Care Career." In C. D. Scott and J. Hawk, *Heal Thyself* (pp. 56–70). New York: Brunner/Mazel, 1986.

Rosenthal, T. L., and Rosenthal, R. H., "Stress: Causes, Measurement, and Management." In K. Craig and R. J. McMahon (Eds.), *Advances in Clinical Behavior Therapy* (pp. 3–26). New York: Brunner/Mazel, 1983.

Sandroff, R., "Is Your Job Driving You Crazy?" *Psychology Today* (July/August 1989): 41–45.

Scheck, Anne, "Physicians Tell How They Avoid Career Apathy." *Clinical Psychiatry News* 17(6, 1989): pp. 3, 23.

Schieber, S. C., and Doyle, B. B. (Eds)., *The Impaired Physician.* New York: Plenum Medical Book Company, 1983.

Seagraves, K., and Seagraves, R. T., "When the Physician's Marriage is in Trouble." *Medical Aspects of Human Sexuality* 21(6, 1987):148–159.

Selye, H., *The Stress of Life.* New York: McGraw Hill, 1978.

Shortt, S. E. D., (Ed.), *Psychiatric Illness in Physicians.* Springfield, IL: Charles C. Thomas, 1982.

Slaby, A. E., "Cancer's Impact on Caregivers." *Advanced Psychosomatic Medicine* 18(1988):135–153.

Tokarz, J. P., Bremer, W., and Peters, K., *Beyond Survival.* Chicago, IL: American Medical Association, 1979.

Twerski, A. J., *It Happens to Doctors, Too.* Center City, MN: Hazeldon, 1982.

41 | Selling or Dissolving a Practice: Assessing the Value of a Practice

JOHN O. GOODMAN

As a starting point for this chapter, the assumption is made that you have already determined that selling or dissolving your medical practice is a necessary or desirable action.

Once this decision has been made, a host of factors must be examined to determine if the practice should be sold as a complete entity or if it should be dissolved and liquidated by asset category—for instance, equipment, accounts receivable, and patient charts. In this chapter, focus will be placed on the components that must be evaluated in order to make these crucial decisions as well as on the strategies and techniques that can then be utilized as part of the actual selling or dissolution process.

As might be imagined in light of today's complex medical environment, selling or dissolving a practice has become an extremely challenging undertaking. To better understand how this contemporary challenge evolved, it is instructive to look back at how these situations were handled in years past.

Reflecting back to the 1940s and 1950s, for example, a striking difference from today's medical practices is readily apparent. Specifically, during this period the majority of physicians could be found in solo practices or, at most, two-person groups. Typically, these practices were not sold. Rather, they were transferred from the departing physician to the new physician. The doctor that was leaving usually would collect his or her own accounts receivable, and any equipment would be sold wholesale to the incoming doctor. Further, the departing physician generally would not charge the new physician for leasehold improvements, the value of medical charts, or any goodwill the practice carried with it.

In fact, the concept of goodwill was almost nonexistent until the early 1960s. This was because practices continued to be solo or no more than two-physician groups and the majority of revenue was received directly from patients. As a result, goodwill was part of the relationship between a specific patient and a specific doctor and was thus not transferrable to a new physician.

Entering the late 1960s and early 1970s, this picture began to change as professional practice brokerage firms became prevalent. In particularly competitive markets, such as California and New York, it was not long before practices no longer needed to be liquidated, but rather could be sold in their entirety. During this period, medical practice revenues began to rise as a result of the emergence of Medicare as well as the growth of third-party payors. As reimbursement increased, so did the size of U.S. medical groups.

In 1980, there were approximately 8000 U.S. medical groups composed of eight or more physicians. By 1985, this number had grown to 15,000, and today, it is estimated that there are 30,000 U.S. medical groups with eight or more doctors.

As a result of their larger size, enhanced revenue potential, and greater capital investments, medical practices of today are valued at much higher levels than were their counterparts of just a few decades ago. The way in which they are valued also has changed significantly. Today, for example, consideration is given to such factors as patient mix, reimbursement mix, physician's income, and physician's benefits aside from direct compensation and goodwill, to cite just a few of the components. What was once a simple transfer is today an intricate business transaction.

Indeed, it is a changed medical world—one that brings with it a host of new challenges and rewards in relation to selling or dissolving a practice.

Selling or Dissolution Considerations

There should first be a clear understanding of the differences between selling and dissolving a practice.

Selling involves the actual transfer of an entity—in this case a medical practice—from one party to another. What is particularly unusual about selling a medical practice is that the whole—that is, the financial value assigned to it—often exceeds the sum of its tangible parts. The reason for this is that the value of a medical practice reflects many intangible factors, such as goodwill, location, facility access, and staff efficiency. When a selling price is assigned to a practice, that total reflects a host of tangible and intangible strengths and weaknesses.

In contrast, when a medical practice is dissolved, values are attached only to tangible assets such as equipment and furniture on an item-by-item basis. The amount received for each item may or may not reflect its actual value.

With these differences in mind, the decision must then be made whether the practice in question should be sold or dissolved. In large part, this should be determined based on the physician's specific circumstances.

For example, if the entity is a solo practice, it is usually advantageous to sell the practice. In this way, the departing physician is able to make an orderly transfer of patients to the purchasing doctor of his or her choice. This method reduces disruption to patients and office staff. It also enables components such as accounts receivable to remain undisturbed. The departing doctor's approval of the new physician can be formally expressed through written communications to patients. Events such as open houses also can be held. In this way, the likelihood of patient retention is increased significantly.

For any of this to occur, however, the departing physician must be both physically and mentally fit and thus capable of assisting the new physician in an orderly transfer of the practice.

However, if the physician in question becomes disabled or passes away and the entity has not been sold within a 90-day period, it is recommended that the practice be dissolved. After 90 days a host of difficulties often comes into play. For example, it becomes more difficult to secure medical coverage. Patient retention starts to fall, and accounts receivable collection similarly begins to slide. To avoid these situations, a practice should ideally be sold within 30 to 60 days of becoming available.

In almost every instance, a practice that is sold will generate more money than a practice that is dissolved.

In today's complex medical environment, it is essential for every practice to have a buy/sell agreement firmly in place. This type of agreement enables a medical group to continue functioning regardless of who joins or leaves the group. If a buy/sell agreement is not in place, a group's existence could easily be threatened if one or more physicians becomes dissatisfied and requests dissolution through the courts.

To prevent this from occurring, the buy/sell agreement should cover a broad range of subjects, including how a new physician becomes an owner and how departing doctors sell their interest in the group. The agreement also should delineate the method by which the practice will be evaluated, the assets and liabilities to be included in the evaluation, the buyout terms for a departing physician, and the terms for resolving any disputes that might arise between the departing doctor and the group. In light of its complexity, it is important that the expertise of both an accountant and attorney be utilized to develop the buy/sell agreement. Once it has been drafted, this document should be reviewed annually and amended as needed.

When determining a practice's value, it should be noted that each specialty brings with it differing characteristics that must be considered in the evaluation process. For example, some practices require an equity approach, others necessitate a patient source approach, and still others focus on income generation.

As might be guessed, an *equity approach* focuses on tangible assets—for instance, equipment, leasehold improvements, and the physical size of the practice and its location. In contrast, a *patient source approach* to valuing a practice relates to patient/payor mix—for example, private pay vs. managed care—as well as patient referral sources. Is the practice's referral base horizontal (composed of a variety of referral sources) or more vertical in nature (consisting primarily of managed care contracts)?

Income generation is a third consideration when determining a practice's value. Following this approach, emphasis is placed not on tangible assets or patient sources, but rather on the departing physician's personal income.

Each of these approaches—equity, patient source, and income generation—will play a different role when determining the value of individual practices. For example, a multiphysician family practice group that has a substantial amount of equipment will be valued quite differently from an orthopedic practice with an equivalent number of physicians. A cardiovascular surgery group, with the same number of physicians as both the family practice and orthopedic practices, will be valued in an entirely different manner as well.

The family practice group, will generate considerably less revenue than both the orthopedic and cardiovascular surgery groups. The family practice group, however, is likely to have substantially more investment in equipment, leasehold improvements, and other tangible assets. As a result, it is common to evaluate family practice groups on an equity basis, with income generation as a secondary consideration.

In contrast, the average cardiovascular surgery practice generally will have limited capital investments, but the income generated per physician will exceed that of many other specialties. Not surprisingly, the value of a cardiovascular surgery group is usually focused on income generation versus equity.

In the case of an orthopedic practice, there is likely to be both substantial capital investment and significant income generation. As a result, such a practice must be evaluated in terms of its equity position as well as its income potential.

In terms of income potential, the average family practice physician generally has base earnings of $120,000 to $130,000 annually, compared with $400,000 to $500,000 for the average orthopedist and $600,000 to $750,000 for the typical cardiovascular surgeon.

During the course of an evaluation, if a practice is found to be generating substantially more income than is typical for its specialty, then the goodwill value of that practice would increase as a result of these elevated incomes. Conversely, if a practice's revenue is found to be below the average for its specialty, the practice's goodwill value and hence, its overall value, would be reduced.

Although many factors may figure into the decision of whether to sell or dissolve a practice, the pivotal issue is the individual physician's specific circumstances. Once the sell-versus-dissolve decision is made, attention must be paid to the particular value-related characteristics associated with each specialty.

Evaluation Components

Regardless of specialty, numerous tangible and intangible components must be evaluated when any practice is being sold or dissolved. The value of these components can often be misleading. It is not unusual for an intangible asset to carry greater value than a tangible one.

For example, a successful practice situated in a good geographic location will command greater value than will an equally successful practice located in a less desirable area. In this case an intangible component sets the two practices apart.

Specifically, the following intangible components should be reviewed as part of any practice evaluation process.

Location

As alluded to previously, location is an intangible value that relates to a practice's geographic situation. It also refers to the practice's location in the building in which it is housed.

From a geographic perspective, for example, a practice located in Los Angeles will probably have a higher value than a similar practice located in a midwestern city. Even within Los Angeles, however, practice values vary significantly according to location. A successful practice in Beverly Hills will probably be valued much higher than a comparable practice located in East Los Angeles. Even third-party payors adjust their reimbursement rates for practices in these different geographic locations.

As is apparent, specific location can play a major role in determining practice value, even when practices are located in the same county.

Office Staff

A medical practice's office staff brings with it many potential points of value, including length of service, individual capabilities, and patient relationships. All of these factors will affect the degree to which a practice can successfully be transferred and thus will affect the practice's overall value.

Facility Appearance

Attention must be paid to the practice's actual physical appearance. This includes its decor, the condition of equipment, and its general expandability. Each of these characteristics affects the practice's income-earning potential and thus the practice's value.

Patient Charts

It is not unusual to assign a monetary value to the number of patient charts that are being transferred to a purchaser. For example, an internal medicine practice typically would place a value of from $130 to $200 on each active patient chart.

The value of patient charts increases if the practice has a method of recalling patients on a regular basis, thereby enhancing the charts' activity. Such charts would be of greater value than charts that represented only episodic care. The more active charts bring with them a greater potential of retention for the purchasing physician.

Goodwill

This is probably the most misunderstood component in the entire practice evaluation process. For years, in fact, court battles have been waged to determine if goodwill is a factor that can in fact be transferred from one practice to another.

Goodwill can vary dramatically between specialties. For example, a primary care group with a broad base of self-referred private-pay patients who are accustomed to seeing different physicians will command substantial goodwill value based on these highly transferable characteristics. In contrast, a solo peripheral vascular surgeon who relies on several physicians for referrals, and who has virtually no self-referrals, is unlikely to command any goodwill value.

Although goodwill is a factor that must be determined individually on a practice-by-practice basis, some consistent standards can be followed. A general rule of thumb for valuing goodwill related to a family practice group is 30% to 50% of the practice's gross receipts for the previous 12 months. In contrast, a general surgery practice may have a goodwill value that is not more than 15% of the previous 12 months' gross receipts.

In addition to these intangible factors, several tangible components also must be considered when determining a medical practice's value.

Accounts Receivable

The accounts receivable of a medical practice should be evaluated based on their full value minus the receivable's projected uncollectible portion.

Typically, accounts receivable should represent 150% to 300% of the practice's average monthly charges in order to achieve an optimum collectible accounts receivable ratio. For example, if a physician's average monthly charges are $30,000, this doctor's accounts receivable should not exceed 300% of these monthly charges, or $90,000 per month. If receivables surpass this amount, it is appropriate to adjust the receivables' value downward based on the probability that those receivables exceeding the 300% range will be uncollectible.

Although some variation is based on specialty, the average physician's accounts receivable today possesses a 72% to 81% likelihood of being collectible.

Medical and Office Equipment

The value of both medical and office equipment should be determined by comparing the items' current fair market value with their original cost. As a general rule of thumb, equipment should be priced at its appraised value or 50% of its original cost, whichever figure is greater.

Leasehold Improvements

The value of leasehold improvements frequently are overlooked by physicians selling or liquidating their practices.

Specifically, the value of leasehold improvements should reflect their original cost, which is then amortized over the remaining term of the lease. For example, if a physician has a five-year lease, has spent $50,000 on leasehold improvements, and is selling three years into the lease, it is reasonable to assert that the physician's leasehold improvements are worth 40% of their original cost. The only exceptions to this assertion might be if the leasehold improvements were subject to extreme wear and tear or had become obsolete.

Medical and Office Supplies

Medical and office supplies should be inventoried and valued at their actual cost less any adjustment required because of change of circumstance. An example of the change of circumstance would be the fact that a departing physician's letterhead will have no value if it cannot be utilized by the purchasing physician.

Marketing Materials

Like leasehold improvements, marketing materials are a commonly overlooked asset. For example, if a practice has developed patient-information or other types of brochures, these materials should be valued at their actual cost. Again, however, adjustments must be made if there is any change of circumstance.

Summary

Evaluating a medical practice in preparation for selling or dissolving clearly is a complex undertaking.

Certainly, departing physicians will want to maximize the value of their assets. To accomplish this, all of the components addressed in this chapter should be considered, as should the revenue an incoming physician can expect to earn from the practice. To ensure that the valuation includes all appropriate factors, it is strongly recommended that the services of both an accountant and attorney who specialize in medical practice evaluations be engaged.

Although this chapter has outlined a variety of components that should be considered as part of any standard valuation process, this process is an individual one, and as a result each practice must be evaluated based on its own unique characteristics.

A physician's practice is more than bricks and mortar. It represents time, energy, personal devotion—a career. As such, it deserves careful, concerted attention when the decision is made to sell or dissolve.

42 | Preparing for Retirement from Medical Practice

ROBERT H. COOMBS, PHD AND
BERNARD B. VIRSHUP, MD

Relatively little is known about physician retirement—how well physicians adjust to this new phase of life, what they do with their time, and how happy they are. Only a few studies have been conducted with retired doctors.

To learn more about physician retirement, we sent a six-page questionnaire to a random sample of retired physicians in Los Angeles County. One hundred physicians returned forms. Supplementing this information, we tape-recorded interviews with 20 of these physicians queried in small groups about their retirement experiences.

Most physicians were unprepared for the kind of life they lead in retirement. Both their expectations and fears of retirement were generally unfounded. Despite some problems, most of the physicians greatly enjoyed their new freedom.

Most physicians are introverts (that is, they derive their energy mostly from within themselves, rather than from others) and were unprepared for the close and demanding emotional connection patients expect of them. Most coped successfully by developing an emotional and intellectual distance from their patients and enjoying a relationship in which they saw themselves as helpers. At retirement, few missed their patients as people; typically they experienced relief or only a mild regret.

What they missed most upon retiring was a feeling of being valuable. They experienced difficulty feeling worthwhile when they no longer were helping patients; an intrinsic sense of worth rarely survived retirement intact.

Retired physicians spoke disparagingly and yet wistfully of the loss of a certain godlike image given them by their former patients. They spoke sadly, for example, of now being addressed by their first names.

Some found difficulty shifting to a nonmedical perception of themselves and prolonged the transition by keeping in touch with their former colleagues, eating breakfast at the hospital, and going to lectures. Other retired physicians deprecated this behavior, believing that it was important for the physician to transfer his or her interests to other areas of life.

Many reported that their family relationships suffered during their careers but saw this as a necessary part of the job. Some experienced family breakups. On retirement, some still found it difficult to connect with spouses and children. Most, however, welcomed the improved temporal and emotional closeness with their family and, despite fears to the contrary, were warmly welcomed home. Physicians who had managed to spend adequate time with their family members during their careers strongly advised that others do the same.

Poor health was mentioned as a factor in retirement by almost half the physicians, yet within their limitations, this did not prevent most from enjoying themselves. They deplored their medical conditions, but not their retirement; they generally said only that they would enjoy retirement more if they were healthier.

Finances were of interest to many but not a source of anxiety or concern. Some would have liked a bigger income, but almost all adjusted well and felt comfortable living within the income they had.

Fears of boredom were realized by only a few. Most retirees became involved in one or many of the myriad aspects of life, some that were not experienced while they were in practice.

Retirement—Culmination of Career Experiences

Physician retirement is best understood as the culmination of a long process that began before medical school. As medical students 30 to 40 years ago, they came from middle- to upper-class homes, were mostly white, mostly men, and had high expectations of themselves and of medicine. They were generally intelligent, good learners, and well motivated. A majority were introverts, willing to spend long solitary hours in the library with a minimum of human interaction. They were less experienced socially than were most undergraduates. Their wish to spend the rest of their lives in a profession that involved close, helping relationships with others was based on idealism with little idea of what that implied. Their sense of self was largely based on intellectual achievements and academic rewards. In general they were unprepared for and naive about the nature of medical school and medicine.

Medical school introduced them to medicine by the study of anatomy. On the first day of school, with minimal psychological preparation, they were confronted with the task of skinning a dead person who had been preserved with formalin. Some dropped out that week; those who remained usually handled the emotional turmoil silently, hoping that their feelings did not show, pretending casualness and indifference. They retreated into intellectuality and morbid attempts at humor.

At the same time, their sense of self was threatened by being expected to master more material than it is possible to learn in a limited time. By the first examination they were in a state of desperate anxiety. These feelings were exacerbated when they learned that honors and As, their criteria for self-esteem, were reserved for those few who could achieve what they could not. B grades were perceived as labeling them second-class physicians; worse yet, C's, received for the first time in their lives, brought humiliation and shame, labeling them (in their own eyes) as inadequate people. At that time, as much as 25% of some classes flunked; they dropped out of sight by the end of the first year and were replaced by graduates of two-year medical schools (a practice that fortunately has ceased).

By the second year, some had burned out. Motivation had dropped to the point where studying was a difficult and onerous task, performed only because of the dreaded consequences of not passing exams. Many perceived themselves as inadequate and incompetent, not knowing as much as they should; they were generally unable to express their feelings or share them with their classmates and others. Their personal relationships (for those few who had them) were rocky because of their own emotional disarray, their lack of time, and the demands they made on others. Visits to a counselor were nonexistent. To their teachers and classmates, they pretended all was well, lest they be perceived by others as inadequate.

Their clinical education (limited to the third and fourth years) was mostly Socratic in nature; the student presents a case to a resident or fellow, who then questions, discusses, and critiques. Unprepared for this role, even the well-meaning instructor (and there were some who were not) often created feelings of anger and humiliation in the student. By the third and fourth years of school, the students developed a psychological armoring that was thin but rigid. It provided the ability to get the maximum amount of information from a patient in a minimum of time, without forming an emotional connection. Attempts to show interest and concern for their relationships with their patients were rarely rewarded, and sometimes actively discouraged. Far from enjoying their contact with patients, students learned to see them as problems that were often unpleasant and potential sources of difficulty and conflict.

The residency years further emphasized the importance of data collection, developing skills, and mastering technology and the efficient use of time and contributed to an ever-increasing emotional alienation. The young physicians developed the ability to continue working long past their personal threshold of exhaustion and burnout, and they were encouraged to develop a sense of responsibility that overwhelmed personal concerns.

By the time they entered practice, they had developed a sense of being special, different, of being set apart from and somewhat above the general run of human beings. This was acknowledged and accepted not only by their patients, but by their spouses and families as well. In general, they worked long hours, enjoyed their autonomy and responsibility, accepted the adulation of their patients, and expected dinner to be kept warm. They were buoyed by these feelings of specialness. Failures and feelings were never discussed. Those who succumbed to the pressure by suicide or addiction were largely ignored or served as reminders of the importance of emotional strength and character.

These retired physicians have also lived through some serious changes and dislocations. When they began practice, it was common for physicians to tailor their charges to their clientele and locale—the same visit and procedure could cost someone who could afford it 10 times what another physician charged—but both donated time to a clinic, and either did not charge or reduced charges for poorer patients. This practice was considered by some to be demeaning to those who did not wish to be considered "charity patients," and so the right to medical care paid for by the state for those indigent or aged became established. With it came the image of the physician as provider and patients as consumers, and as the cost mounted, so did government and insurance controls and restrictions. Technological advances progressed faster and faster, and mounting malpractice suits and insurance fees underscored the slide of the physician's prestige and self-esteem. Physician impairment was identified as a widespread problem.

Whereas retirement a generation ago was rarely considered an alternative except when physically mandated, more and more physicians began to save for their retirement, with one eye on inflation and the other on their investments.

Cognizant of their needs, the American Association of Senior Physicians was formed and began a series of seminars for those considering retirement and for those already retired. The seminars are conducted by an attorney and investment and financial advisers, and for the three-day preretirement seminar, subjects listed include "What income is needed to retire," "Social Security entitlements," "What does your standard of living cost?" "Will your assets cover the cost of retirement?" "Constructing a retirement portfolio," "Concepts of investment, risk, and return," and so on. For the fully retired couple, a 1½-day seminar includes "Achieving maximum yield from a retirement portfolio," "Concepts of investment risk and return," "Meaningful volunteer activities," "Avoiding boredom in retirement," and "Finding travel bargains." The brochure adds, "Physicians in retirement are happiest when retiring from something to something, a second career if you will, so that a sense of identity and usefulness remains."

Reasons for Retiring

A number of factors contributed to the decision to retire. Almost half the surveyed retirees cited health as a factor, but even so, they were also emotionally ready for retirement. The practice of medicine had lost its appeal. One said, "I asked myself, 'why do I need this?' It wasn't so much aggravating, but just that there wasn't the fun that I had had before. It wasn't the same." Another said, "Practice was a joy in the beginning, but I gradually came to dislike what I was doing."

The increased difficulty in relating to and enjoying patients contributed to retirement. "The milieu of medicine is getting uglier all the time," one observed. "I hadn't planned on retiring, but I reassessed everything and decided it was time for me and I quit." "The attitude of the public has changed," another remarked. "The expectations of patients are different now, and they are more contentious and argumentative."

The new economics also contributed. "Medicine has become a business rather than a profession, and I really resent this," one complained. "I remember practicing in the Golden Age of Medicine—me and the patient. It was marvelous. But now it is the doctor, the patient, and the third party." The latter has become overbearing, intrusive, and manipulative, others note. "They've skewed the process, and the patients' best interests, the bottom line, has been lost." "I intensely disliked the pressures, anxieties, and frustrations progressively placed upon me by third-party interference," another added. "It took one-half day a week just looking at the mail every morning, time that could have been spent more fruitfully helping patients."

Some blamed the government. "The rules being imposed upon doctors by the government took the pleasure out of medicine. I was very unhappy with the government telling me that I must agree with this DRG—you can't put this guy in the hospital, you can't use this medicine," one complained. "There are so many regulations by city, state, and federal organizations that now interfere with the right of the physician and the patient to make decisions together on how to proceed. This has become a real nuisance."

The increasing malpractice crisis also contributed. "The malpractice threat took all the fun out of my work," one said. "In 1976–77, my insurance escalated from $6000 to $12,000 to $28,000," one complained. "When it escalated so quickly, I suddenly had to be concerned. I used to take lots of time to listen to patients talk about their problems, but I could no longer do that because I had to increase the volume to pay my insurance premiums. So I said, 'This is not for me. I will not write another $28,000 check,' and I just quit."

One physician described an episode that triggered his retirement: "I had a malpractice suit that was utterly baseless. This case took eight years, filling my life with anxiety the entire time. When it finally got to court, it took only 15 minutes; it was thrown out and that was the end of it! All of a sudden, my patients became potential risks and I was less open to them. It made me disenchanted with medicine."

Others felt less competent because the technology had gotten away from them. "After age 60 or so, it's hard to learn new things," one confessed. "I was getting to the point where I backed away from the tough surgery," another noted. "Although I still enjoyed doing what I did, I realized that I should refer these cases to others."

A comparison with younger, more energetic colleagues also accentuated feelings of inadequacy. "One of the physicians in our group seemed to have an incredible facility to be one step ahead of the world of medicine. Here I am using penicillin while he's using the latest. It gave me the feeling that my expertise was less than it should be." Sometimes younger colleagues bluntly pointed out deficiencies. "My younger colleagues felt I was not doing the job," one lamented.

Others found hostile relationships with colleagues: "I was forced out of practice in a power struggle with my group. I was doubled-crossed by my ex-partner."

Although many mentioned the work demands of medicine and enjoyed their absence after retiring, few said they were a reason for leaving practice. Mentioned were the long, irregular, and sometimes exhausting hours, the constant demands on their personal lives, being tied to a telephone 24 hours a day, the need to be up early almost daily, night emergencies, an inability to help patients at times, the constant pressure to read and keep up with recent advances in medicine, having to deal with doctors who are disliked or not respected, filling out forms, being forced to attend meetings, routine boring paperwork, meeting deadlines, and the need to constantly watch income to see if expenses were met with enough left over for a decent salary.

Adjusting to Retirement

Some physicians adjusted readily to retirement. "It took me one minute to make the change," one reported. "I went out from under a cloud into the sunlight. On the morning of January 1, 1978, I was emancipated."

Being out from under the burden of daily work strain was a relief. "My only direct connection with medicine now is with dreams—all unpleasant," one explained. Asked about the disadvantages of retirement, these physicians emphatically reply, "Nothing!"

What physicians like about their retirement include having more time with their spouse, children, and grandchildren; freedom to travel and study the things they want; and leisure time—time to be themselves doing what they want to do when they want to do it, with no telephones, no house calls, no hospital, and no worries. "I live by the acronym, ADIP," one said: "everyday is Another Day in Paradise." "I've never been so happy and contented," another reported. "These are the best days of my life. I like everything about retirement. I don't have to get up early in the morning anymore, I will not make any appointment until 10:00 a.m. or commit myself to anything that imposes a schedule. I just do things on the spur of the moment during the day. There are no longer any hassles."

A contented retiree can be a blessing to one's spouse, as one physician illustrated: "I feel different internally; I'm not itchy-antsy-tense anymore —not the aggressive person I used to be. I'm quite a different person than the SOB I was in those days. Now I am only occasionally an SOB."

Other physicians, however, had a difficult time adjusting to retirement. "I hated it at first," one reported. "I wasn't prepared for it. I was very depressed and angry for a year or two, but with psychotherapy and time I'm very happy now." "I was depressed and had feelings of sleeplessness, insomnia, etc.," another related. "But it is getting much better now. I am sleeping better and the whole thing is starting to come around."

Letting go is difficult for these physicians. They stay close to the hospital or their colleagues or continue to do some medical work. They attend medical seminars to keep up, but as one lamented, "It's not the same."

Some stay in the same routine as when they were practicing. "I've been going to lectures just like I did when I was in practice," one reported. "I get up at 5:30 a.m., do my reading like I used to, go to lectures at 8:00, then work at a free clinic in the mornings." "I have coffee at the hospital every morning and then go to my office," another said. "Though I don't have patients, I do consulting work. We have a group that meets in the morning for coffee and we talk about our problems—the stock market and other topics. Some of the younger doctors come around and listen to our conversations; they want to learn from us old guys." "I keep my license going, although I don't know exactly why. It's a security blanket, I guess." In short, as one said, "I don't want to give up medicine—it's been my lifetime. I want to participate but don't want the financial responsibilities or have to pay the malpractice premiums."

Asked what they miss about medical practice, retirees catalogued some losses. A few mentioned their relationships with patients. "I love them all. Living in a small community, I'm always bumping into them. They greet me and we talk. I enjoy seeing people." Others liked their patients more in retrospect. "I liked my patients very much but I'm not sure I realized this until I left. After I retired, I wrote a little note on every chart for the doctor who took over. After doing this for a week or so, I came to the realization that every note started off the same way ('this lovely woman, bla-bla-bla') and it suddenly dawned on me how much I really liked the people I had taken care of."

An important part of the relationship was the satisfaction that came from helping others. "As trite as it may seem, I felt I gave my patients good care and helped a goodly number on the road to health and life. The satisfaction of being helpful, comforting, reassuring—occasionally curing a disease—was very rewarding. It was satisfying to diagnose quickly and correctly sometimes."

"The longer I've been retired, the more I appreciate and value what I did as a doctor," another noted. "I keep running into people who were my patients and not one of them was unhappy with me. That is very satisfying."

Some enjoyed the professionalism of medicine—its collegiality, prestige, and mutual respect for fellow physicians. "Why do you suppose I stayed at the hospital for 30 years?" one asked rhetorically. "Damn, it was fun. We used to say, 'We ought to be paying the hospital to be allowed to work here.'"

The association with bright, interesting, fellow physicians was stimulating. However, professional collegiality changed after retirement. "I hate to say this but my colleagues were a lot more friendly toward me when I was in active practice and referred patients to them. There was a lot more cordiality, because the bottom line was referrals and money. I used to get invitations to play golf from physicians I referred to. But since I've been retired, the invitations have stopped coming."

Others enjoyed the intellectual stimulation with medicine. They most enjoyed the problem-solving aspects of medicine. "I was constantly learning," one said enthusiastically. "It was constantly challenging, stimulating. There was always more knowledge than I could encompass."

Asked about the downside of retirement, these physicians mentioned the same things that others were eager to leave behind. "I miss the intellectual stimulation; I feel the absence of something important to do, the lack of structure," one said. "There's a lack of goals, a lack of accomplishment," another agreed. "I miss the camaraderie of the surgical lounge, seeing my friends, the fellowship and the stimulus of problem cases, the opportunity to use my skill and experience, the professional, and societal contacts." "I miss doing what I was trained to do and was good at," another added. "There isn't enough to do now; I miss being with people and would like to do more. I feel at times like I am wasting my training, talent, and abilities. I miss my patients and work. At times I'd like to get back to work."

Maintaining Interests and Activities Outside Medicine

Boredom was a major fear of many physicians considering retirement. They worried about the transition from "full throttle" to "idle," as these comments illustrate! "One guy I knew came back to practice. He got bored." "Another doctor went crazy because he had nothing else of interest." "I have watched great doctors try to retire but can't find things to do. So they go back and practice again."

And indeed, boredom *was* a problem for some. "The problem I have now is that I'm not doing anything important. I've got to get into something. I have only medical interests. I play golf about three times a week, do some writing, and watch lots of television. But that's not enough."

The most successful retirees develop and maintain other interests before retiring. "My list of interests is so long it is astounding. There are so many enjoyable things to do there just isn't enough time," one said enthusiastically. "There are so many activities that I've never had time for that I'm spoiled with so many choices." "Looking back I don't know how I found time to practice medicine! I'm mixed up with so many projects that keep me busy. I'm an inventor and that keeps me very busy. I always have about three inventions I'm trying to sell."

These physicians looked with pity upon those who, having devoted themselves fully to their practice, "haven't taken full advantage of the other wonderful things in life." "There are other vistas but I find that many doctors are not interested in what goes on in the world; they're so preoccupied with medicine their interest in other things is zero." "Medicine isn't the alpha and omega of life," one chided. "There are so many other things in which I am interested—medicine was just the way I financed it, and I loved doing it." "Doctors who devote themselves to their careers don't realize that when they die, society won't skip a beat. No one's going to be missed." Their devotion is admirable, but they are not indispensable.

Exploring intellectual avenues occupied some physicians. "For anyone who has a mind that has been working all his life, the mind keeps working.

You don't have to have a hobby in place, a schedule made up or anything like that." Comparing criminal justice systems throughout the world occupied the time of one retiree. "If I told someone that that was my interest, they would look at me like I was a nut." Another physician immersed himself in a philosophical society. "I'm totally involved," he reported. "Those who participate are marvelous people. My circle of lifelong friends palls compared to this bunch. They have enlarged my life and constitute my most important associates."

Other physicians lose themselves in hobbies such as gardening, redecorating houses, and renovating automobiles; serving on boards and service groups for groups such as the mentally retarded; attending plays, musicals, and classes; reading, playing golf, and traveling. "I'm busy all the time," one reported. "I control my own time and it is wonderful." "I am so busy that I don't have time to do nothing!"

Achieving Self-Worth Outside Medicine

One of the most frequently mentioned difficulties that retirees experienced was the loss of self-worth that came when giving up the healer role. Their self-image relied solely on career attainment. "When I retired I was at a loss; my self-esteem took a real beating," one confessed. "I wasn't doing anything of much significance and no one came to me for advice or looked up to me. What am I worth now? I went from being almost worshipped to just an ordinary guy." Another said, "I lost my place and importance in the world. I was so involved in medicine that it was hard to give up my lofty role. In practice, people look up to you almost as a god. They know that you are not, but they hope when they are sick you can perform a miracle."

Giving up the title, "Doctor," was a big part of the adjustment. Most physicians had signed their names with "M.D." as though this title was an integral part of their personality. "Being an M.D. gave me instant prestige and recognition. It was a big plus. It made me feel good and important. But I feel that I have lost my identification as a doctor." "It was hard changing from being 'Doctor so-and-so' to just 'Tom' or 'Fred'—just an ordinary person."

The letdown was pronounced when forced to do "scut work around the home." One said, "When I was practicing, I never picked up a dish at home and took it over to the sink, but now that I'm retired, I'm expected to do my share. It's quite an adjustment from giving orders to underlings to *being* the underling." "Doing household chores and pulling a few weeds in the front yard isn't quite as important as sewing up somebody's wound," another lamented. "It bothered me for a while, but now I do my share. I must confess that it bothers me occasionally."

Other physicians made it a point not to let their ego depend solely on their medical practice. "My image wasn't tied up in being a physician," one noted. "I was proud of being a physician, but I tried hard to keep this from becoming my sole source of identity." One physician took "M.D." off his cards. "I try not to let people know that I was a physician, because that orients them in a way that I don't like. My sense of identification doesn't depend on being a physician. So now I have no problem in worrying about how good I am. It has never entered my consciousness."

Others credited their children with bringing them down to size before retirement. "My kids kept lowering my ego," one noted. "They never let me believe I could walk on water." The county hospital prevented another ego from being inflated. "When I finished medical school, I couldn't wait to be called "Doctor," he said. "I interned at the county hospital and I thought others would defer to me because I was a physician with a stethoscope and everything. At the elevator would you think that they would let the doctor on first? Forget it. Janitors and everybody else rush on and I have to do the best I can."

Maintaining Viable Family Relationships

In retrospect, many retirees regretted their neglect of spouses and children. "I was a father who left home at 5:00 a.m. and returned between 8:00 p.m. and midnight—long after the children's bedtime. I wasn't that involved in my children's lives. I was a semistranger to them. I wish I had been there more and given them more support. I have resolved that that won't be the case with my grandchildren." Pleasantly surprised to find that his children had done so well, another regretted that he had missed significant moments. "In retrospect I knew very little about what my kids were doing. I rarely ate a meal with them. I was gone when they got up and they were down when I got home. I remember when my oldest son graduated from high school and won all the awards. I was the most surprised person there. I had no idea about his status in school or anything. It came as quite a shock to me that all this had been going on and I had missed it all."

Neglected marital relationships created problems in retirement. "I found that if you don't love your wife when you retire, you are in a mess. As long as you have love between you and get along, you are all right," one observed. "My first wife felt that I should have given her more support," another acknowledged. "I didn't pay enough attention to the things that troubled her. She was a psychologically oriented person who sought conversation. But I was interested only in my profession and couldn't tolerate such talk. I couldn't take her seriously or follow it. I didn't listen to what was troubling her and paid the consequences. I could have done better."

Friction occurred in some marriages when the doctor suddenly started being around the home. "My wife has had a real problem with me," one confessed. "She used to be in charge of her day, and I would come home at night for a brief visit. But now I'm there all day. Who's in charge?" "When you've been gone so much, it's quite an adjustment for your spouse to have you around 24 hours at a time," one explained. "My wife says, 'For better or worse, but not for lunch every day.' " "Even if your wife loves you, it's a big adjustment for her to have an autocrat at home now running her household.

You say, get so-and-so on the phone, and she says, 'I'm not your slave!' In medical practice I had a 'slave' all those years, but now I have to use the telephone book myself."

Conflicts are resolved in various ways. "We've made a resolution: I don't get in her way. We go our own ways and meet in the middle." Others resolve differences by mutual agreement; each contracts for part of the workload. "She does the gardening, mowing, etc., and I wash the dishes."

Doctors who cultivated their marital relationships throughout the years welcomed the additional time to spend together. In retirement, their relationship even improved. "She's one remarkable person," one doctor acknowledged. "I've been fortunate. I honestly look forward to the free time that we spend together." "My wife is one fantastic woman, really! I don't know how the hell I got that lucky." "I live with the woman I love. She seems to want to have me around and doesn't like me going back to the hospital." "My wife is much happier since I retired," another noted.

Some spouses were pleasantly surprised at the improvements that came over their doctor spouses at retirement. "My wife is enthralled with what happened to me since I retired. She can't believe that it worked out so well. What pleases her the most is that I'm different. She has very positive feelings about me now."

The greatest achievement in life, some physicians claim, is the love and rapport with family members gained and maintained in the years of their busy practice. "I always made breakfast for the kids," one boasted. "When my grandkids come over, they always want grandpa's eggs."

These physicians simply made time for family. "First things first!" one said. "I decided early that I have a responsibility to my family and that they come first. Most of my activities have been with my children. I was a sailor, and all my kids were good sailors and never got busted for drugs or drunk driving or other problems. Being a father is more important than medicine. They are still with you when medicine is gone. Sometimes it takes a while to learn this—sometimes too late."

The simplest and most profound way to maintain one's mental health while actively involved in a demanding, open-ended career is to establish and cultivate a viable relationship with a caring, emotionally expressive spouse. The lack of such a companion is an interpersonal deficit that makes one vulnerable to stress. At work, one is judged primarily on the basis of one's achievements. Mates and other family members, however, place more emphasis on *who you are* than on *what you can do*. Unlike "roadside romances" that quickly flourish and wither like flowers along the freeway, long-term, good relationships do not develop quickly and are not maintained successfully without effort. Like careers, they must be carefully nurtured, and like gardens, they can become unsightly when neglected. Retirees who have taken time to maintain their "interpersonal gardens" enjoy the benefits in their declining years.

A senior physician expressed it this way: "Most doctors don't realize what is happening to their marriages until they get to their forties, and by that time they've lost contact with their families. Upon seeing that the road to glory is going to end and that they are achieving the thing that they have striven to, their disappointment is bitter to find success is really cotton candy; there is no substance to it. The thing that is really important—their interpersonal relationship with family members—has gone down the drain."

Prescription for a Successful Retirement

In Maslow's Hierarchy of Human Needs, the need for love and belonging immediately follows that of food and shelter. Of the various mechanisms that society has established to meet this need, marriage and family are the most universal and can be, with planning and effort, the most fulfilling. Retired physicians engaged in a happy, emotionally expressive marriage generally have a pleasant and satisfying retirement. The experiences of retired physicians suggest that the adjustment to retirement is facilitated when the practicing physician (1) regularly invests time and energy in maintaining viable family relationships, (2) achieves feelings of self-worth for areas outside his or her career, (3) develops and regularly maintains activities and friendships outside medicine, (4) has developed good, nonaddictive psychological coping behaviors, (5) has good health-maintenance habits, and (6) has an adequate financial base for the remainder of his or her life.

Suggested Reading

Coombs, R. H., "Structured Strain in the Medical Marriage." In R. H. Coombs, D. S. May, and G. W. Small (Eds.), *Inside Doctoring: Stages and Outcomes in the Professional Development of Physicians* (pp. 183–190). New York: Praeger Publishers, 1986.

Coombs, R. H., and Fawzy, F. I., "Medical Marriage as Prevention for Physician Impairment." *California Academy of Family Practitioners* 33(1982):14–18.

Farley, Gerald, Executive Director, American Association of Senior Physicians, 515 North State Street, Chicago, IL.

Graver, H., and Cambell, N. M., "The Aging Physician and Retirement." *Canadian Journal of Psychiatry* 28(1983):552–554.

Rowe, M. Laurens, "Health, Income, and Activities of Retired Physicians." *New York State Journal of Medicine* 89(1989):450–453.

Index